Pharmacology in Respiratory Care

NOTICE

Pharmacology in Respiratory Care

STUART R. LEVINE, PharmD

Director of Pharmacy Services, Alfred I. du Pont Hospital for Children, Wilmington, Delaware
Associate Professor, Temple University School of Pharmacy, Philadelphia, Pennsylvania
Adjunct Instructor, Respiratory Care Degree Program, Delaware Technical and Community
College, Wilmington, Delaware

ARTHUR J. McLAUGHLIN, Jr, MS, CRT

President, A. J. McLaughlin and Associates, Dover, Delaware
Former Director of Respiratory Care, Wilmington Medical Center
Former Adjunct Instructor, Respiratory Care Degree Program, Delaware Technical and
Community College, Wilmington, Delaware

CHAPTERS ADAPTED FROM *BASIC PHARMACOLOGY*
BY HENRY HITNER, PhD, AND BARBARA NAGLE, PhD

THE McGRAW-HILL COMPANIES
MEDICAL PUBLISHING DIVISION

New York   Chicago   San Francisco   Lisbon   London   Madrid   Mexico City
Milan   New Delhi   San Juan   Seoul   Singapore   Sydney   Toronto

McGraw-Hill

*A Division of The **McGraw·Hill** Companies*

Pharmacology in Respiratory Care

Copyright © 2001 by The McGraw-Hill Companies. All rights reserved. Printed in the United States of America. Except as permitted under the United States Copyright Act of 1976, no part of this publication may be reproduced or distributed in any form or by any means, or stored in a data base or retrieval system, without the prior written permission of the publisher.

1234567890   DOCDOC   09876543210

ISBN 0-07-134727-5

This book was set in New Baskerville by Rainbow Graphics. The editors were Sally J. Barhydt and Karen G. Edmonson. The index was prepared by Kathryn Unger. The production supervisor was Richard C. Ruzycka. The text was designed by Robert Freese. R.R. Donnelley & Sons Company was the printer and binder.

This book is printed on acid-free paper.

LIBRARY OF CONGRESS CATALOGING-IN-PUBLICATION DATA
Levine, Stuart R. (Stuart Robert), 1950–
    Pharmacology in respiratory care / authors, Stuart R. Levine ... [et al.].
        p. ; cm.
    Includes bibliographical references.
    ISBN 0-07-134727-5
    1. Respiratory agents.   2. Respiratory therapy.   I. Title
    [DNLM: 1. Respiratory System Agents—pharmacology.   2. Respiratory Therapy. QV
120 L665p 2001]
    RM388 .L485 2001
    615'.72

                                                                                00-045240

Dedication

To our wives, Sally and Susan, for their patience and support for all the time we spent writing this book. We also dedicate this book to our friends and family members who suffer from asthma, in the hope that increasing the knowledge of respiratory care practitioners will improve the quality of their care and their lives.

Contents

PREFACE   xiii
ACKNOWLEDGMENTS   xv

1 Introduction to Pharmacology   **1**
HENRY HITNER, PhD, AND BARBARA NAGLE, PhD

2 Biological Factors Affecting the Action of Drugs   **17**
HENRY HITNER, PhD, AND BARBARA NAGLE, PhD

3 Math Review and Dosage Calculations   **43**
HENRY HITNER, PhD, AND BARBARA NAGLE, PhD

4 Preventing Medication Errors   **63**
STUART LEVINE, PharmD

5 Autonomic Nervous System   **69**
HENRY HITNER, PhD, AND BARBARA NAGLE, PhD

6 Drugs Affecting the Sympathetic Nervous System   **77**
HENRY HITNER, PhD, AND BARBARA NAGLE, PhD

7 Drugs Affecting the Parasympathetic Nervous System   **95**
HENRY HITNER, PhD, AND BARBARA NAGLE, PhD

8 Drugs Affecting the Autonomic Ganglia   **109**
HENRY HITNER, PhD, AND BARBARA NAGLE, PhD

9   Skeletal Muscle Relaxants   **115**
HENRY HITNER, PhD, AND BARBARA NAGLE, PhD

10   Local Anesthetics   **131**
HENRY HITNER, PhD, AND BARBARA NAGLE, PhD

**11   Introduction to the Central
Nervous System**   **143**
HENRY HITNER, PhD, AND BARBARA NAGLE, PhD

12   Sedative-Hypnotic Drugs and Alcohol   **151**
HENRY HITNER, PhD, AND BARBARA NAGLE, PhD

13   General Anesthetics   **167**
HENRY HITNER, PhD, AND BARBARA NAGLE, PhD

**14   Narcotic (Opioid) Analgesics
and Antitussives**   **181**
HENRY HITNER, PhD, AND BARBARA NAGLE, PhD

15   Cardiac Physiology and Pathology   **201**
HENRY HITNER, PhD, AND BARBARA NAGLE, PhD

**16   Cardiac Glycosides and the Treatment
of Congestive Heart Failure**   **209**
HENRY HITNER, PhD, AND BARBARA NAGLE, PhD

17   Anticoagulants and Coagulants   **217**
HENRY HITNER, PhD, AND BARBARA NAGLE, PhD

18   Antiallergic and Antihistaminic Drugs   **235**
HENRY HITNER, PhD, AND BARBARA NAGLE, PhD

**19   Bronchodilator Drugs and the Treatment
of Asthma**   **253**
HENRY HITNER, PhD, AND BARBARA NAGLE, PhD

20   Adrenal Steroids   **271**
HENRY HITNER, PhD, AND BARBARA NAGLE, PhD

21 Antibacterial Agents   **289**
     HENRY HITNER, PhD, AND BARBARA NAGLE, PhD

22 Antiseptics and Disinfectants   **311**
     HENRY HITNER, PhD, AND BARBARA NAGLE, PhD

**23 Herbal Remedies
     for Respiratory Diseases**   **323**
     ELLEN FEINGOLD, MD, MPH

24 Antiviral Drugs   **335**
     HENRY HITNER, PhD, AND BARBARA NAGLE, PhD

25 Mechanical Ventilation   **351**
     VINAY NADKARNI, MD, AND STUART LEVINE, PharmD
     ADAPTED FROM *ESSENTIALS OF MECHANICAL VENTILATION* BY DEAN HESS, PhD, RRT,
     FAARC, AND ROBERT KACMAREK, PhD, RRT, FAARC

**26 New Treatments in Respiratory Care
     Pharmacology**   **357**
     BARBARA NAGLE, PhD, AND STUART LEVINE, PharmD

**Appendix I: Regulatory Issues
                 in the Practice
                 of Respiratory Care**   **367**
     ROBERTO PALERMO, MBA, RRT, AND ARTHUR J. McLAUGHLIN, JR, MS, CRT

**Appendix II: Compatibility Chart
                 for Nebulized Respiratory
                 Medications** (COURTESY OF
     KEVIN HILLEGASS, PharmD CANDIDATE)   **371**

Index   **373**

Contributors

Ellen Feingold, MD, MPH
Director of the Homeopathy Center of Delaware, Wilmington, Delaware

Dean Hess, PhD, RRT, FAARC
Assistant Director, Department of Respiratory Care, Massachusetts General Hospital
Assistant Professor of Anesthesia, Harvard Medical School Boston Massachusetts

Henry Hitner, PhD
Professor, Department of Biomedical Sciences, Philadelphia College of Osteopathic Medicine, Philadelphia, Pennsylvania

Robert M. Kacmarek, PhD, RRT, FAARC
Director of Respiratory Care, Massachusetts General Hospital
Associate Professor of Anesthesia, Harvard Medical School, Boston, Massachusetts

Vinay Nadkarni, MD
Associate Professor of Pediatrics, Thomas Jefferson School of Medicine
Medical Director, Pediatric Intensive Care Unit, Alfred I. du Pont Hospital for Children, Wilmington, Delaware

Barbara Nagle, PhD
Vice President, Clinical Operations, InKine Pharmaceutical Company, Inc., Philadelphia, Pennsylvania

Roberto Palermo, MBA, RRT
Director of Outpatient Services, Union Hospital, Elkton, Maryland

Preface

As teachers, we are of course concerned about the quantity and quality of knowledge that our students acquire during their training. The ease with which our students learn and the amount that they retain will, in part, determine their abilities as respiratory care practitioners.

In the past, we have used available texts in our classes that have provided more depth in the science of pharmacology than we need and more than our students can absorb in one short course. We have developed this book in order to provide a text that contains the basic pharmacological information for beginning students in the field of respiratory care.

This book utilizes a format that can be understood by students with limited or no background in pharmacology. We believe that we have reached a balance in this book, providing both the appropriate depth of knowledge and ease of use for respiratory care practitioners in all practice settings.

This book contains a number of chapters that have been adapted from *Basic Pharmacology* by Hitner and Nagle. For this book, the original authors adapted these chapters, and then the chapters were further refined to closely target the specific needs of respiratory care students.

In addition, we have included chapters written by other experts in areas of pharmacology that in our experience are particularly important in the practice of respiratory care today.

We believe that we have achieved our goal of providing a more student friendly, yet complete textbook, and hope that it provides a good foundation for your careers. Learning is a never-ending pursuit. New medications and techniques will continue to be developed throughout your career. We hope that the knowledge you gain from this book will be a building block that will serve as a base throughout your careers.

Stuart R. Levine

Arthur J. McLaughlin, Jr.

Acknowledgments

We would like to acknowledge some whose efforts made this book a reality. At McGraw-Hill, we would like to thank first Steve Zollo, who brought this project to us initially, and Sally Barhydt, who patiently helped us with editorial guidance.

We thank Rodney Washington, CRCST, for reviewing the chapter on Antiseptics and Disinfectants, and Tim Cox, RRT, and Bert Palermo, RRT, for technical review of respiratory care therapeutic techniques.

Finally, we thank Susan Carr McLaughlin, MS, who supervised the organization of electronically transmitted documents, and Debbie Poore, who once again provided us with the organizational and word-processing skills that resulted in a final manuscript.

Pharmacology in Respiratory Care

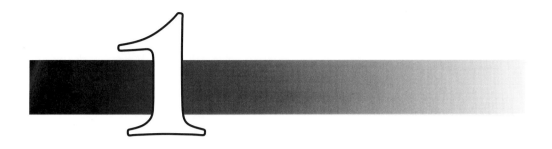

Introduction to Pharmacology

HENRY HITNER, PhD
BARBARA NAGLE, PhD

Chapter Focus

This chapter provides an introduction to basic pharmacology. It also describes the properties of drugs, their sources, how drugs produce effects, and drug nomenclature.

Chapter Terminology

adverse effect: General term for undesirable and potentially harmful drug effect.

agonist: Drug that binds to its receptor and produces a drug action.

antagonist: Drug that binds to its receptor and prevents other drugs or substances from producing an effect.

chemical name: Name that defines the chemical composition of a drug.

contraindications: Situations or conditions when a certain drug should not be administered.

controlled substance: Drug that has the potential for abuse and thus is regulated by law.

dose: Exact amount of a drug that is administered in order to produce a specific effect.

drug: Chemical substance that produces a change in body function.

drug indications: Intended or indicated uses for any drug.

ED50:   Effective dose 50, or dose that will produce an effect that is half of the maximal response.

generic name: Nonproprietary or common name of a drug.

LD50:   Lethal dose 50, or dose that will kill 50% of the animals tested.

mechanism of action: Explanation of how a drug produces its effects.

nonprescription, over-the-counter (OTC) drug: Drug that can be purchased without the services of a physician.

pharmacology: Study of drugs.

potency: Measure of the strength, or concentration, of a drug required to produce a specific effect.

prescription drug: Drug for which dispensing requires a written or phone order that can only be issued by or under the direction of a licensed physician or other person authorized by their state to write for such drugs.

receptor: Specific location on a cell membrane or within the cell where a drug attaches to produce its effect.

response: The effect that a dose of a drug produces.

Schedule I drug: Drug with high abuse potential and no accepted medical use.

Schedule II drug: Drug with high abuse potential and accepted medical use.

Schedule III drug: Drug with moderate abuse potential and accepted medical use.

Schedule IV drug: Drug with low abuse potential and accepted medical use.

Schedule V drug: Drug with low abuse potential and accepted medical use.

side effect: Drug effect other than the therapeutic effect that is usually undesirable.

site of action: Location within the body where a drug exerts its therapeutic effect, often a type of specific receptor.

therapeutic effect: Desired drug effect to alleviate some condition or symptom of disease.

therapeutic index (TI):   Ratio of the LD50 to the ED50.

toxic effect: Undesirable drug effect that implies drug poisoning; can be very harmful or life-threatening.

trade name: Patented proprietary name of a drug sold by a specific drug manufacturer.

Chapter Objectives

After studying this chapter, you should be able to:

- Define pharmacology and its major subdivisions.
- Describe what a drug is and explain the differences among therapeutic effects, side effects, and toxic effects.

Table 1-1
Major Areas of Pharmacology

Area	Description
Pharmacodynamics	Study of the action of drugs on living tissue
Pharmacokinetics	Study of the processes of drug absorption, distribution, metabolism, and excretion
Pharmacotherapeutics	Study of the use of drugs in treating disease
Pharmacy	Science of preparing, dispensing, and monitoring drugs to assure their proper and safe use
Posology	Study of the amount of drug that is required to produce therapeutic effects
Toxicology	Study of the harmful effects of drugs on living tissue

- Identify a drug receptor and trace how agonists and antagonists interact with receptors.
- Explain the relationship between drug dosage and drug response, and the relationship between drug response and time.
- Explain drug safety and therapeutic index.
- Describe three names by which drugs are known.
- List two common drug reference books.
- Describe three sources of medications.

Pharmacology is the study of drugs. A drug can be any substance that, when administered to living organisms, produces a change in function. Thus, substances such as water, metals (iron), or insecticides can be classified as drugs. However, the term **drug** commonly means any medication that is used for treating disease.

Pharmacology refers to a very broad area of study. It can be broken down into several topics, each one a major subject area of study. Table 1-1 lists some of these areas. Throughout this book, tables organize information so that the pharmacology of each drug class can be easily understood.

Drug Sources

A logical question to ask about pharmacology is, "Where do drugs come from?" There are several sources of drugs. In the early days of medicine, most drugs were obtained from plant or animal sources. Plants and living organisms contain active substances that can be isolated, purified, and formulated into effective drug preparations. Examples of drugs derived from plants that are still widely used today include the analgesics morphine and codeine, which were obtained from the poppy plant *(Papver somniferum);* the heart drug digitalis, which was obtained from the purple foxglove *(Digitalis purpurea);* and the antimalarial drug quinine, which was obtained from the bark of the cinchona tree. Recently, a new anticancer drug, paclitaxel, was isolated from the yew tree. The search for new plant drugs is still very active.

It is also interesting that many of the drugs of abuse such as cocaine, marijuana, mescaline, heroin, and others are derived from plants. Most of these drugs were used for hundreds of years by many different cultures in their religious and ritual ceremonies. Drugs obtained from living organisms include hormones such as insulin (pig) and growth hormone from pituitary glands. In addition, antibiotics such as cephalosporins and aminoglycosides have been derived from bacteria.

The early history of pharmacology is filled with many interesting stories of discovery and medical experimentation. Textbooks devoted to the history of medicine and pharmacology are the best sources for additional information. Despite the many examples of drugs obtained from plants and living organisms, the main source of new drugs today is chemical synthesis. Also, many of the drugs that once were obtained from plants and animals are now chemically synthesized in pharmaceutical laboratories. Within recent years, researchers have been able to train bacteria to produce specific proteins that are used as drugs in the treatment of diseases. This process is known as genetic engineering and produces most of the insulin used today.

Terminology Related to Drug Effects

Another basic question that should be answered is, "What actually is a drug?" Every pure drug is a chemical compound with a specific chemical structure. Because of its structure, a drug has certain properties that are usually divided into chemical properties and biological properties. The properties of any drug determine what effects will be produced when the drug is administered. An important fact to remember is that, structurally, the human body is composed mostly of cells, even though these cells are highly organized into tissues, organs, and systems. Consequently, drugs produce effects by influencing the function of cells. Figure 1-1 illustrates the chemical structures of some common drugs.

Pharmacologists know that all drugs produce more than one effect. Every drug produces its intended effect, or **therapeutic effect,** along with other effects. The therapeutic use(s) of any drug is referred to as the **drug indication,** meaning indications for use. The term **contraindication** refers to a situation or circumstance when a particular drug should not be used. Some drug effects, other than therapeutic effects, are described as undesirable. Undesired drug effects are categorized as side effects, adverse effects, and toxic effects.

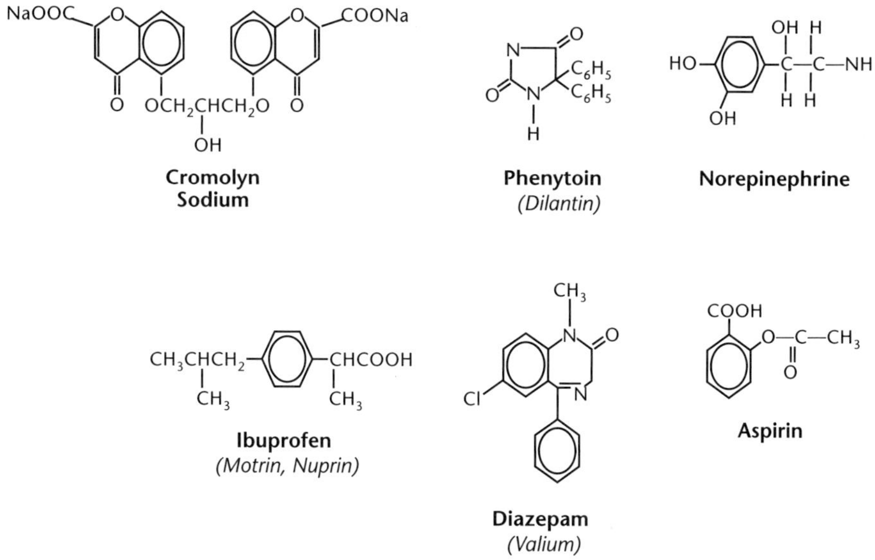

Figure 1-1
The chemical structures of several drugs.

SIDE EFFECTS

Many **side effects** are more of a nuisance than they are harmful. The dry mouth and drowsiness caused by some antihistamine drugs are an example. In many cases, drug side effects must be tolerated in order to benefit from the therapeutic actions of the drug.

ADVERSE EFFECTS

Adverse effects are also undesired effects, but these are effects that may be harmful (persistent diarrhea, vomiting, or CNS disturbances such as confusion) or that, with prolonged treatment, may cause conditions that affect the function of vital organs such as the liver or kidneys. Reduction of dosage or switching to an alternative drug will often avoid or minimize these harmful consequences.

TOXIC EFFECTS

Toxic effects or **toxicity** implies drug poisoning; the consequences can be extremely harmful and may be life-threatening. In these situations, the drug must be stopped, and supportive treatment and the administration of antidotes may be required.

The term most frequently used to describe the undesirable effects of drugs is adverse effects. However, you should be familiar with the other terms because they are used and, if used correctly, describe the nature and potential severity of undesired drug effects.

Most drugs will cause all three types of undesired effects, depending on the dose administered. At low doses, side effects are common and often expected. At higher doses, additional adverse effects may appear. At very high doses, toxic effects may occur that can be fatal. Consequently, the undesired effects produced by most drugs are often a function of dosage, which is why a well-known physician from the Middle Ages, Parcelsus (1493–1541), made the famous statement, "Only the dose separates a drug from a poison," and we could add, "a therapeutic effect from a toxic effect." Respiratory care practitioners spend the majority of their time in patient contact. Therefore, they have an important responsibility to observe the undesired effects of drugs, to recognize the side effects, which are often expected, and to identify and report the adverse and toxic effects that are potentially harmful and that often require medical attention.

Basic Concepts in Pharmacology

As in any subject, fundamental principles and concepts form the basis on which additional information can be added. Pharmacology is no exception, and the following basic concepts apply to any drug.

SITE OF ACTION

The **site of action** of a drug is the location within the body where the drug exerts its therapeutic effect. The site of action of some drugs is not known; however, the site of action for most drugs has been determined. For example, the site of action of aspirin to reduce fever is in an area of the brain known as the hypothalamus. Within the hypothalamus, the temperature-regulating center controls and maintains body temperature. Aspirin alters the activity of the temperature-regulating center so that body temperature is reduced. Throughout this book, when the site of drug action is known or suspected, it will be presented.

MECHANISM OF ACTION

Mechanism of action explains how a drug produces its effects. For example, local anesthetic agents produce a loss of pain sensation by interrupting nerve conduction in sensory nerves. In order for nerve impulses to be conducted, sodium ions must pass through the nerve membrane. Local anesthetic agents attach to the nerve membrane and prevent the passage of sodium ions. Consequently, sensory nerve impulses for pain are not conducted to the pain centers in the brain. Knowledge of the sites and mechanisms of action of drugs is essential to understanding why drugs produce the effects that they do.

RECEPTOR SITE

Drug action is usually thought to begin after a drug has attached itself to some cell membrane. For a few drugs and for some normal body substances, there seems to be a specific location on certain cells. This area is referred to as the **receptor** site.

The attachment, or binding, of a drug to its receptors begins a series of cell changes referred to as the drug action.

When a specific receptor site for a drug is known, that receptor site becomes the site of action for that particular drug. Morphine, an analgesic drug, is an example of a drug that binds to specific receptors. The receptors for morphine are located in the brain and are known as the opioid receptors. When morphine binds to its receptors, it produces cell changes that reduce the perception of pain. There are many different pharmacological receptors, and they will be described in the appropriate chapters.

AGONISTS AND ANTAGONISTS

Drugs that bind to specific receptors and produce a drug action are called **agonists.** Morphine is an example of an agonist. Drugs that bind to specific receptors but do not produce any drug action are called **antagonists.**

Antagonists are also known as blocking drugs. Usually, antagonists bind to the receptors and prevent other drugs or body substances from producing an effect. Naloxone, a morphine antagonist, is administered to prevent, or antagonize, the effects of morphine in cases of morphine overdose. There are many examples in pharmacology where drug antagonists are used to prevent other substances from exerting an effect.

When both agonist and antagonist drugs are administered together, they compete with each other for the same receptor site. This effect is known as competitive antagonism. The amount of drug action produced depends on which drug (agonist or antagonist) occupies the greatest number of receptors. The actions of a drug agonist and antagonist are illustrated in Figure 1-2.

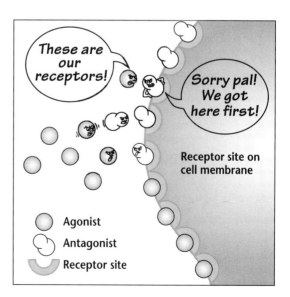

Figure 1-2
Competitive antagonism at work.

DOSE-RESPONSE CURVE

A fundamental principle of pharmacology is that the response to any drug depends on the amount of drug given. This principle is known as the dose-response relationship. A **dose** is the exact amount of a drug that is administered in order to produce a specific effect. The effect is referred to as the **response.** When the relationship between the dose and the response is plotted as a graph, it is referred to as a dose-response curve.

Figure 1-3 illustrates the appearance of a typical dose-response curve for two similar drugs. The main feature of the dose-response relationship is that a drug response is proportional to the dose. As the dose increases, so does the magnitude of the response. Eventually, a maximal response is usually attained (100% response); further increases in dose do not produce any greater effect. This point on the graph is known as the ceiling effect. The ceiling effect reflects the limit of the ability of some drug classes to produce a particular effect. Above a certain dosage, no further increase in effect is observed. Doses above those needed to produce the ceiling effect usually cause other, undesired, often toxic, drug effects. Drugs within a drug class that are more potent than other drugs in the same class will produce the ceiling effect at a lower dosage, but they will not "raise the ceiling." Drugs that continue to cause an increased effect as long as the dose is increased do not have a ceiling effect.

A graded dose-response curve can be used to evaluate drug response among different drugs. In a graded dose-response curve, the increases in drug dosage are plotted against the increases in drug response. For example, dose-response curves are used to compare the potency of similar drugs. **Potency** is a measure of the strength, or concentration, of a drug required to produce a specific effect. The dose that will produce an effect that is half of the maximal response is referred to as the effective dose 50, or **ED50.**

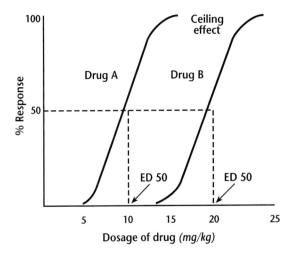

Figure 1-3

A typical dose-response curve.

The ED50 can be used to compare the potency of drugs that produce the same response. In Figure 1-3, the ED50 of drug A is 10 mg, and the ED50 of drug B is 20 mg. Therefore, drug A is twice as potent as drug B. Twice the concentration of drug B is needed to produce the same response as drug A.

Quantal (referred to as all-or-none) dose-response curves are used to show the percentage of a human or animal population that responds to a specific drug dosage. This information is important for determining the dosages that are recommended for various treatments. Quantal dose-response curves require an understanding of mathematical statistics that is beyond the scope of this textbook.

TIME-RESPONSE CURVE

The relationship of the drug response and time (duration of action) is known as the time-response relationship. Duration of action is the length of time that a drug continues to produce its effect. Most drugs produce effects over a relatively constant period of time. When the relationship between time and response is plotted on a graph, it is known as a time-response curve. Figure 1-4 illustrates the appearance of a typical time-response curve. In this example, the drug response being measured is the plasma concentration of the drug. After drug administration, a certain amount of time is required before a drug will produce an observable effect.

The time from drug administration to the first observable effect is known as the onset of action. The drug response will continue as long as there is an effective concentration of the drug at the site of action. As the drug is metabolized and excreted, the response gradually decreases because the drug level is decreasing. Eventually, the response will no longer be observed. Time-response curves are used for predicting the frequency with which a drug must be administered in order to maintain an effective drug response.

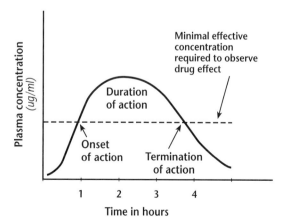

Figure 1-4
A typical time-response curve.

Drug Safety

The Federal Food and Drug Administration (FDA) has established guidelines that govern the approval and use of all drugs. Every drug must fulfill two major requirements before it can be approved for use in human beings: efficacy (proof of effectiveness) and safety. The drug must be effective in the disease state for which it has been approved. Approved drugs must satisfy specific safety criteria as determined by extensive animal testing and controlled human testing. As discussed, the dose separates therapeutic effects from toxic effects.

Drug safety receives much attention today. It is a constant source of concern and debate because the public is more aware than in the past of the potential dangers of drugs. In order to receive approval for use in humans, a drug must undergo several years of animal testing and evaluation. Several animal species must be used in order to evaluate the effectiveness and toxicity of a drug. One of the first tests that is performed is the lethal dose 50, or **LD50.** The LD50 is the dose that will kill 50% of the animals tested. The results of the LD50 and other tests are used to predict the safety of a drug.

THERAPEUTIC INDEX

The **therapeutic index** (TI) is the ratio of the LD50 to the ED50 of a drug. It gives an estimate of the relative safety of a drug. The equation is expressed as TI = LD50/ED50 = 1000 mg/100 mg = 10.

In this example, the therapeutic index is 10. This index indicates that 10 times as much drug is needed to produce a lethal effect in 50% of the animals as is needed to produce the therapeutic effect in 50% of the animals. The therapeutic index is used only in animal studies to establish dosage levels for other testing procedures. The goal of drug therapy is to achieve therapeutic effects in all individuals without producing any harmful effects.

ADVERSE EFFECTS

All drugs produce adverse and toxic effects if taken in excess. Most adverse effects are dose dependent, which means the higher the dose, the greater the chances of producing an adverse effect. Certain tissues are more frequently affected than others. Oral drugs often cause nausea, vomiting, and diarrhea as a result of gastrointestinal (GI) irritation. The liver, kidneys, brain, and cardiovascular system may be adversely affected because these organs are exposed to the highest concentrations of the drug. Drugs that produce birth defects, such as thalidomide, are known as teratogens. Drugs that promote the growth of cancerous tumors are called carcinogens.

A few adverse effects are not dose dependent. These effects, such as drug idiosyncrasy and drug allergy, are determined by individual variation. Although all human beings are basically similar, there may be minor variations in certain enzymes or other body proteins. These variations may produce changes in drug metabolism that lead to unusual responses to a particular drug. An individual reaction to a drug with an unusual or unexpected response is known as an idiosyncrasy.

Drug allergy occurs when an individual becomes sensitized to a particular drug and produces antibodies against the drug (antigen). Subsequent administration of the drug leads to an antigen-antibody reaction. Antigen-antibody reactions involving drugs usually cause the release of histamine from cells known as mast cells. Histamine produces the characteristic symptoms of allergy, which include rashes, hives, itching, nasal secretion, decrease in blood pressure, and difficulty in breathing.

In serious allergic reactions, the symptoms may be so severe that death may occur. The term anaphylaxis is used to describe these serious allergic reactions.

Drug Nomenclature

All drugs are chemicals, and many have long **chemical names.** As a result, all drugs are given a shorter name, known as the nonproprietary name, which is usually a contraction of the chemical name. The nonproprietary name is more commonly referred to as the **generic name.**

When the drug is marketed by a pharmaceutical company, it is given a third name, known as the proprietary name or **trade name.** Because several different pharmaceutical companies may market the same generic drug, there may be several different trade names for any one drug. Figure 1-5 gives three names of a commonly prescribed drug.

Drugs are also divided into prescription and nonprescription drugs. **Prescription drugs** require a written or phone order (the prescription), which can be issued only by or under the direction of a licensed physician, dentist, veterinarian, or, depending on the state, physician assistant, advanced practice nurse, or pharmacist. The prescription is a legal document that contains instructions for the pharmacist, who is licensed to dispense prescription medications (Table 1-2). **Nonprescription drugs,** usually referred to as **"over-the-counter" (OTC) drugs** (such as aspirin, antacids, cold remedies), can be purchased anywhere and do not require the services of a physician or pharmacist.

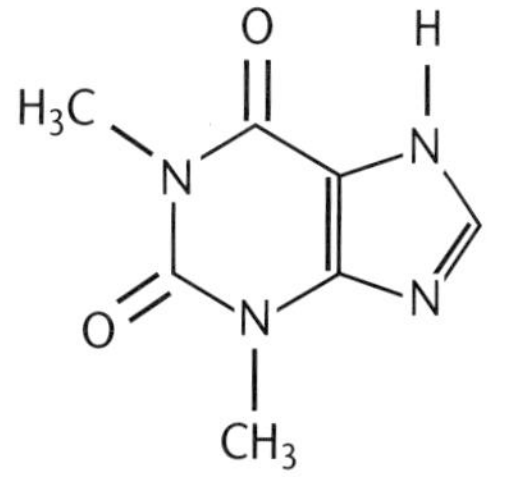

Figure 1-5
Drug nomenclature.

Chemical name: 1,3 dimethylxanthine
Nonproprietary name: Theophylline
Proprietary name: Theaduv
(Trade name)

Table 1-2
Elements of a Prescription

1. Patient's name
2. Name of drug
3. Strength of drug
4. Units to be dispensed
5. Full directions
6. Prescriber
7. Refills
8. Date

DRUG REFERENCES

Medical libraries, hospital libraries, and educational institutions that provide medical education generally stock one or more drug reference books that provide drug information.

The *United States Pharmacopeia/National Formulary (USP/NF)* is the official drug list recognized by the US government. It provides information concerning the physical and chemical properties of drugs. The *USP/NF* is revised every 5 years and is used primarily by drug manufacturers to ensure drug production according to official government standards.

The *Physician's Desk Reference (PDR)* is the reference widely used by physicians, pharmacists, and nurses for information relating to the use of drugs in the practice of medicine. It is updated yearly and provides information on indications for use, dosage and administration, contraindications, and adverse reactions. You should learn how to look up drugs in the *PDR*.

Drug Facts and Comparisons is a loose-leaf index and drug information service subscribed to by most medical libraries. Drug information and new drug additions are updated monthly. This index provides the most current drug information on a regular basis.

The United States Pharmacopeial Convention, Inc. publishes a series of volumes under the general title of *United States Pharmacopeia Dispensing Information (USP DI)* that are updated yearly. Volume I, *Drug Information for the Health Care Professional,* provides in-depth information about prescription and over-the-counter medications and nutritional supplements. Volume II, *Advice for the Patient,* provides drug information for the patient.

Drug Information—American Hospital Formulary Service provides detailed drug information. Drugs are organized according to therapeutic use and classification; it is updated yearly. Other references are available in hard copy, CD ROM, and online. Pediatric information is available from both *Harriet Lane Handbook* and the *Pediatric Dosage Handbook.*

CONTROLLED SUBSTANCES ACT

The Federal Comprehensive Drug Abuse Prevention and Control Act of 1970 is designed to regulate the dispensing of certain drugs that have the potential for abuse. These **controlled substances** are assigned to one of five schedules, depending on their medical usefulness and potential for abuse. Table 1-3 describes the schedules and provides examples of some controlled substances.

Table 1-3

Drug Schedules Defined in the Federal Comprehensive Drug Abuse Prevention and Control Act

Schedule	Definition	Controlled Drugs
Schedule I	Drugs with high abuse potential and no accepted medical use	Heroin, hallucinogens, marijuana; these drugs are not to be prescribed
Schedule II	Drugs with high abuse potential and accepted medical use	Narcotics (morphine and pure codeine), cocaine, amphetamines, short-acting barbiturates; no refills without a new written prescription from the physician
Schedule III	Drugs with moderate abuse potential and accepted medical use	Moderate- and intermediate-acting barbiturates, glutethimide, preparations containing codeine plus another drug; prescription required, may be refilled five times in 6 months when authorized by the physician
Schedule IV	Drugs with low abuse potential and accepted medical use	Phenobarbital, chloral hydrate, antianxiety drugs (Librium, Valium); prescription required, may be refilled five times in 6 months when authorized by the physician
Schedule V	Drugs with limited abuse potential and accepted medical use	Narcotic drugs used in limited quantities for antitussive and antidiarrheal purposes; drugs can be sold only by a registered pharmacist; buyer must be at least 18 years old and show identification. This varies from state to state.

Chapter 1 Review

UNDERSTANDING TERMINOLOGY

Match the definition in the left column with the appropriate term in the right column.

1. The study of the amount of drug that is required to produce therapeutic effects.

2. The study of the harmful effects of drugs on living tissue.

3. The study of the action of drugs on living tissue.

4. The study of drugs.

5. The science of preparing, dispensing, and monitoring drugs to assure their proper and safe use.

6. The study of the process of drug absorption, distribution, metabolism, and excretion.

7. The study of the use of drugs in treating disease.

a. pharmacodynamics

b. pharmacokinetics

c. pharmacology

d. pharmacotherapeutics

e. posology

f. pharmacy

g. toxicology

Answer the following questions.

8. Define a drug.

9. Differentiate among therapeutic effect, side effect, and toxic effect.

10. What is the difference between site of action and mechanism of action?

11. What is the relationship among ED50, LD50, and therapeutic index?

12. Explain the differences among a prescription drug, OTC drug, and a controlled substance.

13. Explain the difference between idiosyncrasy and drug allergy.

14. Write a short paragraph describing the following terms: receptor site, binding, drug action, agonist, antagonist, and competitive antagonism.

ACQUIRING KNOWLEDGE

Answer the following questions.

15. Examine a copy of the *Physicians' Desk Reference (PDR)*. In the beginning of the book are different groups of colored pages. Briefly describe the information found in the white, pink, and blue pages. How might the information in the glossy gray pages be helpful?

16. Look up the popular decongestant pseudoephedrine in the pink pages of the *PDR*. What is your conclusion based on the available trade names?

17. What is a dose-response curve, and what information is given by a dose-response curve?

18. What is the importance of a time-response curve? How often would you estimate that a drug should be administered per day if the drug is eliminated in 4 hours? In 24 hours?

19. It is interesting that a drug can produce a therapeutic effect and an undesired side effect in one situation and that the same side effect may be considered a therapeutic effect in another situation. Explain this phenomenon using the drug promethazine (Phenergan) as an example.

APPLYING KNOWLEDGE ON THE JOB

After reading this chapter, you should be able to answer the following questions:

20. Obtain a copy of the *PDR* from your school, patient care unit, or clinic and use it to do some sleuthing. Find the drugs that solve the following "medical mysteries."

    a. Dan is currently taking the drugs Mephyton, Biaxin, and Entex LA for his chronic celiac disease and acute sinusitis. He was just prescribed Coumadin for thrombosis, and it had no therapeutic effect. Dan's doctor suspects it's a case of drug antagonism. Which drug is Dan taking that is antagonistic with Coumadin?

    b. Mary's grandfather just came home from the doctor with a prescription for Accolate, and he has already forgotten why he is supposed to take it. Explain what this drug is, its indications, and the most common adverse effects.

    c. Bill's young wife was just prescribed Vibra-Tabs for a respiratory infection. Bill asks you what this drug is, and is it safe for his wife to take because she may be pregnant. Is it safe?

21. Assume that your employer has asked you to help screen patients for potential prescription drug problems. Look up the following frequently prescribed prescription drugs in the *PDR*, and fill in the information requested in the spaces provided.

    a. Indocin: What would tip you off that a patient was showing adverse effects to the drug?

    b. Bicillin: Describe symptoms of a patient who is allergic to this drug.

    c. Inderal: For whom is this drug contraindicated?

22. A patient calls with a minor problem. While traveling, she got her medications mixed together. She needs to take her Singulair tablet but isn't sure which one it is. Can you please describe it to her?

23. A physician wants to know the available forms and strengths of Ventolin. Using one of your resources, look up the available forms, strengths, and package sizes. Compare two different resources and see which one is more comprehensive.

Internet Activities

There are a number of internet Web sites that provide drug information. One of these is **Rx List (http://www.rxlist.com).** Rx List has information and drug monographs on the top 200 drugs, based on prescriptions filled, in the United States. When you reach the Web site, click on the heading Top 200. What is the top drug for 1999? Notice that this drug reappears on the list several times under a different trade name. Click on this drug heading and explore the information presented. Notice the number of different trade names that this drug is sold under. Select another drug that you may be familiar with and survey the information. This Web site can be useful throughout your course when additional drug information is needed.

Another Web site is the **Food and Drug Administration (http://www.fda.gov).** Listed are topics on foods, cosmetics, animal and human drugs, and tobacco. Click on some of these headings to familiarize yourself with the FDA.

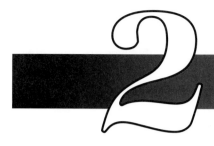

Biological Factors Affecting the Action of Drugs

Henry Hitner, PhD
Barbara Nagle, PhD

Chapter Focus

This chapter provides a description of the basic principles of pharmacokinetics, or the study of what happens to a drug after it is administered. It also describes how different dosage forms, individual variations, drug interactions, and drug dependency affect drug response.

Chapter Terminology

bioavailability: Percentage of the drug dosage that is absorbed.

drug absorption: Entrance of a drug into the bloodstream from its site of administration.

drug addiction: Condition of drug abuse and drug dependence that is characterized by compulsive drug behavior.

drug dependence: Condition of reliance on the use of a particular drug, characterized as physical and/or psychological dependence.

drug distribution: Passage of drug from the blood to the tissues and organs of the body.

drug microsomal metabolizing system (DMMS): Group of enzymes located primarily in the liver that function to metabolize (biotransform) drugs.

enzyme induction: Increase in the amounts of drug-metabolizing enzymes after repeated administration of certain drugs.

half-life: Time required for the body to rid itself of half of the drug dosage that was absorbed (percentage bioavailability).

individual variation: Difference in the effects of drugs and drug dosages from one person to another.

intramuscular (IM) injection: Route of drug administration; drug is injected into gluteal or deltoid muscles.

intravenous (IV) injection: Route of drug administration; drug is injected directly into a vein.

loading dose: Initial drug dose administered to rapidly achieve therapeutic drug concentrations.

maintenance dose: Dose administered to maintain drug blood levels in the therapeutic range.

oral administration: Route of drug administration by way of the mouth through swallowing.

parenteral administration: Route of drug administration that involves injection of a sterile product.

Topical application: Medications applied to the surfaces of the body.

Chapter Objectives

After studying this chapter, you should be able to:

- List different forms of drug products and the routes by which they are administered.
- Explain the processes of pharmacokinetics.
- Identify how half-life, blood drug level, and bioavailability relate to drug response.
- List several factors of individual variation that can alter drug response.
- Understand the drug factors that relate to pediatric drug administration.
- Define the different types of drug interaction.
- Explain the basic terminology of chronic drug administration and drug dependence.

The familiar saying, "No two people are exactly alike," applies well to the effects produced by drugs. An identical drug and dose may produce an intense response in one individual and no observable effect in another. The major reason for these differences is **individual variation.** Individual variation occurs as a result of several factors, any of which can influence the pharmacological response to drugs. There are also factors that determine how fast a drug reaches its site of action (receptors), how long it remains there, and how long the body takes to eliminate the drug. These important pharmacological considerations are understood by examining the biological factors that affect drug action.

One of the factors that affects drug action is the route of drug administration. The route determines the rate of drug absorption. **Drug absorption** refers to the entrance of a drug into the bloodstream, where it is distributed (**drug distribution**) to the various tissues of the body. The intensity of drug action depends primarily on the rate of drug absorption and distribution. The duration of drug action depends primarily on the rate of drug metabolism and drug excretion. Figure 2-1 shows the interrelationship of these processes.

Individual variation is caused by a number of physical and psychological factors, including age, sex, weight, genetic variation, emotional state, patient expecta-

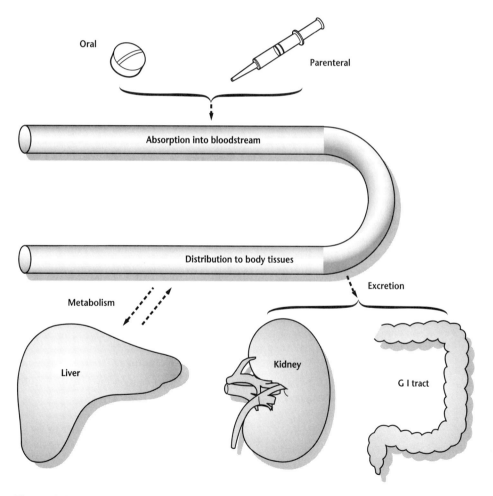

Figure 2-1
Movement of a drug in the body.

tions (placebo effect), and the presence of other disease conditions (pathology) or other drugs. The remainder of this chapter will describe what happens to a drug between its administration and its elimination from the body. The interplay among the various biological factors determines the actual drug response.

Drug Forms

Drugs are prepared in various forms for administration. The physical and chemical properties of a drug usually determine which form will be most effective. In addition to the drug, most drug products contain other ingredients that facilitate the administration and absorption of the drug. Drug preparations should always be taken exactly as prescribed. Some of the more common drug forms and preparations follow.

AQUEOUS PREPARATIONS

Syrups are commonly used aqueous preparations. A syrup is a solution of water and sugar to which a drug is added. Addition of flavoring agents eliminates the bitter taste of many drugs.

ALCOHOLIC PREPARATIONS

Elixirs, spirits, tinctures, and fluid extracts are drugs dissolved in various concentrations of alcohol, usually in the range of 5% to 20%.

SOLID AND SEMISOLID PREPARATIONS

The solid type of preparation is most common. A number of different kinds for different purposes are available.

Powders   Powders are drugs or drug extracts that are dried and ground and micronized into fine particles. Powders can be dissolved and taken orally or administered into the nasal or respiratory tract.

Tablets   Tablets are drug powders that have been compressed into a convenient form for swallowing. They usually disintegrate in the stomach more rapidly than most other solid preparations.

Troches and Lozenges   These flattened tablets are allowed to dissolve in the mouth. They are commonly used for colds and sore throats.

Capsules   Gelatin capsules are used to administer drug powders or liquids. Gelatin capsules dissolve in the stomach, thereby releasing the drug.

DELAYED-RELEASE PRODUCTS

These are usually tablets or capsules that are treated with special coatings so that various portions of the drug will dissolve at different rates. Delayed-response products usually contain the equivalent of two or three single-dose units. They are designed to produce drug effects over an extended time.

ENTERIC-COATED PRODUCTS

Some drugs are very irritating to the stomach. Also, the gastric juices of the stomach can inactivate certain drugs. In these cases, the drug tablet or capsule is coated with an acid-resistant substance that will dissolve only in the less acidic portions of the intestines. Enteric-coated products should be taken on an empty stomach with water, either 1 hour before or 2 hours after meals.

SODAS

SODAS refers to the spheroidal oral drug-absorption system, which allows less frequent dosing. This is a system of administering pellets covered in a gelatin capsule. Each pellet slowly releases the drug and is not affected by food or the environment of the gastrointestinal (GI) tract.

GITS

GITS refers to the GI therapeutic system, which is composed of a two-compartment tablet. Within the GI tract, water is drawn into the tablet, which then forces the drug out of the tablet. This system is used to deliver drugs at a constant rate over extended periods of time.

SUPPOSITORIES

These are drugs mixed with a substance (cacao butter) that will melt at body temperature. Suppositories are intended for insertion into the rectum, urethra, or vagina.

OINTMENTS

Ointments or salves are soft oily substances (petrolatum or lanolin) containing a drug that is applied to the skin or, in the case of ophthalmic ointments, to the eye.

TRANSDERMAL PRODUCTS

Transdermal products are administered through a bandage or patch system. The drug is slowly released through a membrane in the patch and is then absorbed through the skin into the systemic circulation. This method provides a continuous source of the drug over 24 hours or more. Nitroglycerin, estrogen, and clonidine are drugs available in this form.

AEROSOLS, SPRAYS, AND GASES

Drugs administered by spray or inhalation via the nasal and respiratory tracts are intended for both local action within the nasal and respiratory tracts (allergy, asthma, obstructive pulmonary disease) and systemic action throughout the body (general anesthetic gases). Nasal sprays, metered-dose inhalers, nebulizers, and positive-pressure breathing apparatus are common methods of administration into the nasal and respiratory tracts.

Routes of Administration

ORAL ADMINISTRATION

The most common routes of drug administration are oral (PO) and parenteral. **Parenteral administration** is any route that involves the injection of a sterile product. The **oral administration** route is the safest and the most convenient method. Oral administration usually requires 30 to 60 minutes before significant absorption from the GI tract occurs; therefore, the onset of drug action is delayed.

Although some drugs are irritating to the stomach and may cause nausea, heartburn, and vomiting, administration of such drugs with sufficient amounts of water or with meals minimizes gastric irritation. However, food also delays drug absorption and, therefore, delays the onset of drug action.

Besides convenience, another advantage of oral administration is that drugs given orally can be removed (within the first few hours) by gastric lavage or induced vomiting. This procedure is often employed in drug overdose (sleeping pills) or accidental poisoning.

PARENTERAL ADMINISTRATION

The most common routes of parenteral administration include intramuscular injection and intravenous injection. **Intramuscular (IM) injections** are usually delivered into the gluteal or deltoid muscles. Extreme caution should be observed with gluteal injections, so that injury to the sciatic nerve is avoided. The onset of action with IM administration is relatively short, usually within several minutes. **Intravenous (IV) injection** is usually restricted to use in the hospital. The IV injection offers the fastest means of drug absorption because the drug is delivered directly into the circulation; therefore, the onset of drug action is almost immediate. However, there is some degree of risk, because the drug cannot be withdrawn once it has been injected. Dosage miscalculations resulting in overdose can produce serious, even fatal, consequences. **Topical application** of creams and ointments is used for local effects in the skin and in certain conditions for systemic effects, as with nitroglycerin ointment for the treatment of angina pectoris.

INHALATION

Inhalation involves administration of drug through the nose or mouth and into the lungs during respiratory inspiration. The lungs (alveoli) are highly vascularized and have a large surface area, which contributes to rapid drug absorption from the lungs to the general circulation. Two important factors that determine the effectiveness of this route are aerosol droplet size and patient inhalation technique.

Only about 10% of an inhaled drug dose reaches the respiratory airways. Most of the drug is deposited on the inhalation device and within the oral cavity. Drug deposited in the oral cavity is subsequently swallowed into the GI tract. Particle size is very important for the proper distribution and deposition of inhaled aerosol particles into the lower airways. Drug particles greater than 10 μm are usually trapped in the upper respiratory tract. Particles 2–10 μm reach the bronchi and bronchioles, and only particles less than 1 μm pass directly to the alveoli for immediate absorption into the bloodstream. Tobacco smoke containing nicotine is an example of a particle that is less than 1 μm. Spacer devices can be used to decrease the deposition of drug within the oral cavity. Spacers are extension tubes that fit into the inhaler and into the mouth to direct more of the drug directly into the airways.

Drug preparations intended for local effects within the respiratory tract contain small drug dosages in particle sizes (2–8 μm) that provide rapid drug onset and minimal systemic drug absorption. The most common drug delivery devices are nebulizers, metered-dose aerosol inhalers, and dry powder inhalers. Nebulizers use air or oxygen to convert a drug solution into an aerosol that is then inhaled via a mouthpiece or mask. Metered-dose inhalers consist of an aerosol drug solution that is mixed with liquefied chlorofluorocarbon (Freon®) or other propellants under high pressure. Dry powder preparations are encapsulated solid drug particles that are inhaled with a special device. This device, either a Spinhaler or Rotohaler, pierces the capsule and withdraws the drug into the respiratory system when the patient inhales. More recently, other inhalers that utilize dry powders have been developed. These are in response to the need to eliminate the use of Freon in our environment. Some of these inhalers are called Rotadisks or Turbuhalers. Proper patient education on the correct use of inhalers is essential for obtaining maximum drug effects.

Gases (oxygen), volatile general anesthetics, and other volatile drugs (nicotine, crack cocaine) are rapidly absorbed from the lungs into the general circulation and provide a rapid onset of systemic drug action.

INTRANASAL ADMINISTRATION

Drugs are administered into the nasal cavity primarily to produce local effects within the nasal cavity and the nasal sinuses that drain into it. The nose is highly vascularized and possesses a series of bone plates (turbinates) that increase nasal surface area. Nasal preparations are administered as drops or fine aerosol sprays. Because most drug absorption occurs from the posterior portion of the nasal cavity, it is important to extend the head backward during administration in order to maximize drug absorption.

Several other routes of administration are used in specific situations. The most commonly used routes are listed in Table 2-1 with examples of their indications for use. Other routes will be presented in the appropriate chapters.

Table 2-1
Routes of Drug Administration

Route	Approximate Onset of Action	Indications	Examples
Oral (PO)	30 to 60 minutes	Whenever possible, the safest and most convenient route	Most medications— aspirin, sedatives, hypnotics, antibiotics
Sublingual	Several minutes	When rapid effects are needed	Nitroglycerin in angina pectoris
Buccal	Several minutes	Convenient dosage form for certain drugs	Androgenic drugs
Rectal	15 to 30 minutes	When patient cannot take oral medications and parenteral is not indicated, also for local effects	Analgesics, laxatives
Transdermal	30 to 60 minutes	Convenient dosage form that provides continuous absorption and systemic effects over many hours	Nitroglycerin, estrogen
Subcutaneous (SC)	Several minutes	For drugs that are inactivated by the GI tract	Insulin, heparin
Intramuscular (IM)	Several minutes	For drugs that have poor oral absorption, when high blood levels are required, and when rapid effects are desired	Narcotic analgesics, antibiotics
Intravenous (IV)	Within 1 minute	In emergency situations, where immediate effects are required, also when medications are administered by infusion	IV fluids (dextrose), nutrient supplementation, antibiotics
Intraarterial	Within 1 minute	For local effects within an internal organ	Cancer drugs
Intrathecal	Several minutes	For local effects within the spinal cord	Spinal anesthesia with lidocaine
Inhalation	Within 1 minute	For local effects within the respiratory tract	Antiasthmatic medications such as albuterol
Topical	Within 1 hour	For local effects on the skin, eye, or ear	Creams and ointments
Vaginal	15 to 30 minutes	For local effects	Creams, foams, and suppositories

Drug Absorption

Drug absorption refers to the entrance of a drug into the bloodstream. In order for absorption to occur, the drug must be dissolved in body fluids. With the exception of intravenous or intraarterial administration, drugs must pass through membranes of the GI lining and blood vessels before they gain access to the blood. Cell membranes are composed of lipids and proteins, which form a semipermeable barrier.

Cells have special transport mechanisms that allow various substances (including drugs) to pass through the cell membrane. These mechanisms include filtration, passive transport, and active transport. Most drugs pass through membranes by passive transport. An important principle in passive transport is that the concentration of drug on each side of the membrane differs. In passive transport, drug molecules pass from an area of high concentration to an area of low concentration (Law of Diffusion).

For example, following oral administration, there is a large amount of drug in the GI tract and no drug in the blood. Consequently, the drug molecules have a natural tendency to diffuse from the GI tract into the blood. The speed or rate of drug absorption also depends on the chemical properties of the drug and the site of administration. The properties of the drug that most determine absorption are lipid (fat) solubility of the drug and the degree of drug ionization.

LIPID SOLUBILITY

Cell membranes are composed of a significant amount of lipid material. In general, the more lipid-soluble a drug is, the faster it will pass through a lipid substance such as the cell membrane. With the exception of general anesthetics (highly lipid soluble), most drugs are primarily water soluble and only partially lipid soluble. Many water-soluble drugs are weak acids or bases that can form charged particles or ions (ionization) when dissolved in body fluids. The absorption of water-soluble drugs is mainly influenced by the degree of drug ionization.

DRUG IONIZATION

Many drugs exist in two forms, ionized and un-ionized. Like electrolytes (Na^+ and Cl^-), ionized drugs are charged molecules because their atomic structure has lost or gained electrons, leaving the molecules either positively or negatively charged. In general, ionized drug molecules do not readily cross cell membranes. The un-ionized (uncharged) form of the drug is required in order for absorption to occur.

The first generalization is that acid drugs (aspirin) are mostly un-ionized when they are in an acidic fluid (gastric juice). Consequently, drug absorption is favored. Conversely, acid drugs are mostly ionized when they are in an alkaline fluid; therefore, absorption is not favored and occurs at a slower rate and to a lesser extent.

The second generalization is that basic drugs (streptomycin, morphine) are mostly un-ionized when they are in an alkaline fluid (lower GI tract after rectal administration). Conversely, these drugs are mostly ionized when they are dissolved in an acidic fluid as found in the upper GI tract. This is the reason why morphine is usually administered parenterally. In the stomach (pH 1 to 3) and upper intestinal tract (pH 5 to 6), basic drugs such as morphine are absorbed more slowly and to a lesser extent than acidic drugs because they are primarily in an ionized form.

The acid and base nature of drugs may be useful in treating drug toxicity (overdose). Drugs are generally excreted by the kidneys in an ionized form. To increase drug excretion, the pH of the urine can be altered. For example, to increase the renal excretion of an acid drug (aspirin), the urine is alkalinized (pH > 7). In an alkaline urine, acidic drugs are mostly ionized and more rapidly excreted. In the same manner, basic drugs are more rapidly excreted by acidifying the urine (pH < 7).

DRUG FORMULATION

Drugs must be in solution before they can be absorbed. Tablets and capsules require time for the dissolution to occur. For this reason, liquid medications are generally absorbed faster than the solid forms. Drug particles can be formulated into different sizes, such as crystals, micronized particles, or ultramicronized particles. The smaller the drug particle, the faster are dissolution and absorption.

Drug Distribution

After a drug gains access to the blood, it is distributed to the various tissues and organs of the body. Several factors determine how much drug reaches any one organ or area of the body. The main factors are plasma protein binding, blood flow, and the presence of specific tissue barriers.

PLASMA PROTEIN BINDING

Several different proteins (albumin and globulins) are present in the plasma and form a circulating protein pool. These plasma proteins help regulate osmotic pressure (oncotic pressure) in the blood, which determines whether water is kept in or lost from the bloodstream. These plasma proteins transport many hormones and vitamins. In addition, many drugs are attracted to the plasma proteins, especially albumin. The result is that some drug molecules are bound to the plasma proteins, although some drug molecules remain unbound (free in the circulation). Only the unbound or free drug molecules can exert a pharmacological effect. The ratio of bound to unbound drug molecules varies with the drug used. Some drugs are highly bound (99%), and other drugs are not bound to any significant degree.

Occasionally, there is competition between drugs or other plasma substances for the same plasma protein binding site. In this situation, one drug may displace another. The result is that the concentration of free drug of one of the drugs increases, and this concentration can lead to increased pharmacological and adverse effects similar to overdosage.

BLOOD FLOW

The various organs of the body receive different amounts of blood. Organs such as the liver, kidneys, and brain have the largest blood supply. Consequently, these organs are usually exposed to the largest amount of drug. Some tissues, such as adipose tissue, receive a relatively poor blood supply and, as a result, do not accumulate large amounts of drug. However, highly lipid-soluble drugs can enter adipose tissue easily, where they can accumulate and remain for an extended period of time.

BLOOD–BRAIN BARRIER

In the case of the brain, an additional consideration is the blood–brain barrier. This barrier is an additional lipid barrier that protects the brain by restricting the passage of electrolytes and other water-soluble substances. Because the brain is composed of a large amount of lipid (nerve membranes and myelin), lipid-soluble drugs pass readily into the brain. As a general rule, then, a drug must have a certain degree of lipid solubility if it is to penetrate this barrier and gain access to the brain.

Drug Metabolism

Whenever a drug or other foreign substance is taken into the body, the body attempts to eliminate it. This usually involves excretion by one of the normal excretory routes (renal, intestinal, or respiratory). Some drugs can be excreted in the same chemical form in which they were administered. Other drugs, however, must be chemically altered before they can be excreted by the kidneys. Drug metabolism, also referred to as biotransformation, is the chemical alteration of various substances (drugs and foreign compounds) in the body. Proteins that function as enzymes are an essential part of the metabolic process.

The liver is the main organ involved in drug metabolism. Within the cells of the liver are a group of enzymes that specifically function to metabolize foreign (drug) substances. These enzymes are referred to as the **drug microsomal metabolizing system (DMMS).** The main function of this system is to take lipid-soluble drugs and chemically alter them so that they become water-soluble compounds. Water-soluble compounds can be excreted by the kidneys. Lipid-soluble compounds are repeatedly reabsorbed into the blood. Although most drugs are inactivated by metabolism, a few are initially converted into more pharmacologically active drugs. This conversion increases the duration of drug action.

An interesting phenomenon occurs with some drugs, especially the barbiturates and other sedative-hypnotic drugs. When these drugs are taken repeatedly, they stimulate the **DMMS.** By stimulating this system, the drugs actually increase the amount of enzymes in the system; this process is referred to as **enzyme induction.** With an increase in the amount of enzymes, there is a faster rate of drug metabolism. Consequently, the duration of drug action is decreased for all drugs metabolized by the microsomal enzymes. This change occasionally produces serious adverse interactions with other drugs that must be metabolized by the drug microsomal metabolizing system.

After oral administration, all drugs are absorbed into the portal circulation, which transports the drugs to the liver before they are distributed throughout the body. Some drugs are metabolized significantly as they pass through the liver this first time. This effect is referred to as first-pass metabolism. It can significantly reduce the amount of active drug that reaches the general circulation. This is the reason that some oral doses must be greater than parenteral doses.

Drug Excretion

The common pathways of drug excretion are renal (urine), GI (feces), and respiratory (exhaled gases). Although the liver is the most important organ for drug metabolism, the kidneys are the most important organs for drug excretion.

RENAL EXCRETION

After the blood is filtered through the glomerulus of the kidneys, most of the filtered substances are eventually reabsorbed into the blood. The exceptions to this are the urinary waste products and anything else that is in a nonabsorbable form. In order for drug excretion to occur, the drug or drug metabolite must be water soluble and preferably in an ionized form. As mentioned, acid drugs are mostly ionized in alkaline urine, and basic drugs are mostly ionized in an acid urine. In the case of barbiturate or aspirin overdose (acid drugs), alkalinization of the urine with sodium bicarbonate will hasten elimination of either drug in the urine.

GI EXCRETION

After oral administration, a certain portion of drug (unabsorbed) passes through the GI tract and is excreted in the feces. The amount varies with the particular drug used.

In addition, there is another pathway involving the intestinal tract, the enterohepatic pathway. Certain drugs (fat-soluble drugs) can enter the intestines by way of the biliary tract. After the drug is released into the intestines (in the bile), it may be absorbed into the blood again. This is referred to as the enterohepatic cycle. The duration of action of a few drugs is greatly prolonged because of this repeated cycling of the drug (liver → bile → intestines → blood → liver).

RESPIRATORY EXCRETION

The respiratory system does not usually play a significant role in drug excretion. However, some drugs are metabolized to products that can be exchanged from the blood into the respiratory tract. General anesthetic gases are not totally metabolized, and a significant fraction of these drugs are eliminated by the lungs.

MISCELLANEOUS

Some drugs and drug metabolites also can be detected in sweat, saliva, and milk (lactation). Infants can be exposed to significant amounts of certain drugs after nursing (see the section on drug exposure during nursing later in this chapter).

Half-Life

The **half-life** of a drug is the time required for the blood or plasma concentration of the drug to fall to half of its original level. It is important in determining the frequency of drug administration. The major factors that determine half-life are the rates of drug metabolism and excretion. The half-life of any drug is relatively constant if the individual has normal rates of drug metabolism and excretion. It can be prolonged when liver or kidney disease is present. In these situations, the dose or the frequency of administration can be reduced.

Blood Drug Levels

The intensity of drug effect is mainly determined by the concentration of drug in the blood or plasma. The amount of drug in the plasma is determined by an interplay of all the pharmacokinetic processes (absorption, distribution, metabolism, and excretion). These processes occur together. As a drug is absorbed and distributed, the liver and kidneys begin the processes of metabolism and excretion. The plasma level of the drug is constantly changing, as illustrated in Figure 1-4. In the beginning, absorption and distribution predominate, and the plasma level increases. Later, drug metabolism and excretion predominate, and the plasma level decreases.

Drug monitoring, the periodic measurement of blood drug levels, is performed to ensure that the level of drug in the blood is within the therapeutic range. Drug levels below the therapeutic range will not produce the desired drug effect, whereas levels above the therapeutic range cause increased side effects and toxicity. This concept is illustrated in Figure 2-2.

There are some drugs that require several dosages or several days or weeks to reach the desired drug effect. In some clinical situations, it may be necessary to reach therapeutic drug levels as rapidly as possible. In these cases, a loading dose may be administered. A **loading dose** is usually an initial higher dose of drug, often administered IV, to rapidly attain the therapeutic drug level and drug effects. Loading doses are usually followed by **maintenance doses** that are smaller and calculated to maintain the drug level within the therapeutic range.

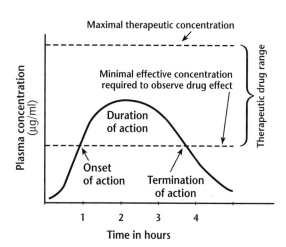

Figure 2-2

Illustration of therapeutic drug range.

STEADY STATE

In order to get the benefit of a medication, we usually must take the medicine on a regular schedule. You might take a medicine once a day, twice a day, or more often. The question is, when do we get the full effects of a medicine? There are a number of factors, but the primary one is when the levels of the medicine reach **steady state.** Steady state is the condition in which there is a balance between absorption and elimination that occurs over time. After one dose we will reach a balance, but before the medicine is totally eliminated, we get the next dose, so there is a steady increase in the level of medicine over time. The point at which levels of medicine reach their full potential is referred to as steady state.

As a rule, steady state occurs after 5 half-lives. The same rule applies in the case when a medicine is discontinued, and we want to know when the effects of the drug will be gone. It takes 5 half-lives to totally remove the drug from the body. Figure 2-3 illustrates this principle.

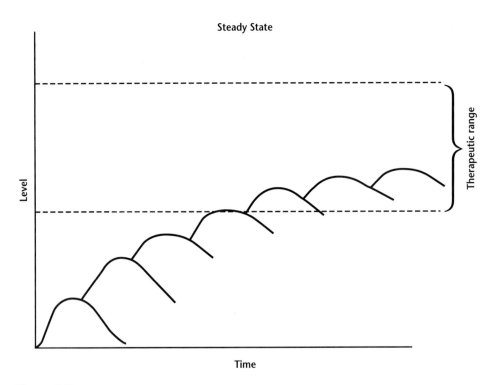

Figure 2-3
Steady state.

Bioavailability

Bioavailability is the percentage of the dose of a drug that is actually absorbed into the bloodstream. Differences in drug formulation, route of administration, and factors that affect GI absorption can influence bioavailability. A particular drug may be manufactured by many different drug companies and sold under different trade names. In these situations, the amount of drug may be the same in each product, but the product may be different because of particle size, binders, fillers, and tablet coating. These differences may alter bioavailability. There have been examples of this in the past. Now, however, the Food and Drug Administration (FDA) regulates and requires bioavailability testing.

Factors of Individual Variation

Many factors affect individual variation. These factors include age, weight, sex, genetic variation, emotional state, placebo effect, the presence of disease, and patient compliance.

AGE

The effects of drugs in different age groups is of particular importance. Infants, children, and the elderly are generally more sensitive to the actions of drugs than younger adults. Drug considerations during pregnancy on fetal development, during the infant nursing period, and in infants and children are discussed below. Drug considerations for the elderly are presented in the section on geriatric drug considerations later in this chapter.

WEIGHT

Most adult dosages are calculated for the average adult weight, 150 lb between the ages of 16 and 65. Obviously, all adults are not 150 lb. In small individuals (100 lb), the dose may have to be reduced. In larger individuals (200 to 300 lb), the dose may have to be increased. However, this approach does not always hold true because many other factors are involved.

SEX AND PERCENT BODY FAT

Women possess a higher percentage of body fat and a lower percentage of body water than do men of equal weight. Consequently, women may experience a greater drug effect than do men because the drug is dissolved in a smaller volume of body fluid. Women also possess more body fat than men. Lipid-soluble drugs are more widely distributed and may produce longer durations of action than in men. This same concept also applies to the differences in body fat composition between members of the same sex.

GENETIC VARIATION

Individuals tend to inherit the proteins and enzyme patterns of their parents. There is significant genetic variation in some of the drug-metabolizing enzymes, so individual differences can occur. If the difference affects the rate of drug metabolism, there may be a difference in the effects produced by the drug. An enzyme may be missing, in which case drug metabolism is extremely slow. A slowed metabolism rate may result in increased and prolonged drug effects that can lead to serious consequences. Examples of genetic variation will be discussed in specific chapters.

EMOTIONAL STATE

Differences in drug effects can be caused by the emotional state of the individual. For example, an individual who is excited or extremely anxious may require larger doses of hypnotic or tranquilizer drugs than an individual who is not emotionally stimulated but who still has difficulty sleeping.

PLACEBO EFFECT

Patients come to physicians and hospitals with varying expectations. It has been observed that if patients have a positive attitude and think that a drug or treatment will help, chances are the patients will claim an improvement whether there actually is one or not.

In some studies, patients have been unknowingly given sugar pills or placebos instead of an actual drug. A large percentage of these patients claim an improved condition even though they received no real drug. Likewise, patients with hostile or negative attitudes, who feel that nothing will help their condition, usually say that they feel no difference or even worse after a specific treatment or medication. The influence of one's mind on the course of treatment is referred to as the placebo effect. This phenomenon can be used by the medical and nursing staff to enhance the positive attitude of patients. Thus, the patients stand a better chance of responding successfully to therapy.

PRESENCE OF DISEASE

The presence of other diseases that are debilitating or that decrease the function of some vital organ usually makes an individual more susceptible to the effects and adverse reactions of the drug therapy. As mentioned, the liver and kidneys are especially important because these two organs are exposed to the highest drug levels. For this reason, liver and kidney function are often adversely affected by drugs. Patients with hepatic or renal disease suffer a greater incidence of adverse drug effects because they are unable to eliminate the drug and its metabolites effectively. Consequently, plasma drug levels are much higher in these patients as a result of an accumulation of the drug in the plasma.

PATIENT COMPLIANCE

Drug compliance refers to taking a drug exactly as prescribed. If doses are forgotten or skipped, the drug effects will be reduced or absent. This is referred to as noncompliance. Noncompliance is often a problem in geriatric patients, who may have memory difficulties and who are easily confused by complicated dosing schedules, especially when several different drugs are involved. Particular care and sufficient patient instruction and training must be given to ensure that all patients understand dosing instructions.

Pediatric Drug Considerations

FETAL PERIOD DURING PREGNANCY

Before birth, the developing fetus will be exposed to most drugs taken during pregnancy. The placenta is not a drug barrier, and drug absorption and distribution to the fetus follow the same principles as with other maternal organs (passive diffusion based on lipid solubility and ionization). Although there are relatively few drugs that have been proven to be teratogenic (cause birth defects), it is recommended that drug exposure during pregnancy be avoided if possible. This is especially true during the first trimester, when organogenesis, the formation of body organs, is occurring. Drugs that are teratogens may cause spontaneous abortion, growth retardation, birth defects, or carcinogenesis (development of cancer). The Food and Drug Administration has established guidelines, the FDA Pregnancy Categories (see Table 2-2), that classify drugs based on fetal risk. Table 2-3 lists some drugs that have been associated with teratogenicity in humans.

DRUG EXPOSURE DURING INFANT NURSING

Drugs administered to nursing mothers appear in breast milk to varying degrees. Unfortunately, there is a lack of controlled studies and reliable information in this area. The major concern is that the drug concentration in the milk will be high enough to produce undesired or harmful effects in the infant. Generally, the recommendation is to avoid unnecessary drug administration. Usually, the infant experiences the same pharmacological effects as appear in the mother. For example,

Table 2-2

Description of FDA Pregnancy Categories

Category	Description
Pregnancy Category A	Drug studies in pregnant women have not yet demonstrated risk to the fetus.
Pregnancy Category B	Drug studies have not been performed in pregnant women; animal studies have not demonstrated fetal risk.
Pregnancy Category C	Drug studies have not been performed in pregnant women or in animals, or animal studies have revealed some teratogenic potential, but the risk to the fetus is unknown.
Pregnancy Category D	Drug studies have revealed adverse risk to the fetus. The benefit-to-risk ratio of the drug must be established before use during pregnancy.
Pregnancy Category X	Drug studies have revealed teratogenic effects in women and/or animals. Fetal risk clearly outweighs benefit. Drug is contraindicated in pregnancy.
Pregnancy Category NR	Drug has not yet been rated by FDA.

Table 2-3

Examples of Drugs with Demonstrated Teratogenic Risk in Humans

Drug	Teratogenic Effect
Androgens (male hormone)	Masculinization of female fetus
Carbamazepine	Craniofacial and fingernail deformities
Diethylstilbestrol	Vaginal tumors and genital malformations in offspring
Estrogen (female hormone)	Feminization of male fetus
Lithium	Cardiac defects
Phenytoin	Craniofacial and limb deformities, growth retardation
Retinoic acid	Craniofacial, cardiac, and CNS defects
Thalidomide	Phocomelia (limb deformities)
Warfarin	Facial, cartilage, and CNS defects

when taken by the mother, laxatives may cause infant diarrhea, and sedatives and hypnotics will cause drowsiness and lethargy. Other drugs, such as anticancer agents or drugs with increased toxicities, are contraindicated unless the benefit to the mother clearly outweighs the risk to the infant. Table 2-4 lists some of the drugs that appear in breast milk.

Table 2-4

Examples of Drugs That Cross into Breast Milk Following Maternal Use

Drug Class	Examples
Antibiotics	Ampicillin, erythromycin, penicillin, streptomycin, sulfa drugs, tetracyclines
Antiepileptic agents	Phenytoin, primidone
Antithyroid agents	Thiouracil
CNS stimulants	Nicotine
Laxatives	Cascara, danthron
Narcotic analgesics	Codeine, heroin, methadone, morphine
Nonnarcotic antiinflammatory agents	Phenylbutazone
Sedative-hypnotic agents	Barbiturates, chloral hydrate
Tranquilizers (antipsychotic agents)	Chlorpromazine, lithium

PEDIATRIC CONSIDERATIONS

There are a number of pharmacokinetic and pharmacodynamic differences between pediatric and adult patients. Neonates (0–1 month), infants (1–12 months), and children of increasing age are not simply "small adults." There are a number of factors that must be considered that generally require reduction in dosage beyond the obvious difference in body weight. These differences tend to decrease with advancing age, especially after the first year of life.

DRUG ADMINISTRATION AND ABSORPTION

Neonates and infants have a small skeletal muscle mass. In addition, limited physical activity results in a lower blood flow to the muscle. Therefore, absorption after IM injections is slower and more variable. There is also increased risk of muscle and nerve damage with IM injections. In serious situations, the IV route is more reliable and generally preferred. The skin of neonates and infants is thinner, and topically applied drugs are more rapidly and completely absorbed into the systemic circulation. With regard to oral administration, the gastric pH of premature babies and neonates is less acidic. This could result in decreased bioavailability and lower blood levels of orally administered drugs that are acidic in nature.

DRUG DISTRIBUTION

Pediatric patients possess a higher percentage of body water and a lower percentage of body fat. These differences decrease the distribution of lipid-soluble drugs to body tissues and organs. This tends to cause higher drug blood levels. Water-soluble drug distribution is increased (greater peripheral drug distribution), which tends to lower drug blood levels. These effects are all in comparison to the adult. Although pediatric patients have higher percentages of water, they are more easily dehydrated by vomiting and diarrhea. The resulting reduction of body fluids will increase drug concentrations and drug effects.

Plasma protein levels are also lower, especially in neonates. This results in lower plasma protein binding of drugs and, therefore, greater amounts of unbound or "free" drug. Because only the unbound drug exerts an effect, there will be a greater intensity of drug effect.

DRUG METABOLISM AND EXCRETION

There is a reduced capacity for drug metabolism and drug excretion during the first several years of life. Consequently, drug elimination occurs more slowly, and the duration of drug action is prolonged. The decreases in drug metabolism and excretion are most evident in the neonate and infant. After the first year, drug metabolism and excretion gradually become proportional to those of the adult. There are some exceptions where the metabolism is increased and drug dosage needed to be increased during this period.

DOSAGE ADJUSTMENT

Dosage calculations in pediatrics are based mainly on age, body surface area, and body weight. The rules and formulas used for these calculations are presented in Chapter 3, Math Review and Dosage Calculations.

GERIATRIC DRUG CONSIDERATIONS

Concerns about medication use in geriatric patients are actually very similar to those for pediatric patients. Rather than being concerned about maturing systems, we need to be concerned with systems that no longer function at full capacity.

With age, there is a decrease in the body's ability to absorb medications from the GI tract in geriatric patients. This results in delays in the onset of action as well as decreases in the peak levels.

A change in body composition also occurs over time. Our bodies have more fat, less water, and less lean muscle as we age. This changes the distribution characteristics of many drugs depending on their lipid or water solubility.

Our metabolism decreases as the blood flow to the liver decreases, and the production of enzymes for metabolism of the drug also decreases.

Elimination is also reduced as the body ages. Decreased blood flow also reduces drugs passing through the kidney, and the functioning units of the kidney no longer work at full capacity.

There is also a change in our response to drugs. As we age, we lose certain receptors, and this results in a decreased response to the dose of medicine that worked well when we were younger.

β_2-Agonists, which are used to dilate the respiratory passages, no longer work at the same level because of decreased sensitivity of the receptors. In addition, elderly patients are more likely to experience side effects such as increased heart rate and decreased potassium levels.

For geriatric patients who take high doses of inhaled steroids, there may be an increased incidence of cataracts, osteoporosis, and reduced control of diabetes.

As we age, we also lose the ability to learn new things, and our coordination decreases. Generally, it is more difficult for a geriatric patient to learn how to use a metered dose inhaler (MDI) than it is for a younger patient. It is also more difficult for the elderly to grip the inhaler and press the actuator with decreased grip strength that relates to arthritis. As many as 40% of geriatric patients do not use an inhaler correctly.

Drug Interactions

Drug interaction refers to the effects that occur when the actions of one drug are affected by another drug. There are many different types of drug interactions. Some drugs interfere with each other during GI absorption and, therefore, should not be administered at the same time. Other drugs may interfere with plasma protein building, drug metabolism, or drug excretion. Throughout this book, the common drug interactions will be given. Table 2-5 explains the general terms that are associated with drug interactions.

Table 2-5
Terminology of Common Drug Interactions

Term	Explanation
Incompatibility	Usually refers to physical alterations of drugs that occur before administration, when different drugs are mixed in the same syringe or other container
Additive effects	When the combined effect of two drugs, each producing the same biological response by the same mechanism of action, is equal to the sum of their individual effects
Summation	When the combined effect of two drugs, each producing the same biological response but by a different mechanism of action, is equal to the sum of their individual effects
Synergism	When the combined effect of two drugs is greater than the sum of their individual effects
Antagonism	When the combined effect of two drugs is less than the sum of their individual effects

Terminology Associated with Chronic Drug Use and Abuse

The chronic use of certain drugs results in a number of physiological and pharmacological changes in drug response. The development of drug tolerance and drug dependence are two important phenomena involved in chronic drug use.

TOLERANCE

Tolerance is defined as a decreased drug effect that occurs after repeated administration. In order to attain the previous drug effect, the dosage must be increased. This is a common occurrence in individuals who abuse drugs such as cocaine, barbiturates, morphine, and heroin. There is also the phenomenon of cross-tolerance, which is the tolerance that exists between drugs of the same class. Tolerance is caused by changes or adaptations that occur in response to repeated drug exposure. The main types of tolerance are referred to as metabolic tolerance and pharmacodynamic tolerance. Metabolic tolerance is caused by enzyme induction; the drug increases the drug-metabolizing enzymes (DMMS), and the dose must be increased in order to attain the same previous effect. Pharmacodynamic tolerance is caused by the ability of some drugs to decrease the number of drug receptors. This usually takes several weeks or months and is referred to as "down-regulation." With the reduction in drug receptors, there is a reduction in intensity of drug effect.

DRUG DEPENDENCE

Drug dependence is a condition in which reliance on the administration of a particular drug becomes extremely important to the well-being of an individual. Drug dependence is usually characterized as psychological and/or physical. When the drug is used repeatedly for nonmedical purposes, the term drug abuse is implied. Any activity that is repeated and that provides pleasure involves a psychological component of behavior. The smoking of tobacco, for example, is an activity associated with psychological dependence. Deprivation of smoking causes some unpleasant feelings but does not result in serious medical consequences. All drugs that are abused have varying degrees of psychological dependence associated with them. Many abused drugs also produce physical dependence when taken for prolonged periods of time and usually at increasing dosages. Deprivation of these drugs leads to a physical withdrawal syndrome that is very unpleasant, characterized by measurable changes in many bodily functions, and that may cause serious medical consequences. The withdrawal reactions from alcohol, barbiturates, and opiate drugs are examples of this type of reaction. When drug dependence is particularly severe, and compulsive drug behavior dominates all other activities, the term **drug addiction** is used.

Chapter 2 Review

UNDERSTANDING TERMINOLOGY

Match the description in the left column with the appropriate term in the right column.

1. When the combined effect of two drugs, each producing the same biological response by the same mechanism of action, is equal to the sum of their individual effects.

2. When the combined effect of two drugs, each producing the same biological response but by a different mechanism of action, is equal to the sum of their individual effects.

3. When the combined effect of two drugs is greater than the sum of their individual effects.

4. When the combined effect of two drugs is less than the sum of their individual effects.

5. Usually refers to physical alterations of drugs that occur before administration when different drugs are mixed in the same syringe or other container.

6. Decreased drug effects after chronic administration.

a. additive effects
b. antagonism
c. incompatibility
d. summation
e. synergism
f. tolerance

Answer the following questions.

7. Differentiate among the following terms: parenteral administration, oral administration, intramuscular injection, and intravenous injection.

8. What is the main disadvantage to the IV method of drug administration?

9. By what method of cell transport are most drugs absorbed? What are the main requirements for drug absorption?

10. Explain why alkalinization of the urine increases the rate of excretion of drugs such as aspirin or phenobarbital.

11. Briefly describe the main factors that determine drug distribution.

12. What is the major requirement for a drug if it is to gain access to the brain?

13. What is the drug microsomal metabolizing system, and what is its main function?

14. List the major pathways of drug excretion.

15. Why is the plasma drug concentration important? What are the main factors that determine plasma concentration?

16. List the factors that can contribute to individual variation in drug response.

ACQUIRING KNOWLEDGE

After reading this chapter, you should be able to answer the following questions:

17. A single IV injection of 100 mg of a drug with a half-life of 4 hours is administered to a young adult. Approximately how many hours will it take to totally eliminate this dosage from the body?

18. A drug has a bioavailability of 70% after oral administration. How many milligrams of drug will be absorbed following a dose of 200 mg? What would be the expected effect on bioavailability if a large meal were ingested just before administration?

19. Your grandmother has just been prescribed a very lipid-soluble drug. Would you expect her dosage to be larger or smaller than that for a younger adult? Explain.

20. Rifampin is a drug that causes enzyme induction. Would you have to increase or decrease the dosage of another drug taken concurrently if it required drug metabolism for elimination? What change in dosage would a very water-soluble drug require?

21. Individuals who become dependent on drugs such as alcohol or narcotics require a steady supply of drug for administration, or they will experience unpleasant and potentially harmful effects. Individuals with diabetes require insulin injections on a daily basis, or they will experience potentially harmful effects. Are the individuals taking insulin dependent on the drug? Is there a difference between the dependence on insulin and that on alcohol? Explain.

APPLYING KNOWLEDGE ON THE JOB

After reading this chapter, you should be able to answer the following questions:

22. Assume that your new job in a neighborhood health clinic is to identify individual patient factors that might affect the bioavailability of drugs

prescribed for the patients. Five of the clinic's patients whom you dealt with this morning are described below. For each patient, identify one factor that could affect drug bioavailability and explain how dosage could be changed to compensate for it.

a. Jonathan is a 35-year-old man with a medical history of stomach complaints but no evidence of ulcer. When Jonathan visited the clinic this morning, he weighed in at 324 lb. He presented with upper respiratory symptoms attributable to allergy and was prescribed a decongestant and an antihistamine.

Factor:

Dosage change:

b. Lisa is a 25-year-old woman weighing 103 lb. She is in good health. At her clinic visit this morning, she complained of muscle pain caused by moving furniture into her new apartment. She was prescribed a muscle relaxant and a pain reliever.

Factor:

Dosage change:

c. Al is a 50-year-old male alcoholic weighing 150 lb. His history reveals long-term alcohol abuse. Liver function tests run last month showed some enzyme abnormalities. Al's visit to the clinic this morning was for a sinus infection. He was prescribed an antibiotic and a decongestant.

Factor:

Dosage change:

d. Janet is a 49-year-old woman weighing 130 lb. Her visit to the clinic this morning was for insomnia, which she has suffered since her husband's death 2 weeks ago. It was clear from her behavior at the clinic today that she's still emotionally distraught. She was prescribed a mild sedative.

Factor:

Dosage change:

e. Jessie is a 5-year-old girl weighing 43 lb. She presented at the clinic this morning with an upper respiratory virus and strep throat. She was prescribed an antibiotic for the strep throat and pediatric ibuprofen for fever and discomfort.

Factor:

Dosage change:

23. Assume that you have volunteered to work a nonprescription-drug hotline. Your job is to give people who call assistance with over-the-counter drugs. How would you react, and why, to the following anonymous callers?

a. Caller A is worried about taking too much aspirin. She didn't realize until after she took the capsules that they were double the dose of the product she usually takes. She wants to know if there's something she might have on hand at home that she could take to counter the effects of the extra aspirin in her system.

    b. Caller B wants to know if it's all right to take a laxative while she is breast-feeding her baby.

Additional Reading

Blodget JB. Managing injection reactions. *Nursing* 1995;25(9):46.

Carr DS. New strategies for avoiding medication errors. *Nursing* 1989;19(8):38.

Cirone N, Schwartz N. Finding the balance for drug therapy. *Nursing* 1996;26(3):40.

Cohen MR, Cohen HG. Medication errors: Following a game plan for continued improvement. *Nursing* 1996;26(11):34.

Crane R. Intermittent subcutaneous infusion of opioids in hospice home care. *Am J Hospice Palliative Care* 1994;11(1):8.

Hahn K. Brush up on your injection technique. *Nursing* 1990;20(9):54.

Hussar DA. Helping your patient follow his drug regimen. *Nursing* 1995;25(10):62.

Kean MF. Get on the right track with Z-track injections. *Nursing* 1990;20(8):59.

Konich-McMahan J. Full speed ahead with caution: Rushing intravenous drugs. *Nursing* 1996;26(6):26.

McGovern K. Ten golden rules for administering drugs safely. *Nursing* 1988;18(8):34.

McLean J. The placebo effect: Magic pills. *Nurs Times* 1990;86(28):28.

Wichowski HC, Kubsch S. Improving your patients' compliance. *Nursing* 1995;25(1):66.

Math Review and Dosage Calculations

Henry Hitner, PhD
Barbara Nagle, PhD

Chapter Focus

This chapter reviews basic mathematical operations required for drug calculation. It also provides examples that clearly show how to set up and solve different types of dosage problems necessary for proper drug administration.

Chapter Terminology

decimal: Another way to write a fraction when the denominator is 10, 100, 1000, and so on.

denominator: Bottom number of a fraction, which shows the number of parts in a whole.

fraction: Part of a whole.

improper fraction: Fraction that has a value equal to or greater than 1.

mixed number: Number written with both a whole number and a fraction.

numerator: Top number of a fraction, which shows the part.

percent: Decimal fraction with a denominator of 100.

proper fraction: Fraction that has a value less than 1.

proportion: A mathematical equation that expresses the equality between two ratios.

ratio: The relationship of one number to another expressed by whole numbers (1:5) or as a fraction (1/5).

solute: Substance dissolved in a solvent; usually present in a lesser amount.

solution: Homogeneous mixture of two or more substances.

solvent: Liquid portion of a solution that is capable of dissolving another substance.

Chapter Objectives

After studying this chapter, you should be able to:

* Solve basic arithmetic problems involving fractions, decimals, and percentages.
* Perform conversions from one metric unit of measure to another.
* Set up ratio and proportion equations and solve for the unknown term.
* Solve drug problems involving solutions and solid dosage forms.
* Solve problems involving pediatric dosing.

Because the intensity of drug response is directly related to dosage (dose-response relationship), administration of the proper drug dosage is essential to the practice of medicine. Drugs whose names look alike or sound alike (for example, Isordil/Isuprel) can cause improper drug selection. Mistakes in dosage calculation can cause insufficient drug response or excessive and potentially harmful drug effects. Consequently, it is essential for anyone responsible for administering medication to understand the proper procedures for dosage calculation.

Fractions, Decimals, and Percents

A brief review of fractions, decimals, and percentages is presented to refresh the memory for the basic arithmetic procedures used in dosage calculation.

FRACTIONS

When something is divided into equal parts, one of the parts is referred to as a **fraction** (part of the whole). A fraction is composed of two numbers, a numerator and a denominator. The **numerator** is the top number of a fraction. It indicates how many parts are being referred to. The **denominator** is the bottom number of a fraction. It indicates how many parts something has been divided into *(see Figure 3-1)*.

Proper Fractions   Fractions whose values are less than 1 (the numerator is smaller than the denominator) are called **proper fractions.** The following are examples of proper fractions:

1/4, 2/3, 7/8, 9/10

The Fraction $\frac{2}{3}$

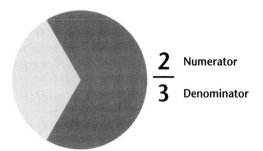

$$\frac{2}{3} \quad \begin{matrix} \text{Numerator} \\ \\ \text{Denominator} \end{matrix}$$

Figure 3-1
The fraction ⅔ represents two of three equal-sized pieces of a whole.

Improper Fractions Fractions whose values are equal to or greater than 1 (the numerator is equal to or greater than the denominator) are called **improper fractions.** The following fractions are improper:

$$5/5, 7/5, 11/6, 15/8$$

An improper fraction can be written as a **mixed number,** which is a whole number plus the fractional remainder. This is calculated by dividing the denominator of the improper fraction into the numerator and placing any remainder over the original denominator. The following improper fractions have been changed to mixed numbers:

$$5/5 = 1; 7/5 = 1\tfrac{2}{5}; 11/6 = 1\tfrac{5}{6}; 24/8 = 3$$

The terms of a fraction can be changed without changing its value. Multiplying or dividing the numerator and the denominator of a fraction by the same number does not change the value of the fraction, as shown in the following examples:

$$\frac{2 \div 2}{4 \div 2} = \frac{1}{2} \qquad \frac{2 \times 3}{4 \times 3} = \frac{6}{12}$$

Fractions are generally written in their reduced or lowest terms. For example:

$$\tfrac{6}{12} = \tfrac{1}{2}$$

Reducing Fractions to Their Lowest Terms Reduce a fraction to its lowest terms by dividing the numerator and denominator by the largest number that will divide into both of them evenly. For example:

$$\frac{15}{20} \div \frac{5}{5} = \frac{3}{4} \qquad \frac{35}{49} \div \frac{7}{7} = \frac{5}{7}$$

Multiplying Fractions   Multiply fractions by multiplying the numerators together and the denominators together and reducing to lowest terms. For example:

$$\tfrac{2}{3} \times \tfrac{3}{4} = \tfrac{6}{12} = \tfrac{1}{2}$$

If the fractions involve large numbers, reduce the numbers by dividing any numerator and any denominator by the same number. Repeat this cancellation process as often as possible. For example:

$$\frac{\overset{1}{\cancel{9}}}{\underset{2}{\cancel{18}}} \times \frac{\overset{1}{\cancel{27}}}{\underset{2}{\cancel{54}}} = \frac{1}{4}$$

$$\frac{\overset{1}{\cancel{4}}}{\underset{1}{\cancel{6}}} \times \frac{\overset{2}{\cancel{12}}}{\underset{\cancel{4}\,2}{\cancel{16}}^{\,1}} = \frac{1}{2}$$

To multiply a whole number by a fraction, place the whole number over a denominator of 1; then multiply numerators and denominators. For example:

$$10 \times \tfrac{1}{2} = \tfrac{10}{1} \times \tfrac{1}{2} = \tfrac{10}{2} = 5$$

Dividing Fractions   Dividing one fraction by another is similar to multiplying fractions. However, first you must invert the divisor before multiplying the numerators together and the denominators together. For example:

$$\frac{2}{3} \div \frac{3}{4} = \frac{2}{3} \times \frac{4}{3} = \frac{8}{9}$$

If the divisor is a whole number, place it over 1, invert it, and then multiply as before. For example:

$$\frac{3}{3} \div 4 = \frac{3}{4} \div \frac{4}{1} = \frac{3}{4} \times \frac{1}{4} = \frac{3}{16}$$

DECIMALS

Any whole number may be divided into tenths (0.1), hundredths (0.01), thousandths (0.001), and so on. These divisions of a number by orders of 10 (10, 100, 1000, etc.) are known as decimal fractions or **decimals.** Decimals are another way of expressing fractions. For example:

$$1/10 = 0.1 \qquad 1/100 = 0.01 \qquad 1/1000 = 0.001$$

To change a fraction to a decimal, simply divide the numerator by the denominator. Note that you may need to add zeroes after the decimal point in the dividend. For example:

$$\frac{1}{4} = 4\overline{)1.00}^{\,0.25} = 0.25$$

To change a decimal to a fraction, place the decimal number over the order of 10 (10, 100, 1000, etc.) that corresponds to the last place of the decimal and reduce to lowest terms. For example:

$$0.5 \text{ (tenths)} = \frac{5}{10} = \frac{1}{2}$$

$$0.25 \text{ (hundredths)} = \frac{25}{100} = \frac{1}{4}$$

$$0.005 \text{ (thousandths)} = \frac{5}{1000} = \frac{1}{200}$$

Multiplying Decimals   Multiplying decimals is similar to multiplying whole numbers except for the placement of the decimal point. After multiplying the two decimal numbers, add the total number of decimal places (places to the right of each decimal point) and count off the total number of decimal places in the answer (product). Count from right to left, and put the decimal point in front of the last number you count. For example:

$$
\begin{array}{r}
1.25 \text{ (2 decimal places)} \\
\times\ 0.25 \text{ (2 decimal places)} \\
\hline
625 \\
250 \\
\hline
0.3125 \text{ (4 decimal places)}
\end{array}
$$

When an answer has fewer numbers than total decimal places, add zeros as placeholders to make up the difference.

$$
\begin{array}{r}
0.5\ \text{ (1 decimal place)} \\
\times\ 0.1\ \text{ (1 decimal place)} \\
\hline
0.05 \text{ (2 decimal places)}
\end{array}
$$

Dividing Decimals   When dividing decimals, move the decimal place in the divisor to the far right and then move the decimal place in the number being divided by the same number of places. For example:

$$25 \div 0.05 = 0.05\overline{)25.000}^{\,500.0}$$
$$\text{(2 places)}\quad\text{(2 places)}$$

$$0.010 \div 0.5 = .5\overline{)0.010}^{\,0.02}$$
$$\text{(1 place)}\qquad\text{(1 place)}$$

PERCENTS

Percent means per hundred, so **percents** are decimal fractions with denominators of 100. See the following examples:

$$10\% = \frac{10}{100} = 0.10$$

$$25\% = \frac{25}{100} = \frac{1}{4} = 0.25$$

Multiplying Percentages   Change the percent to a decimal (in hundredths) and multiply. For example:

15% of 75

$$
\begin{array}{r}
75 \\
\times\, 0.15 \text{ (2 decimal places)} \\
\hline
375 \\
75 \\
\hline
11.25 \text{ (2 decimal places)}
\end{array}
$$

0.2% of 50

$$
\begin{array}{r}
50 \\
\times\, 0.002 \text{ (3 decimal places)} \\
\hline
0.100 \text{ (3 decimal places)}
\end{array}
$$

Dosage Calculations

Health professionals today are very fortunate because pharmaceutical manufacturers prepare and market most drugs in convenient dosage forms. The metric system has essentially replaced the apothecaries' system, so mathematical conversions are rarely necessary. Also, the concept of unit dose packaging eliminates much of the time that was previously required for drug calculation and preparation. However, in certain situations, drug calculations are still required. These situations primarily involve the preparation of a drug dosage from a stock solution, vial, scored tablet, or calculation of dosage based on body weight or other body measurement.

BASIC CALCULATIONS

Ratio is the relationship of one number to another expressed by whole numbers (1:5) or as a fraction (1/5). The lowest form of the ratio is determined by dividing the smaller number into the larger number. In this example, the ratio would be 5:1.

Proportion is a mathematical equation that expresses the equality between two ratios. For example:

25:5 = 50:10

The first (25) and last terms (10) are called the extremes. The second (5) and third terms (50) are called the means. The product (multiplication) of the extremes must equal the product of the means. An example follows:

$$\overset{\text{Means}}{25:\!\overset{\downarrow\ \ \downarrow}{5 = 50}:\!10}$$
$$\underset{\text{Extremes}}{\nwarrow\ \ \ \ \ \ \ \ \nearrow}$$

$$25 = 10 = 5 = 50$$

$$250 = 250$$

When one of the numbers in the proportion is not known, the proportion equation can be solved for the unknown (referred to as x).

> *EXAMPLE*   There are 10 milligrams (mg) of drug per milliliter (mL) of solution. How many milliliters must be administered in order to provide 65 mg of drug?

$$10 \text{ mg}:1 \text{ mL (what you know)} = 65 \text{ mg}:x \text{ mL (what you need to know)}$$

$$10x = 65$$

$$x = 6.5 \text{ mL}$$

Remember, the smaller known ratio is put to the left of the equals sign, and the unknown ratio is put to the right of the equals sign. Solve for x by multiplying the means and the extremes.

Systems of Measurement

METRIC SYSTEM

The metric system is the preferred system for scientific measurement. The units of measure for the metric system are meter (length), gram (weight), and liter (volume). A convenient feature of the metric system is that measurements are in decimal progression, so that 10 units of one size equals 1 unit of the next-higher size.

The names of the metric system are formed by joining Greek and Latin prefixes with the terms **meter** (m), **gram** (g), and **liter** (L):

$$\text{milli- } \frac{1}{1000} \ (0.001)$$

$$\text{centi- } \frac{1}{100} \ (0.01)$$

$$\text{deci- } \frac{1}{10} \, (0.1)$$

deka- 10

hecto- 100

kilo- 1000

APOTHECARY SYSTEM

The apothecary system is an older system of measurement that is rarely used today. The basic unit of measurement is the grain (gr). Only a few conversion values are included to show the relationship to the metric system.

HOUSEHOLD SYSTEM

The household system is a less accurate system of measurement. It is mainly used in the home, where dosages can be expressed in terms of common household measurements: teaspoon (tsp), tablespoon (tbsp), and liquid ounces (oz).

Tableware should never be used as a means of measuring medication. The average household teaspoon is only 3.7 mL. If oral dosing syringes or measured containers are not available, then use graduated measuring spoons, those used for cooking and baking.

CONVERSION TABLES
Weights

1 kilogram (kg) = 1000 grams (g)

1 gram (g) = 1000 milligrams (mg)

1 milligram (mg) = 1000 micrograms (µg)

1.5 grains (gr, apothecary) = 100 mg

1 grain (gr, apothecary) = 60.0 mg

1/2 gr = 30.0 mg

Volumes

1 liter (L) = 1000 milliliters (mL), 1000 cubic centimeters (cc), or approximately 1 quart

500 mL = approximately 1 pint

250 mL = approximately 8 fluid ounces = 1 cup

30.0 mL = approximately 1 fluid ounce

1.0 mL = 1.0 cc

Approximate Household Measures

60 drops (gtt) = 1 teaspoon (tsp)

1 teaspoon (tsp) = approximately 5.0 mL

1 tablespoon (tbsp) = approximately 15.0 mL

2 tablespoons (tbsp) = approximately 1 fluid ounce (oz)

1 measuring cup = approximately 8 fluid ounces (oz)

Conversions It is frequently necessary to make conversions of solution concentrations from liters (L) to milliliters (mL) and drug weights from grams (g) to milligrams (mg) or micrograms (µg). Knowledge of metric system equivalents is essential to performing these simple conversions. Conversion problems can be set up as a proportion and solved for x.

EXAMPLE Convert 1.5 liters (L) to milliliters.

1 L:1000 mL = 1.5 L:x

1x = 1500 mL

x = 1500 mL

Alternate setup of proportion equation as a fraction:

EXAMPLE Convert 1.5 liters to mL.

1 L:1000 mL = 1.5 L:x

1x = 1000 × 1.5

x = 1500 mL

EXAMPLE Convert 750 mL to liters.

$$\frac{1000 \text{ mL}}{1 \text{ L}} = \frac{750 \text{ mL}}{x \text{ L}}$$

$$1000x = 750$$

$$x = \frac{750}{1000}$$

$$x = 0.75 \text{ L}$$

EXAMPLE Convert 0.25 g to milligrams.

$$\frac{1 \text{ g}}{1000 \text{ mg}} = \frac{0.25 \text{ g}}{x \text{ mg}}$$

$$x = 1000 \times 0.25$$

$$x = 250 \text{ mg}$$

EXAMPLE Convert 350 mg to grams.

$$\frac{1000 \text{ mg}}{1 \text{ g}} = \frac{350 \text{ mg}}{x \text{ g}}$$

$$1000x = 350$$

$$x = \frac{350}{1000}$$

$$x = 0.35 \text{ g}$$

Sometimes, it is necessary to convert from one system of measurement to another.

EXAMPLE Convert 500 mL to fluid ounces.

$$\frac{250 \text{ mL}}{8 \text{ oz}} = \frac{500 \text{ mL}}{x \text{ oz}}$$

$$250x = 500 \times 8$$

$$250x = 4000$$

$$x = 16 \text{ oz}$$

PRACTICE PROBLEMS (ANSWERS IN CHAPTER 3 REVIEW)

Convert the following:
1. 500 mg = ___ g
2. 0.45 g = ___ mg
3. 0.03 L = ___ mL
4. 4 tbsp = ___ mL
5. 60 mL = ___ oz

Solve the following conversions by setting up a proportion equation:

6. 6 teaspoons (tsp) to tablespoons (tbsp)
7. 1.5 pints to milliliters (mL)
8. 5 grains (gr) to milligrams (mg)
9. 500 micrograms (μg) to milligrams
10. 2500 grams (g) to kilograms (kg)

Solutions

A **solution** is a homogeneous mixture of two or more substances. The liquid portion of the solution is known as the **solvent,** and the substance dissolved within the solvent is the **solute.** Solutions are commonly expressed as percentages. There are three types of percentage solutions:

WEIGHT IN WEIGHT (W/W)

Weight-in-weight solutions contain a given weight of drug (or other solute) in a definite weight of solvent so that the final solution is 100 parts by weight.

> *EXAMPLE* A 10% (W/W) solution of sodium chloride would contain 10 g of sodium chloride in 90 g of water.

WEIGHT IN VOLUME (W/V)

Weight-in-volume solutions contain a given weight of solute (drugs, salts) in enough solvent so that the final solution contains 100 parts by volume.

> *EXAMPLE* A 10% (W/V) solution of sodium chloride would contain 10 g of sodium chloride in enough water to make 100 mL of final solution.

VOLUME IN VOLUME (V/V)

Volume-in-volume solutions contain a definite volume of solute added to enough water so that the final solution would be 100 parts by volume.

> *EXAMPLE* A 10% (V/V) solution of glycerin would contain 10 mL of glycerin (100% solution) in enough water to make 100 mL of final solution.

Calculating Dosages

The proportion equation is useful for calculating dosages. Whenever three of the terms of a proportion are known, the unknown term can be determined if the equation is properly constructed.

> EXAMPLE Morphine sulfate injection for intravenous use is available in a concentration of 8 mg/mL of solution. Calculate the number of milliliters required to administer a dosage of 20 mg of morphine sulfate.

$$\frac{8 \text{ mg}}{1 \text{ mL}} = \frac{20 \text{ mg}}{x \text{ mL}}$$

$$8x = 20$$

$$x = 2.5 \text{ mL}$$

> EXAMPLE There is a drug order for 50 mg of secobarbital (elixir). The stock bottle contains 22 mg of secobarbital in 5 mL of solution. How many milliliters should the patient receive?

$$\frac{22 \text{ mg}}{5 \text{ mL}} = \frac{50 \text{ mg}}{x \text{ mL}}$$

$$22x = 50 \times 5$$

$$22x = 250$$

$$x = 11.3636, \text{ or } 11.4 \text{ mL}$$

> EXAMPLE There is a drug order for 75 mg of meperidine (Demerol) to be administered IM. Demerol is supplied in a 5% solution (W/V). A 5% solution (W/V) would be 5 g of Demerol in 100 cc or 50 mg per 1 mL as written on the vial label. How many milliliters of Demerol should be administered to the patient?

$$\frac{50 \text{ mg}}{1 \text{ mL}} = \frac{75 \text{ mg}}{x \text{ mL}}$$

$$50x = 75$$

$$x = \frac{75}{50}$$

$$x = 1.5 \text{ mL}$$

EXAMPLE There is a drug order for 60 mg of drug. The drug is available in 20-mg tablets. How many tablets are required? The problem requires setting up a fraction based on the formula:

$$\frac{\text{desired dosage}}{\text{available dosage}} = \frac{60 \text{ mg}}{20 \text{ mg (1 tablet)}} = 3 \text{ tablets}$$

A variation on this problem could be that 10 mg of a drug is desired

$$\text{desired dosage} = \frac{10 \text{ mg}}{20 \text{ mg (1 tablet)}} = \frac{1}{2} \text{ tablet}$$

The tablet must be scored for breakage.

EXAMPLE An injection of 1000 units of tetanus antitoxin is ordered. The tetanus antitoxin is available in an ampule labeled 1500 units per milliliter. How many milliliters should be injected?

$$\frac{\text{desired dosage}}{\text{available dosage}} = \frac{1000 \text{ units}}{1500 \text{ units}} = \frac{2}{3} \text{ mL} = 0.66 \text{ mL}$$

PEDIATRIC DOSAGE CALCULATIONS

Dosage calculations in pediatrics are based on age, body surface area (BSA), and body weight. Listed below are the formulas used for these calculations.

Young's Rule

$$\frac{\text{age of child}}{\text{age of child} + 12} \times \text{adult dose} = \text{child's dose}$$

Clark's Rule

$$\frac{\text{weight of child}}{150 \text{ lb}} \times \text{adult dose} = \text{child's dose}$$

Fried's Rule

$$\frac{\text{age in months}}{150} \times \text{average adult dose} = \text{child's dose}$$

Body Surface Area Rule

$$\frac{\text{body surface area of child (square meters)}}{1.7} \times \text{adult dose} = \text{child's dose}$$

EXAMPLE Katie just turned 3 years old; she weighs 30 pounds. Her mother wants to know how much cough syrup to give Katie. The directions have worn off the bottle, and she can only make out the dosage for adults: 2 teaspoons every 4 hours. How much should Katie receive?

$$\text{Young's Rule: } 3/(3 + 12) \times 10 \text{ mL} = \text{Katie's dose}$$

$$1/5 \times 10 \text{ mL} = 2 \text{ mL}$$

$$\text{Clark's Rule: } 30/150 \times 10 \text{ mL} = \text{Katie's dose}$$

$$1/5 \times 10 \text{ mL} = 2 \text{ mL}$$

$$\text{Fried's Rule: } 36/150 \times 10 \text{ mL} = \text{Katie's dose}$$

$$0.24 \times 10 \text{ mL} = 2.4 \text{ mL}$$

Dosage Calculations Based on Body Weight   Drug dosages are usually administered on a body weight basis, for example, in milligrams per kilogram. This may require conversion of pounds to kilograms (1 kg = 2.2 lb). The dose per kilogram is then multiplied by the number of kilograms.

EXAMPLE There is a drug order for the antibiotic tobramycin, 2.5 mg/kg, administered via inhalation for a patient weighing 110 pounds. Tobramycin is available as 80 mg/2 mL. How many milligrams of drug is required, and in what volume?

Step 1: Convert pounds to kilograms.

$$110 \text{ lb divided by } 2.2 \text{ lb/kg} = 50 \text{ kg}$$

Step 2: Determine how many milligrams of drug is required.

$$2.5 \text{ mg/kg} \times 50 \text{ kg} = 125 \text{ mg}$$

Step 3: Determine how many milliliters of stock solution contain 125 mg, using the proportion equation method.

$$80 \text{ mg:2 mL} = 125 \text{ mg:} x \text{ mL}$$

$$80x = (125)(2) = 250$$

$$x = 250/80 = 3.1 \text{ mL of solution (rounded to the nearest tenth)}$$

EXAMPLE If the patient in the previous problem were an infant weighing 20 lb with a body surface area of 0.44 square meters, what would be the dose according to the BSA rule?

BSA rule: Child dose is BSA of child (square meters)/1.7 × adult dose.

$$0.44/1.7 \times 125 \text{ mg} = 0.258 \times 125 = 32.4 \text{ or about 32 mg}$$

The vials contain 80 mg/2 mL; calculate volume.

$$80 \text{ mg}/2 \text{ mL} = 32 \text{ mg}/x \text{ mL}$$

$$x = 0.8 \text{ mL}$$

EXAMPLE A loading dose of digoxin capsules (Lanoxicaps), 10 µg/kg, has been ordered for a patient weighing 154 lb. Lanoxicaps are available as 50-µg, 100-µg, and 200-µg capsules. How many capsules should be administered?

Step 1: Convert pounds to kilograms.

$$154 \text{ lb divided by } 2.2 \text{ lb/kg} = 70 \text{ kg}$$

Step 2: Determine how many micrograms are required.

$$70 \text{ kg} \times 10 \text{ µg/kg} = 700 \text{ µg or } 0.7 \text{ mg}$$

Step 3: Determine how many capsules are required.

$$0.2 \text{ mg}:1 \text{ capsule} = 0.7 \text{ mg}:x$$

$$0.2x = 0.7$$

$$x = 3.5 \text{ capsules (3 caps of 200 µg and 1 capsule of 100 µg)}$$

Monitoring Intravenous Infusion Rates

Hospitalized patients often receive drug administration by slow IV infusion. Drugs are added to various sterile IV solutions, such as Sodium Chloride Injection, USP or Dextrose (5%) Injection, USP. Drug concentrations and solutions are prepared by the hospital pharmacy. The IV drug infusion solutions must be prepared under aseptic conditions, the drugs and solutions mixed must be chemically compatible, and often the infusion solution must be adjusted to a specific pH value. Preparation of these solutions should always follow established hospital procedures and be reviewed by a pharmacist.

After establishment of an open IV line, the drug solution is administered according to a specific infusion rate, in drops per minute. Usually there are 15 drops/mL of solution, but this number can vary with the viscosity of different solutions. Because allied health personnel are sometimes called on to monitor IV infusion rates, the following example is presented to illustrate the principles involved.

Formula for adjusting IV infusion rate:

milliliters of IV solution × number of drops per milliliter = drops per minute

hours of administration × 60 = minutes

EXAMPLE An IV infusion of furosemide (Lasix), 2 mg/min for 4 hours, was ordered for a patient with severe edema. The hospital pharmacy prepared the infusion solution by adding 480 mg (2 mg/min x 60 x 4) in 500 mL of Sodium Chloride Injection, USP. How many drops should be administered per minute?

500 ml × 15 drops/mL = 7500 drops = 31.25 drops/min

4 hours × 60 minutes = 240 minutes

Regulate the IV flow by counting the drops (to nearest whole number) for 15 seconds and multiplying by 4 (for 1 minute). Adjust the IV tube clamp until the correct rate is attained.

Chapter 3 Review

UNDERSTANDING TERMINOLOGY

Match the term in the left column with the appropriate set of examples to the right. Use each set of examples only once.

1. Mixed numbers
2. Decimals
3. Proper fractions
4. Denominator
5. Fractions
6. Numerator
7. Improper fractions

a. $\frac{8}{16}$, $\frac{13}{27}$, $\frac{3}{4}$

b. $\frac{15}{12}$, $\frac{4}{3}$, $\frac{39}{18}$

c. $1\frac{1}{2}$, $15\frac{4}{5}$, $\frac{39}{18}$

d. 1.5, 0.75, 12.3333

e. the 3 in $\frac{3}{4}$

f. the 4 in $\frac{3}{4}$

g. $\frac{1}{2}$, $\frac{7}{10}$, $\frac{5}{12}$

After reading this chapter, you should be able to answer the following question:

8. Differentiate between solution, solute, and solvent.

ACQUIRING KNOWLEDGE

After reading this chapter, you should be able to answer the following questions:

9. Convert 0.125 grams to milligrams.

10. Convert 1200 milliliters to liters.

11. Two teaspoons of cough syrup equals how many milliliters?

12. One-quarter grain equals how many milligrams?

13. Four fluid ounces equals how many milliliters?

14. There is a drug order for 2.5 mg of glipizide (Glucotrol). Scored tablets are available in 5- and 10-mg strengths. Calculate the dosage. Why is the drug being given? (Refer to the *PDR.*)

15. After several days, the dosage of glipizide for the patient in Problem 14 has been increased to 7.5 mg. Calculate the dosage.

16. There is an order for 4 mg of Ventolin syrup. The syrup contains 2 mg of Ventolin per 5 mL. Calculate the dosage volume. What is the generic name of the drug? (Refer to the *PDR.*)

17. Several hours later, the patient in Problem 16 complains of difficulty in breathing. The order is changed to 2.5 mg via inhalation. Ventolin is available as 5 mg/mL inhalation solution. Calculate the inhalation volume.

18. A bottle for inhalation is labeled "1 mL contains 5 mg." Calculate the amount required for a 2-mg dose.

ACQUIRING KNOWLEDGE ON THE JOB

After reading this chapter, you should be able to answer the following questions:

19. Assume that you're spending your summer as an intern in a university hospital pharmacy. One of your duties is to prepare desired dosages from available dosages to arrive at the correct weight or number of units of drug for each order the pharmacist fills. Show the calculations for the correct amount of drug for each of the following orders that were filled on your first day of work.

    a. The first order called for 90 mg of drug. The drug is available in 30-mg tablets. How many tablets are required?

    b. The second order called for 2000 units of tetanus antitoxin. The tetanus antitoxin is available in an ampule of 1500 units per milliliter. How many milliliters should be injected?

    c. The third order called for 70 mg of secobarbital. The stock bottle contains 22 mg of secobarbital in 5 mL of solution. How many milliliters should the patient receive?

20. Bert just finished his training as a pharmacist assistant and started working in a nursing home dispensary last week. One of his job duties is to calculate the

number of milliliters of drug for drug orders given in milligrams. Show how you would deal with the following patient orders if you had Bert's job.

a. There's a drug order for 100 mg of Demerol to be administered IM. The label on the stock bottle of Demerol says it's in a 5% solution, or 50 mg/mL.

b. There's an order for a diabetic patient of 30 units of insulin. The stock bottle is labeled U-100, or 100 units per milliliter.

21. There is a drug order for diazepam (Valium), 0.5 mg/kg, administered orally. The patient weighs 110 lb. Valium is available in 2-, 5-, and 10-mg tablets. How many milligrams and what combination of tablets will you administer?

22. Ampicillin (Omnipen) oral suspension is available as 125 mg per 5 mL. There is a drug order for 500 mg qid. How many milliliters will you administer with each dose? How often will you administer the dose?

23. The usual oral dose of ampicillin is 500 mg. How much should a 15-month-old baby receive according to Fried's Rule? A 50-lb child according to Clark's Rule?

ANSWERS TO PRACTICE PROBLEMS IN CHAPTER 3

1. 500 mg is 0.5 g (move decimal 3 places to the left)

2. 0.45 g is 450 mg (move decimal 3 places to the right)

3. 0.03 L is 30.0 mL (move decimal 3 places to the right)

4. 4 tbsp is 60.0 mL

5. 60 mL is 2 oz

6. 3 tsp:1 tbsp = 6 tsp:x tbsp

$$3x = 6$$

$$x = 2 \text{ tbsp}$$

7. 1 pint:500 mL = 1.5 pints:x mL

$$1x = (500 \text{ mL}) \ (1.5)$$

$$x = 750 \text{ mL}$$

8. 1 gr:60 mg = 5 gr:x mg

$$x = (60)(5) = 300 \text{ mg}$$

9. 1 mg:1000 μg = x:500 μg

   $1000x = 500$

   $x = 500/1000 = 0.5$ mg

10. 1 kg:1000 g = x:2500 g

    $1000x = 2500$

    $x = 2500/1000 = 2.5$ kg

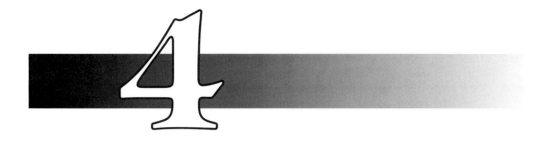

Preventing Medication Errors

STUART R. LEVINE, PHARMD

Chapter Focus

This chapter provides information on potential medication errors that can lead to patient harm. Some methods to reduce the likelihood of errors are reviewed.

Chapter Objectives

After studying this chapter, you should be able to:

- Understand the impact of medication errors on the health care system.
- Understand the need to report all medication errors so that causes can be determined.
- Understand the definition of medication error.
- List four areas of ordering medications that can lead to errors.

Throughout this book you will learn about many medications that are commonly given to people to help them. It is also very important that no harm be done to people who come to you expecting you to make them better. One reason harm may sometimes be done to patients is that medication errors occur. At least 44,000 patients die each year from medical errors that could potentially have been avoided. It is the responsibility of all health care professionals to prevent these errors from occurring. Medication errors are very rarely related to one individual. Most commonly, they are the result of numerous factors that together generate an error. We should encourage people to report errors without fear of personal consequences so that errors can be analyzed and the reasons for their occurrence determined. Only through this type of review can we all help to decrease errors.

What Is a Medication Error?

A medication error is any preventable event that may cause or lead to inappropriate medication use or patient harm while the medication is in control of the health care professional, patient, or consumer. Such events may be related to professional practice, health care products, procedures, and systems, including prescription, distribution, administration, education, monitoring, and use.

Sound-Alike Drug Names

Every day new medications and new names for medications are approved. All of these new medications have generic and brand names. Occasionally, one medication will sound very much like another. This can lead to the wrong medications being prescribed or given to one of your patients. Table 4-1 lists some of the medications that are mistaken for others. This kind of error can occur when orders are given verbally. One way to avoid these errors is by accepting only orders that are written. Alternatively, if you are given a verbal order, be sure to repeat the name of the drug, the dose, and the frequency back to the prescriber to make sure it is correct.

Verbal orders also can be a problem with medications that are available in different dosage forms. There may be syrups, tablets, combination products, or sustained-release dosage forms for the same medication. This can lead to confusion and errors as the information is communicated. Look at the example in Table 4-2. You can see how you might be confused.

Table 4-1
Easily Confused Drug Names

Albuterol	vs.	Alupent
Cerebyx	vs.	Celebrex
Navane	vs.	Norvasc
Prilosec	vs.	Prozac
Zebeta	vs.	Diabeta
Flovent	vs.	Serevent

Table 4-2
Easily Confused Dosage Forms

Claritin Syrup
Claritin Tablets
Claritin Redi-Tabs
Claritin D 12 hour
Claritin D 24 hour

Multiple Concentrations

With numerous dosage forms available, we also see multiple concentrations of liquid and parenteral forms. In the case of some parenteral drugs, there may be concentrates and ready-to-use prediluted forms of the same drug. This is also the reason orders for medications should be given in terms of milligrams and not in milliliters.

Look-Alike Drugs and Labeling

You are driving along, and a billboard catches your eye. It passes quickly, and in that instant you have read and interpreted that message. Sometimes, we read the message so quickly that our brain fills in the blanks to give us what it thinks is a complete picture. Sometimes the picture our brain creates is wrong. Looking at labels can be the same thing. If you use a certain product commonly, and if another new item looks similar, you might assume that the new item is the one you commonly use. For this reason, we have tried to use a number of methods of distinguishing medications that might otherwise look the same. Some medications have color-coded caps, some have different colored labels, and some might have a different-shaped bottle. All of these methods, as well as others, are designed to keep the wrong medication from being picked up by mistake.

Look at the picture in Figure 4-1. This is a photograph of three different drugs manufactured by three different companies. Would you pick the right one?

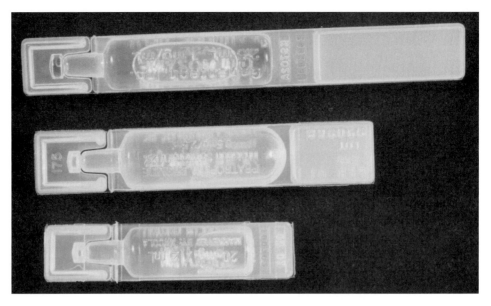

Figure 4-1
Photograph of three commonly used respiratory medications. These drugs are albuterol, cromolyn, and Pulmazyme.

Handwriting and Abbreviations

Everyone always seems to be in a hurry. One way people try to reduce some of their time used in communicating is by using abbreviations. Every profession has its own abbreviations, and as health care professionals, we have developed ours over time. Abbreviations can save time, but only if everyone agrees on what they mean. It doesn't help anyone if you have your own abbreviations but no one but you understands them. Also, it can be a problem if one abbreviation is misinterpreted as another abbreviation or misinterpreted as a number.

Table 4-3 includes those common abbreviations used in health care. You also will see that some words should never be abbreviated. That is because mistakes are commonly made when they are used.

The word "unit" or "units" should never be abbreviated. Many times the "U" is misread as a zero or, if done quickly, can be seen as a "4."

There is no safe abbreviation for daily. QD has been used as an abbreviation. However, QD has been misinterpreted as QID, four times a day, misinterpreted as OD, right eye, or misinterpreted as QOD for every other day.

Do not abbreviate drug names. Does MS or MSO_4 mean morphine sulfate or magnesium sulfate?

Table 4-3
Abbreviations Used in Health Care

BID = twice a day	IV = intravenously
TID = three times daily	IM = intramuscularly
QID = four times daily	IT = intrathecally
Q = every hour	SC = subcutaneously
h = hour	PO = orally
gtt. = drop	NG = nasogastric
a.c. = before meals	NJ = nasaljejunal
p.c. = after meals	ID = intradermal
c̄ = with	PR = per rectum
s̄ = without	IVPB = IV piggyback
q.s. = quantity sufficient	SL = sublingual
p.r.n. = as needed	NEB = nebulization
neb = nebulize	OU = both eyes
Tab = tablet	OS = left eye
Cap = capsule	OD = right eye
mg = milligram	AU = both ears
mL = milliter	AS = left ear
mEq = milliequivalent	AD = right ear
mmole = millimoles	No abbreviations are acceptable for:
μg = microgram	Daily
D = dextrose	Units
NSS = normal saline	Names of medications

Calculation Errors

Performing calculations has always been a problem. Any profession that requires calculations runs a risk of errors. However, in the health care field, errors associated with calculation can be life-threatening. It is not uncommon to find calculations that yield ten times the dose or one tenth the dose. Therefore, always remember that you can't be almost right, or only off by one decimal point. This can mean the patient's life!

Another common error is associated with the use of the "0" and a decimal point. The general rule is, do not use a zero or decimal point after a whole number: 2 mg not 2.0 mg. Many times the decimal is missed and that 2.0-mg dose will be given as 20 mg. On the other hand, always use a zero and decimal point before a fraction: 0.2 mg not .2 mg. If the leading zero is omitted, the decimal point can be missed, and a 2-mg dose can be given.

Five Rights of Drug Administration

It is very important for respiratory care practioners always to follow the prescriber's orders and the established guidelines for the administration of drugs. One practical approach to drug administration is referred to as "the five rights."

This approach advocates that the person administering the drug make a mental checklist that emphasizes giving the:

- Right patient: Check for an ID band if possible.
- Right drug: Check the drug when you pick it up. Check your order, and check again before administering.
- Right dose.
- Right route.
- Right time.

Chapter 4 Review

UNDERSTANDING TERMINOLOGY

1. Define a medication error.
2. Matching abbreviations:

   QID   a. as needed

   gtt   b. four times a day

   qs   c. drop

   PRN   d. quantity sufficient

   BID   e. milliliter

   Q   f. twice a day

   mL   g. every

APPLYING KNOWLEDGE ON THE JOB

1. Review the five rights of drug administration

   a. _____

   b. _____

   c. _____

   d. _____

   e. _____

2. Review three examples of sources of medication errors.

   a. _____

   b. _____

   c. _____

3. Explain when you would use a zero and a decimal point for writing a dose of a medication.

INTERNET CONNECTIONS

Try http://www.ismp.org for information on avoiding medication errors in health care. The Institute for Safe Medication Practices reviews medication errors and potential medication errors from sites around the world.

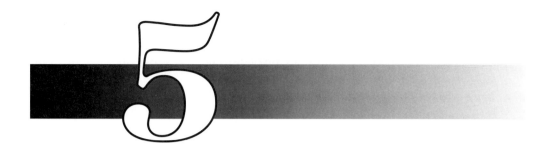

Autonomic Nervous System

Henry Hitner, PhD
Barbara Nagle, PhD

Chapter Focus

This chapter describes the basic organization of the autonomic nervous system (ANS) and how it functions to maintain homeostasis as the body experiences stress. It also explains the role of the sympathetic and parasympathetic divisions of the ANS and how these nerves regulate the activities of the individual body organs.

Chapter Terminology

acetylcholine (ACh): Neurotransmitter of parasympathetic (cholinergic) nerves; stimulates cholinergic receptors.

adrenergic receptor: Receptor located on internal organs that responds to norepinephrine.

afferent nerve: Transmits sensory information to the brain and spinal cord (central nervous system).

autonomic nervous system (ANS): System of nerves that innervate smooth and cardiac muscle (involuntary) of the internal organs and glands.

cholinergic receptor: Receptor located on internal organs that responds to acetylcholine.

efferent nerve: Carries the appropriate motor response from the brain and spinal cord.

epinephrine: Hormone from adrenal medulla that stimulates adrenergic receptors, especially during stress.

fight-or-flight reaction: Response of the body to intense stress; caused by activation of the sympathetic division of the ANS.

homeostasis: Normal state of balance among the body's internal organs.

neurotransmitter: Substance that stimulates internal organs to produce characteristic changes associated with sympathetic and parasympathetic divisions.

norepinephrine (NE):   Neurotransmitter of sympathetic (adrenergic) nerves that stimulates the adrenergic receptors.

parasympathetic: Refers to nerves of the ANS that originate in the brain and sacral portion of the spinal cord; they are active when the body is at rest or trying to restore body energy and function.

sympathetic: Refers to nerves of the ANS that originate from the thoracolumbar portion of the spinal cord; they are active when the body is under stress or when it is exerting energy.

Chapter Objectives

After studying this chapter, you should be able to:

- Describe the two divisions of the ANS and explain how they differ.
- Explain how sympathetic and parasympathetic nerves interact with each other to regulate organ function (maintain homeostasis).
- Describe the fight-or-flight reaction and explain how it affects the activities of the different organs.
- List four effects caused by parasympathetic stimulation.
- List two autonomic neurotransmitters and explain the role of each in the function of the ANS.

The primary function of the nervous system is to control and coordinate the activity of all the systems in the body. The overall activity of the nervous system at any moment depends on neural communication (via nerve impulses) among many areas of the body. Before we discuss the pharmacology of the autonomic division of the nervous system, it is helpful to briefly review the general organization of the nervous system.

Nervous System Organization

The nervous system is an elaborate nerve network that functions at both conscious (under control of the will, or voluntary) and unconscious (not under control of the will, or involuntary) levels.

CENTRAL NERVOUS SYSTEM

The central nervous system (CNS) consists of the brain and spinal cord. The CNS receives and interprets sensory information via peripheral **afferent nerves** and initiates appropriate motor responses via peripheral **efferent nerves.**

SOMATIC DIVISION

The somatic nerves are the branches of the cranial and spinal motor nerves that innervate skeletal muscle (voluntary). These nerves are under conscious, or voluntary, control of the cerebral cortex.

VISCERAL DIVISION (AUTONOMIC NERVOUS SYSTEM)

The visceral nerves are the branches of the cranial and spinal motor nerves that innervate cardiac and smooth muscle (involuntary). The visceral nerves, which are not under conscious control, are regulated by centers in the hypothalamus and the medulla oblongata. The visceral nerves are collectively referred to as the **autonomic nervous system (ANS).**

Physiology and Pharmacology

It is important to emphasize that the physiology and pharmacology of the ANS can be challenging to beginning students. However, understanding the ANS is essential to understanding the actions of many drugs, especially those affecting the cardiovascular and respiratory systems.

The ANS is composed of the nerves that innervate smooth and cardiac muscle. These two types of muscle are found in the walls of the internal organs and possess a special property, autorhythmicity, which allows them to initiate their own contractions. This process can be demonstrated by removing the heart or a piece of intestine from a frog, placing the organ in oxygenated Ringer's solution, and observing the contractions that occur without any stimulation.

If the internal organs can initiate their own contractions, why is the autonomic nervous system needed? The answer is the key to the purpose of the ANS. The ANS functions to regulate the rate at which these organs work, either increasing or decreasing their activity. In this way, **homeostasis,** the normal balance among the body's internal organs, can be maintained.

Whether the activity of an organ increases or decreases depends on body activity. But the question arises, "How can an autonomic nerve going to any visceral organ both increase and decrease the activity of the organ?" The answer is that it cannot. Two different types of autonomic nerves, sympathetic and parasympathetic, innervate most internal organs.

Parasympathetic and Sympathetic Divisions

The ANS has two subdivisions, the parasympathetic and sympathetic divisions. The nerves of the **parasympathetic** division (also known as the craniosacral division) originate from the brain (cranial nerves 3, 7, 9, and 10) and spinal cord (sacral nerves S2 to S4). The nerves of the **sympathetic** division (known as the thoracolumbar division) originate from the thoracic and lumbar spinal nerves (T1 to L3). Figure 5-1 shows how some of these nerves are linked to organs and glands.

As a result, most of the major body organs and glands receive a nerve from each division. There are exceptions: for example, most blood vessels do not receive parasympathetic innervation. In this situation, blood pressure is controlled by either increasing sympathetic activity or decreasing (inhibiting) sympathetic activity. However, the general plan is that one division is responsible for increasing

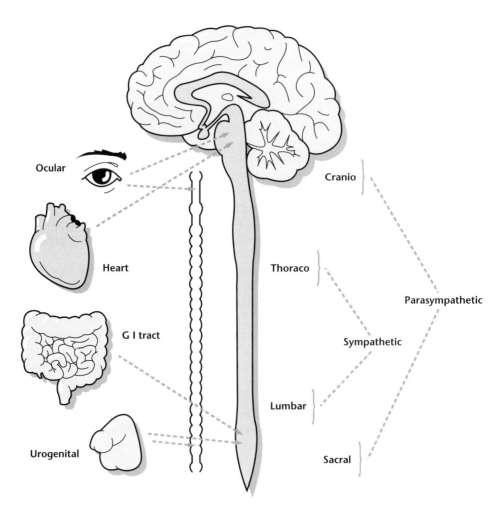

Figure 5-1

The origin and distribution of the autonomic nervous system divisions. Each organ receives two nerves, one from either the cranio (eye, heart) or sacral (GI, urogenital) portion of the parasympathetic division, and one from either the thoraco (eye, heart) or lumbar (GI, urogenital) portion of the sympathetic division. Sympathetic nerves are shown originating from their ganglia along the spinal cord.

the activity of a particular organ while the other division decreases the activity of that organ. Unfortunately, one division does not always increase activity, and the other division does not always decrease activity, in each of the organs. How is the effect of each division predicted? The answer is that sympathetic stimulation produces changes in the body that are similar to changes observed during frightening or emergency situations. These changes are collectively referred to as the **fight-or-flight reaction.**

During the fight-or-flight reaction, the sympathetic division increases the activity of certain organs to allow a greater expenditure of energy for both physical and mental exertion. At the same time, there is a decrease in the activity of the remaining organs, whose functions are not required for the fight-or-flight reaction.

The parasympathetic division is more active during periods of rest and restoration of body energy stores. The parasympathetic nerves regulate body functions, such as digestion and elimination of waste products (urination, defecation).

Normally, we do not experience situations in which we need the fight-or-flight reaction to enable us to fight or run. However, the daily stresses, anxieties, and illnesses we do experience are sufficient to activate the sympathetic system to produce changes that are similar to the fight-or-flight reaction. When the sympathetic division is stimulated, all sympathetic nerves are activated at the same time. Therefore, the whole body is stimulated. With the parasympathetic division, only selected nerves can be stimulated, and the stimulation can be confined to a particular body system, for example, contraction of the urinary bladder during urination. The overall effects of sympathetic and parasympathetic stimulation are summarized in Table 5-1.

Usually in a beginning discussion of the ANS, only the peripheral motor (effer-

Table 5-1

Effects of Sympathetic and Parasympathetic Stimulation

Area	Sympathetic Effect	Parasympathetic Effect
Adrenal medulla	Release of epinephrine	—
Arteries	Vasoconstriction (exceptions are the coronary arteries and arteries to skeletal muscle, which are dilated)	Most arteries are not supplied by parasympathetic nerves
Heart	Increases rate	Decreases rate
	Increases contractility	Decreases contractility
Intestines, GI motility, and secretions	Decreased	Increased
Postganglionic neurotransmitter	Norepinephrine released	Acetylcholine released
Pupil of the eye	Dilation (mydriasis)	Constriction (miosis)
Respiratory passages, lower	Bronchodilation	Bronchoconstriction
Urinary bladder	Relaxation	Contraction
Urinary sphincter	Contraction	Relaxation

ent) nerves are discussed. Peripheral autonomic nerves are the branches of the cranial and spinal nerves that travel to the cardiac muscle and smooth muscle of the internal organs. A typical peripheral nerve is composed of many neurons traveling together to the same destination. In any autonomic nerve, two groups of neurons are linked together by synapses as the nerve travels from the spinal cord to the internal organ. In the peripheral nervous system, a collection of synapses is referred to as a ganglion.

In the ANS, neurons that emerge from the spinal cord form the preganglionic nerve. Neurons that travel from the ganglion to the internal organ form the postganglionic nerve. The ganglion is the collection of synapses between the preganglionic and postganglionic nerve fibers, as illustrated in Figure 5-2.

The main pharmacologic difference between the sympathetic nerves and the

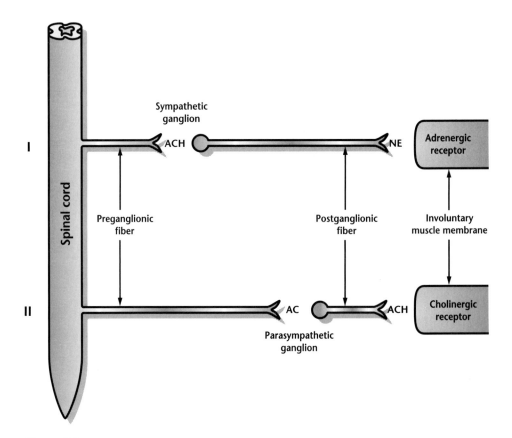

Figure 5-2
A diagrammatic representation of a typical sympathetic and parasympathetic efferent nerve. Above: Sympathetic pre- and postganglionic fibers from the thoracolumbar division. Below: Parasympathetic pre- and postganglionic fibers from the sacral division (ACH, acetylcholine; NE, norepinephrine).

parasympathetic nerves is the **neurotransmitter** released from the postganglionic nerve endings. The neurotransmitter stimulates the internal organs and produces the characteristic changes that are associated with each division of the ANS, as listed in Table 5-1.

In the parasympathetic nervous system, the neurotransmitter released at the ganglia and the postganglionic nerve endings is **acetylcholine (ACh).** In the sympathetic nerves, the neurotransmitter released at the ganglia is ACh, but at the postganglionic nerve endings, it is **norepinephrine (NE).** Nerves that release acetylcholine are referred to as cholinergic, whereas nerves that release norepinephrine are referred to as adrenergic. The cardiac and smooth muscle membrane sites where these neurotransmitters act are known as the **cholinergic receptors** (ACh) and the **adrenergic receptors** (NE), as shown in Figure 5-2.

In summary, the effects of parasympathetic stimulation are produced by the release of acetylcholine, which binds to the cholinergic receptors. The effects of sympathetic stimulation are produced by the release of norepinephrine and epinephrine, which bind to the adrenergic receptors.

Chapter 5 Review

UNDERSTANDING TERMINOLOGY

Test your understanding of the material in this chapter by answering the following questions.

1. What is the difference between an afferent nerve and an efferent nerve?
2. Differentiate between adrenergic receptors and cholinergic receptors.
3. What is the meaning of homeostasis?
4. What terminology is applied to nerves that release acetylcholine?
5. What terminology is applied to nerves that release norepinephrine?

ACQUIRING KNOWLEDGE

Answer the following questions.

6. What are the two main divisions of the autonomic nervous system?
7. What is the main function of each division?
8. From what areas of the CNS does each division originate?
9. What is the significance of "dual autonomic innervation" to most internal organs?
10. What property of smooth and cardiac muscles allows them to initiate their own contractions?
11. Describe what is meant by the fight-or-flight reaction. What conditions activate this reaction?
12. During what body activities is the parasympathetic division active?

13. Think of an emergency situation requiring immediate and intense physical exertion. List as many body organs as you can, and predict the desired level of activity (increased or decreased) for each. Which neurotransmitter would produce this effect? Do your predictions correspond to the fight-or-flight reaction?

APPLYING KNOWLEDGE ON THE JOB

Answer the following questions.

14. Use the *PDR* product category index to look up drugs that mimic (parasympathomimetics) and drugs that inhibit (parasympatholytics) cholinergic activity. List one or two drugs from each category, the main drug effect, and clinical indications. Do your findings correspond to the expected effects of cholinergic stimulation and inhibition?

15. Use the *PDR* product category index to find drugs that mimic (sympathomimetics) and drugs that inhibit (sympatholytics) adrenergic activity. List one or two drugs, the main drug effect, and clinical indications. Do your findings correspond to the expected effects of adrenergic stimulation and inhibition?

Additional Reading

Changeux JP. Chemical signalling in the brain. *Sci Am* 1993;269:58.
Finocchiaro DN, Herzfeld ST. Understanding autonomic dysreflexia. *Am J Nurs* 1990;90(9):56.
Schatz IJ. Autonomic failure and orthostatic hypotension. *Hosp Pract* 32(5):15.

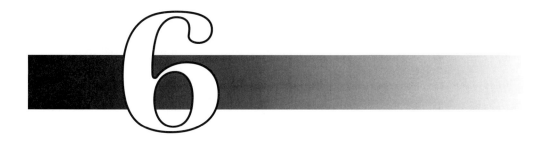

Drugs Affecting the Sympathetic Nervous System

Henry Hitner, PhD
Barbara Nagle, PhD

Chapter Focus

This chapter describes the pharmacology of drugs that affect the sympathetic nervous system. It also explains the ways in which adrenergic drugs (agonists) stimulate adrenergic receptors to increase sympathetic activity and how other drugs (antagonists) block adrenergic receptors to reduce sympathetic activity.

Chapter Terminology

adrenergic neuronal blocker: Drug that acts at the neuronal endings to reduce the formation or release of norepinephrine.

alpha-adrenergic blocker: Drug that blocks the α effects of norepinephrine and epinephrine.

α-adrenergic receptor: Receptor located on smooth muscle that mediates contraction.

β-adrenergic receptor: Receptor located either on the heart (β_1) or smooth muscle (β_2). β_1 stimulation increases heart function, whereas β_2 stimulation relaxes smooth muscle.

catecholamine: Refers to norepinephrine, epinephrine, and other sympathomimetic compounds that possess the catechol structure.

false transmitter: Drug-induced substance in nerve endings that reduces neuronal activity.

nonselective β-adrenergic blocker: Drug that blocks both β_1 and β_2 receptors.

selective β_1-adrenergic blocker: Drug that blocks only β_1 receptors at therapeutic doses.

selective β_2-adrenergic drug: Drug that stimulates only β_2 receptors at therapeutic doses.

sympatholytic: "Blocking" drug or effect that decreases sympathetic nervous system activity.

sympathomimetic: Adrenergic drug or effect that increases sympathetic nervous system activity.

Chapter Objectives

After studying this chapter, you should be able to:

- Explain how the adrenergic nerve endings function both to release and inactivate norepinephrine.
- Name three different adrenergic receptors and describe the actions they mediate.
- Explain the effects of norepinephrine and epinephrine on α and β receptors.
- Name three α-adrenergic agonists and describe the main pharmacologic effects and uses of each.
- Name three β-adrenergic agonists and describe the main pharmacologic effects and uses of each.
- Describe the three major types of adrenergic blocking drugs and the pharmacologic effects produced by each type.

The sympathetic nervous system regulates the activity of the internal organs and glands during physical exertion and other stressful situations. Peripheral sympathetic nerves, known as adrenergic nerves, release the neurotransmitter norepinephrine (NE). The NE binds to its adrenergic receptors and produces the effects that are associated with sympathetic stimulation (fight or flight)

The adrenal medulla releases the hormone epinephrine (EPI), which also stimulates the adrenergic receptors. EPI is released from the adrenal medulla in larger amounts during stress and emergency situations. Norepinephrine and epinephrine are chemically similar and are generally referred to as the **catecholamines.**

Adrenergic Nerve Endings

It is important to have an understanding of how the adrenergic nerve endings function. The nerve endings are mainly concerned with the formation of NE, which is then stored within granules inside the nerve endings. When the adrener-

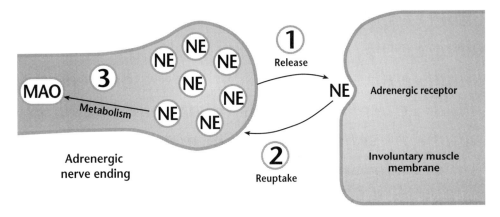

Figure 6-1
The adrenergic nerve ending, illustrating the release, reuptake, and metabolism of norepinephrine (NE).

gic nerves are stimulated, NE is released. NE then travels to the smooth or cardiac muscle membrane, attaches to adrenergic receptors, and produces the sympathetic response. Most of the NE then passes back into the nerve endings (reuptake). Inside the nerve endings, the NE may be reused or may be destroyed by the enzyme monoamine oxidase (MAO). These actions are illustrated in Figure 6-1.

Norepinephrine versus Epinephrine

Although NE and EPI are both adrenergic neurotransmitters, there are some important differences in the effects that each produces. Both NE and EPI stimulate many of the internal organs to increase sympathetic activity. However, EPI causes an inhibition or relaxation of smooth muscle in a few organs. For example, the respiratory airways are relaxed (bronchodilation) by EPI. This effect enhances the fight-or-flight reaction because more oxygen passes into the lungs when the respiratory tract is dilated. Because of the differences in the responses produced by NE and EPI, two main types of adrenergic receptors are believed to exist.

Adrenergic Receptors

The two main adrenergic receptors are known as α- and β-adrenergic receptors. Although some organs contain more than one type of receptor, one receptor type usually predominates and determines the overall response of the organ. **Alpha-**

adrenergic receptors are found predominantly on smooth muscle membranes and when stimulated by NE or EPI, they produce contraction, for example, vasoconstriction of most blood vessels.

Beta-adrenergic receptors are found on both cardiac and some smooth muscle membranes. In the heart, the predominant beta receptors are classified as beta-1 receptors, and when stimulated by NE or EPI, they increase heart rate and force of contraction. In smooth muscle, the predominant beta receptors are classified as beta-2 receptors, and when stimulated by EPI, they produce vasodilation (mainly skeletal muscle blood vessels and coronary arteries) and bronchodilation (relaxation of bronchiolar smooth muscle). NE does not stimulate beta-2 receptors, and this is the main difference between NE and EPI. Note that alpha receptor stimulation causes smooth muscle contraction at some organ sites while beta-2 receptor stimulation causes smooth muscle relaxation at other organ sites. Table 6-1 summarizes the effects of NE and EPI on the adrenergic receptors of several organs.

Although the classification system for the adrenergic receptors seems confusing, it is useful for classifying drugs. There are two main classes of drugs that affect the sympathetic system. The first, adrenergic drugs **(sympathomimetics),** produce effects that are similar to stimulating or mimicking the sympathetic nervous system. There is an increase in blood pressure, heart rate, and diameter of the respiratory passageways (bronchodilation). These responses are clinically useful in patients suffering from shock, cardiac arrest, or respiratory difficulty.

Drugs, including NE and EPI, that produce contraction of smooth muscle by stimulating the α receptors are referred to as α-adrenergic drugs. Drugs, including EPI, that both stimulate the heart (stimulate β_1) and cause relaxation of smooth

Table 6-1

Effects of Norepinephrine and Epinephrine on α and β Receptors

Receptor	Organ	Norepinephrine Effect	Epinephrine Effect
α (contraction of smooth muscle)	Most arteries and veins Pupils of eye	Vasoconstriction Dilation	Vasoconstriction Dilation
β_1 (stimulation of cardiac muscle)	Heart	Moderate increase in heart rate, force of contraction, and atrioventricular conduction	Greater increase in heart rate, force of contraction, and atrioventricular conduction
β_2 (relaxation of smooth muscle)	Bronchiolar smooth muscle Uterus Skeletal muscle vessels and coronary artery vessels	Norepinehrine does not stimulate β_2 receptors	Bronchodilation Relaxation Vasodilation

muscle (stimulate β_2) are referred to as β-adrenergic drugs. Epinephrine is one of the few substances that stimulates both α and β receptors. There are also a few β-adrenergic drugs that selectively stimulate only the β_2 receptors at therapeutic doses. These drugs are referred to as the **selective β_2-adrenergic drugs** and are used primarily as bronchodilators.

The second main class of drugs that affect the sympathetic nervous system is the adrenergic blocking drugs **(sympatholytics).** These drugs produce effects that would be expected by inhibiting or blocking sympathetic activity. Therefore, a decrease in blood pressure and heart rate usually occurs. Clinically, these effects are beneficial in patients with hypertension, angina pectoris, and certain types of cardiac arrhythmias.

Drugs that block the alpha effects of NE and EPI are known as the **alpha-adrenergic blockers.** Drugs that block the beta effects of EPI (beta-1 and beta-2) are known as the **nonselective beta-adrenergic blockers.** Drugs that block only beta-1 receptors are known as **selective beta-1 adrenergic blockers.** The effect of these alpha and beta blockers is to decrease sympathetic activity, especially in the cardiovascular system. The blocking drug competes with NE or EPI for the receptor sites. When the drug occupies the receptors, it prevents NE and EPI from producing an effect. Another method used to inhibit the sympathetic system is to decrease the formation or the release of NE from the adrenergic nerve ending. Drugs that act at the neuronal endings to reduce the formation or release of NE are known as the **adrenergic neuronal blockers.**

α-Adrenergic Drugs

Norepinephrine is considered to be the parent or prototype drug for the α drug class. The α-adrenergic drugs have chemical structures and produce effects that are almost identical to those of NE. The most important clinical effect produced by the α-adrenergic drugs is contraction of smooth muscle. This includes vasoconstriction of most blood vessels, contraction of sphincter muscles in the gastrointestinal (inhibits movement of intestinal contents) and urinary (restricts passage of urine) tracts, and dilation of the pupil of the eye (mydriasis).

CLINICAL INDICATIONS

α-adrenergic drugs are used (usually by IV infusion) in hypotensive states, for example, after surgery, to increase blood pressure and maintain circulation. Vasoconstriction of blood vessels in mucous membranes of the nasal sinuses produces a decongestant effect. Consequently, some of these drugs are included in over-the-counter (OTC) cold and allergy preparations for relief of nasal congestion. A few of the α drugs also are used in ophthalmology to dilate the pupils (mydriatic drug) and as ocular decongestants. α drugs that pass the blood–brain barrier, for example, amphetamines, produce a central effect to suppress appetite. Table 6-2 lists the α drugs and their main uses.

Table 6-2

α-Adrenergic Drugs

Drug (Product Name)	Main Use	Usual Dose*
Ephedrine	To increase blood pressure	15–50 mg PO
Epinephrine (Adrenalin)	To increase blood pressure	0.5–1.0 mL of 1:1000 solution IV
Mephentermine (Wyamine)	To increase blood pressure	15–35 mg IM, IV
	Nasal decongestant	12.5–25 mg PO
Metaraminol (Aramine)	To increase blood pressure	2–10 mg IM
		0.5–5 mg IV
Methoxamine (Vasoxyl)	To increase blood pressure	5–20 mg IM
Norepinephrine (Levophed)	To increase blood pressure	1–10 g/min IV
Phenylephrine (Neo-Synephrine)	To increase blood pressure	1–10 mg IV
	Nasal decongestant	10 mg PO
Pseudoephedrine (many)	Nasal decongestant	30–120 mg PO
Tetrahydrozoline (Visine)	Ophthalmic decongestant	0.05% solution

*_Abbreviations:_ IM, intramuscularly; IV, intravenously; PO, orally.

ADVERSE EFFECTS

The major adverse effects of the α-adrenergic drugs are the result of excessive vaso-constriction of blood vessels. This may result in hypertension, hypertensive crisis, or heart palpitations. In some patients, this can lead either to hemorrhage (usually cere-bral) or to cardiac arrhythmias. Consequently, extreme caution must be observed with hypertensive or cardiac patients. Patients receiving parenteral administration of these drugs should have blood pressure recordings taken at frequent intervals. The most common side effect of decongestant use is irritation of the nasal sinuses or eyes from excessive dryness caused by the vasoconstrictive decrease in blood flow.

CAUTION

The IV needle should be checked frequently to make certain that the drug is not infiltrating the skin. Infiltration by α drugs causes intense vasoconstriction of skin blood vessels, which can lead to death of skin cells and gangrene.

β-Adrenergic Drugs

The β-adrenergic drugs have a selective action to combine with β receptors. With the exception of EPI, most β drugs produce very few α effects.

BETA DRUG EFFECTS

The most important actions of the β drugs are stimulation of the heart ($β_1$) and bronchodilation ($β_2$). Isoproterenol is the most potent β-adrenergic drug that pro-duces both of these effects. This dual action (heart and respiratory system) is the main disadvantage of isoproterenol in treating bronchoconstriction caused by asthma or allergy. With isoproterenol, there is often overstimulation of the heart along with the bronchodilator effect. For this reason, a search was conducted to discover β drugs that would selectively stimulate only the β_2 receptors without causing excessive stimulation of β_1 receptors in the heart. Several of these selective β_2 drugs were discovered and are now widely used as bronchodilators. These β-adrenergic drugs are further discussed in Chapter 19, which discusses the treatment of asthma. Table 6-3 lists the various β drugs and their main clinical uses.

CLINICAL INDICATIONS FOR EPINEPHRINE

Epinephrine is the drug of choice for the immediate treatment of acute allergic reactions such as anaphylaxis. Anaphylaxis can be caused by insect stings, drugs, or other allergens in sensitized individuals. The patient presents with difficulty in breathing situations, EPI (stimulates α and β receptors) administered by subcutaneous injection is the preferred treatment. The α actions of EPI also are used during surgical procedures or in combination with local anesthetics to produce vasoconstriction. The α effect decreases blood flow and bleeding and prolongs the action of local anesthetics at the site of injection. The β effects of EPI are useful for cardiac stimulation (β_1) in emergencies (such as cardiac arrest) and for bronchodilation (β_2) in the treatment of asthma. Both EPI and isoproterenol are available as OTC bronchodilators.

ADVERSE EFFECTS

The β drugs may produce CNS stimulation resulting in restlessness, tremors, or anxiety. The main adverse effect of the older β drugs (EPI or isoproterenol) is

Table 6-3

β-Adrenergic Drugs

Drug (Product Name)	Classification	Main Use
Epinephrine (Adrenalin)	α, β_1, β_2	Vasopressor, cardiac stimulant, bronchodilator
Isoproterenol (Isuprel)	β_1, β_2	Cardiac stimulant, bronchodilator
Isoetharine (Bronkometer)	β_2	Bronchodilator
Metaproterenol (Alupent)	β_2	Bronchodilator
Terbutaline (Brethine)	β_2	Bronchodilator
Albuterol (Proventil, Ventolin)	β_2	Bronchodilator
Levalbuterol (Xopenex)	β_2	Bronchodilator
Fenoterol (Berotec)	β_2	Bronchodilator
Formoterol (Foradil)	β_2	Bronchodilator*
Salmeterol (Serevent)	β_2	Bronchodilator
Bitolterol mesylate (Tornalate)	β_2	Bronchodilator
Pirbuterol acetate (Maxair)	β_2	Bronchodilator
Ephedrine	α, β_1, β_2	Bronchodilator

Pending FDA approval.

overstimulation of the heart, which may result in palpitations or other cardiac arrhythmias. These drugs are used with extreme caution in patients with existing
heart disease. Drugs that produce β_2 effects dilate the blood vessels of skeletal muscle. This dilation may lower blood pressure but rarely results in hypotension. At
higher than therapeutic doses, the selective β_2 drugs can also stimulate cardiac β_1
receptors, which may cause overstimulation of the heart.

Dopamine

Dopamine functions as a neurotransmitter in the brain and is also formed as a precursor in the synthesis of NE in peripheral adrenergic nerve endings. When prepared as a drug (Intropin) and administered intravenously, dopamine produces
several cardiovascular effects that are useful in the treatment of circulatory shock.

At low doses (0.5 to 2.0 µg/kg/min), dopamine stimulates dopaminergic receptors in renal and mesenteric blood vessels, resulting in vasodilation and increased renal blood flow. At moderate doses (2 to 10 µg/kg/min), dopamine also
stimulates β_1 receptors, which increase myocardial contractility and increase cardiac output. Increasing cardiac output and renal blood flow are important actions
during shock, when blood pressure and cardiac function are drastically reduced.
At higher dosages, dopamine stimulates α receptors to produce vasoconstriction.

Dopamine is administered by continuous IV infusion, and the effects disappear
shortly after the infusion is stopped. Adverse effects from overdosage usually involve excessive stimulation of the heart and increased blood pressure (α effect).

Dobutamine (Dobutrex) is a drug similar to dopamine that possesses greater
β_1 effects to increase myocardial contractility. The main use of dobutamine is in
acute heart failure, where it is administered by IV infusion.

α-Adrenergic Blocking Drugs

The α blockers compete with NE for binding to the α-adrenergic receptors. If NE
binds to the receptors, the characteristic effects of NE are produced. When the α
blocker binds to the receptors, it prevents NE from producing sympathetic responses. Consequently, normal sympathetic activity is decreased in organs that
have α receptors. Because the major α organ is the blood vessels, the effect of α
blockade is vasodilation and lowering of blood pressure.

CLINICAL INDICATIONS

The α blockers are widely used in the treatment of hypertension. They are also
used in peripheral vascular conditions (poor blood flow to skin and extremities),
such as Raynaud's disease. In addition, they may be used to diagnose pheochromocytoma, a tumor of the adrenal medulla, which produces excessive catecholamine
levels and causes severe hypertension. The α blockers produce a dramatic reduc-

Table 6-4

α-Adrenergic Blocking Drugs

Drug (Product Name)	Main Use	Usual Daily Dose*
Doxazosin (Cardura)	Treatment of hypertension	1–16 mg PO
	Treatment of benign prostate hyperplasia	1–8 mg PO
Phentolamine (Regitine)	Diagnosis of pheochromocytoma	5 mg IV
Phentolamine (Regitine HCl)	Peripheral vascular disease	50 mg PO, QID
Prazosin (Minipress)	Treatment of hypertension	1–5 mg PO, TID
Terazosin (Hytrin)	Treatment of hypertension	1–20 mg PO
Yohimbine (Yohimex)	Treatment of male impotence	5.4 mg PO, TID

* *Abbreviations:* QID, four times a day; TID, three times a day.

tion in blood pressure in individuals with pheochromocytoma. Table 6-4 lists the α blockers and their main uses.

ADVERSE EFFECTS

Whenever the activity of one division of the autonomic nervous system is blocked (sympathetic), activity in the other division (parasympathetic) appears to increase. After α blockade, when sympathetic activity is blocked, the side effects are similar to an increase in parasympathetic activity in the organs that are blocked. You should note this generalization: that blocking one division of the ANS usually produces some effects that are similar to stimulating the other division. Constriction of the pupils (miosis), nasal congestion, and increased GI activity are commonly experienced after α blockade. Compensatory reflex tachycardia also occurs if the blood pressure is significantly lowered. In addition, the α blockers interfere with normal cardiovascular reflexes. Consequently, some patients experience dizziness, orthostatic hypotension, and fainting.

β-Adrenergic Blocking Drugs

β-blocking drugs bind to β-adrenergic receptors and antagonize the β effects of EPI and NE. Patients with hypertension, angina pectoris, and cardiac arrhythmias often have increased sympathetic activity, with excessive amounts of EPI and NE being released. By occupying β receptors, the β blockers prevent EPI and NE from producing β sympathetic effects. The heart (β_1) is one of the most important β organs, and the main clinical use of β blockers is to decrease the activity of the heart. Blockade of the β_1 receptors produces a decrease in heart rate, force of contraction, and impulse conduction through the conduction system of the heart. There are no specific therapeutic indications for blocking the β_2 receptors.

TYPES OF ß BLOCKERS

The β blockers are divided into the nonselective β blockers (block both $β_1$ and $β_2$ receptors) and the selective $β_1$ blockers. At therapeutic doses, the selective β blockers block only $β_1$ receptors. At higher doses, the selective β blockers may also begin to block $β_2$ receptors. Propranolol was the first β blocker used clinically; it blocks both $β_1$ and $β_2$ receptors. The other β blockers produce similar effects. The major differences among these drugs are the duration of action and the extent of drug metabolism. Table 6-5 lists the β blockers that are currently available.

PHARMACOLOGIC EFFECTS

The main effects produced by propranolol are a decrease in rate, force of contraction, and conduction velocity of the heart. In addition, there is usually a lowering of blood pressure. Reducing the effort and work of the heart causes a decrease in oxygen consumption. This effect is beneficial in the treatment of various cardiovascular conditions, especially when there is hyperactivity of the sympathetic nervous system.

Propranolol is administered either orally or intravenously. After oral administration, the drug is carried directly to the liver by the portal system. With propranolol, there is significant metabolism on the first passage through the liver (first-pass metabolism), which reduces the amount of drug that eventually reaches the systemic circulation.

β blockers also affect carbohydrate and lipid metabolism. Interference with carbohydrate metabolism is usually insignificant; however, diabetic patients may experience hypoglycemia. Serum lipid levels (triglycerides) may be increased by continuous therapy with these drugs.

Propranolol is the most lipid-soluble β blocker and passes into the brain, where

Table 6-5
β-Adrenergic Blocking Drugs

Drug (Product Name)	Main Use	Usual Daily Dose
Nonselective Blockers		
Labetalol (Normodyne)	Hypertension	100–400 mg (divided doses)
Nadolol (Corgard)	Hypertension, angina pectoris	30–240 mg/day (single dose)
Pindolol (Visken)	Hypertension	15–60 mg/day (divided doses)
Propranolol (Inderal)	Hypertension, angina pectoris, arrhythmias, migraine	120–480 mg/day (divided doses)
Timolol (Blocadren)	Hypertension, postmyocardial infarction to reduce mortality	20–40 mg/day (divided doses)
Selective $β_1$ Blockers		
Acebutolol (Sectral)	Hypertension, ventricular arrhythmias	400–1200 mg/day (divided doses)
Atenolol (Tenormin)	Hypertension, angina pectoris	50–100 mg/day (single dose)
Bisoprolol (Zebeta)	Hypertension	2.5–20 mg (single dose)
Esmolol (Brevibloc)	Supraventricular tachycardia	IV infusion
Metoprolol (Lopressor)	Hypertension, angina pectoris	100–450 mg/day (divided dose)

it can exert pharmacologic effects. These effects include CNS sedation, depression, and decreased central sympathetic activity, which may contribute to the lowering of blood pressure in the treatment of hypertension. Nadolol and atenolol are lipid-insoluble (water soluble) β blockers that do not pass into the brain and are excreted mostly unmetabolized in the urine.

CLINICAL INDICATIONS

Propranolol is used in the treatment of angina pectoris, hypertension, and various cardiac arrhythmias. Other uses include the treatment of glaucoma, where it decreases intraocular pressure; treatment of migraine headaches, where it often reduces the number of migraine attacks; and after myocardial infarctions, where, with chronic therapy, β blockers appear to decrease the incidences of additional myocardial infarctions and sudden cardiac death.

Esmolol is a short-acting drug that is administered intravenously in emergency situations. It has a quick onset of action to lower ventricular heart rate in cases of supraventricular tachycardia.

ADVERSE EFFECTS

Common side effects of propranolol include nausea, vomiting, and diarrhea. More serious adverse effects occur when heart function is excessively reduced. This reduction usually produces bradycardia and may lead to congestive heart failure or cardiac arrest. In general, propranolol should not be used in patients with asthma or other respiratory conditions. By blocking β_2 receptor sites, propranolol and other nonselective blockers may cause bronchoconstriction in individuals with asthma or other respiratory conditions. This bronchoconstriction may precipitate a respiratory emergency. The selective β_1 blockers have less of a tendency to do this. However, at higher than therapeutic doses, they may also begin to block β_2 receptors and cause bronchoconstriction. β blockers that gain access to the brain may cause drowsiness, mental depression, and other CNS disturbances.

DRUG INTERACTIONS

The most serious drug interactions involve therapy in which β blockers are used with other drugs that decrease cardiovascular function. These include cardiac glycosides, antiarrhythmic drugs, and calcium blockers. These drug interactions usually lower heart rate and cardiac output, which can lead to hypotension and drug-induced congestive heart failure.

Adrenergic Neuronal Blocking Drugs

The main activity that occurs inside the adrenergic nerve endings is the formation and storage of NE. Norepinephrine is synthesized from amino acids, either phenylalanine or tyrosine. Several drugs interfere with the formation or storage of NE. Such drugs are called **adrenergic neuronal blockers.** Figure 6-2 shows the bio-

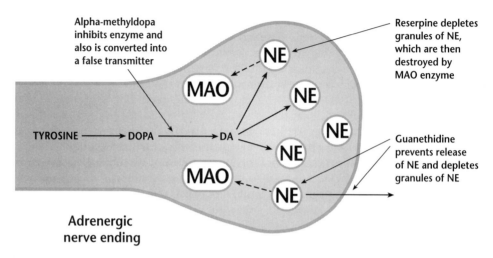

Figure 6-2
Synthesis of norepinephrine (NE) and the sites of action of the adrenergic neuronal blockers.

chemical steps in the synthesis of NE and the specific sites of action of the neuronal blocking drugs.

METHYLDOPA

Methyldopa (α-methyldopa, Aldomet) interferes with the synthesis of NE in the nerve endings and greatly reduces the amount of NE that is formed. Consequently, less NE is released, and the activity of the sympathetic system is decreased. There is evidence that the adrenergic nerve endings convert methyldopa into α-methylnorepinephrine, which is stored and released by the nerve endings like NE. The term **false transmitter** is used to describe drugs that produce neurotransmitter-like substances but that reduce neuronal activity.

The main use of methyldopa is in the treatment of hypertension to lower blood pressure. The most important site of action of methyldopa to reduce blood pressure is in the vasomotor center of the medulla oblongata (central effect). In the medulla, the formation and release of α-methylnorepinephrine lead to a decrease in sympathetic activity to vascular smooth muscle, which produces vasodilation and a lowering of blood pressure. The usual oral dose is 250 to 2000 mg/day (divided doses).

During initial treatment with methyldopa, many patients experience drowsiness and/or sedation, but these effects tend to disappear as drug treatment continues. Other side effects include nausea, vomiting, diarrhea, nasal congestion, and bradycardia. In some patients, adverse reaction may cause one or more of the following: drug fever, liver dysfunction, hemolytic anemia, or a lupus-like syndrome resulting in skin eruptions and symptoms of arthritis.

RESERPINE

Reserpine (Serpasil) is obtained from a plant, *Rauwolfia serpentina,* found mainly in India. The site of action of reserpine is the adrenergic nerve endings. Within the nerve endings, reserpine prevents the storage of NE inside the storage granules. Consequently, the adrenergic nerve endings are depleted of NE. When this occurs, the level of sympathetic activity is greatly reduced.

The most important clinical use of reserpine is in the treatment of hypertension. By reducing sympathetic activity, reserpine produces vasodilation and a lowering of blood pressure. Reserpine is usually administered in combination with a diuretic in the treatment of hypertension.

In addition to its antihypertensive effect, reserpine produces CNS sedation and tranquilization. Before the introduction of the modern antipsychotic drugs, reserpine was widely used to treat psychoses. Today, reserpine is primarily reserved for patients who have not responded to other antipsychotic drugs.

Most of the side effects of reserpine are caused by the decreased sympathetic activity. Side effects are similar to parasympathetic stimulation and include increased salivation, diarrhea, nasal congestion, bradycardia, and excessive hypotension. In the CNS, reserpine may produce excessive sedation, psychic disturbances such as confusion and hallucinations, or mental depression. The mental depression may lead to suicide attempts. At high doses, reserpine may produce symptoms of parkinsonism, which include tremors and muscular rigidity.

GUANETHIDINE

Guanethidine (Ismelin) is a potent adrenergic neuronal blocker. There are two main actions that guanethidine exerts on the nerve endings. First, guanethidine prevents the release of NE from the nerve endings, and second, guanethidine depletes the NE storage granules similarly to reserpine. These two effects produce a significant reduction of sympathetic activity.

The main clinical use of guanethidine is to treat severe hypertension; the usual oral dose is 25 to 300 mg/day. The half-life of guanethidine is relatively long. Therefore, the effects of guanethidine continue for up to 10 days after drug treatment is terminated.

The main adverse effects of guanethidine are caused by the decreased sympathetic activity and include diarrhea, nasal congestion, bradycardia, orthostatic hypotension, and impotence in males.

GUANADREL

Guanadrel (Hylorel) produces effects similar to those produced by guanethidine. It is used in the treatment of hypertension and generally produces a lower incidence of adverse effects than does guanethidine.

Summary of Sites of Action for Adrenergic Drugs

Figure 6-3 provides a diagrammatic summary of typical adrenergic nerve fibers, adrenergic receptors, and representative drugs that act on each receptor site.

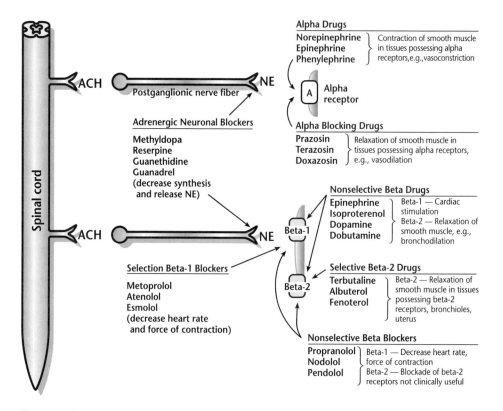

Figure 6-3

Diagrammatic summary of adrenergic receptor sites and sites of action of adrenergic drugs and adrenergic blocking drugs.

Chapter 6 Review

UNDERSTANDING TERMINOLOGY

Match the definition or description in the left column with the appropriate terms in the right column.

1. Drug that blocks or decreases sympathetic nervous system activity.

2. Drug that acts at the neuronal endings to reduce the formation or release of NE.

3. Mediates contraction, located on smooth muscle.

a. adrenergic neuronal blocker

b. α blocker

c. α receptor

d. β receptor

e. catecholamine

f. epinephrine

g. nonselective β blocker

4. Adrenergic receptor located on either the heart or smooth muscle.

5. Drug that blocks the β effects of EPI.

6. Drug that blocks the α effects of NE and EPI.

7. Norepinephrine and epinephrine.

8. Adrenergic drug or effect that increases sympathetic nervous system activity.

9. Hormone released from the adrenal medulla that stimulates the sympathetic nervous system.

h. sympatholytic

i. sympathomimetic

ACQUIRING KNOWLEDGE

Test your understanding of the material in this chapter by answering the following questions.

10. What is the main function of the sympathetic nervous system?

11. List the different types of adrenergic receptors and relate them to specific organ functions.

12. What two neurotransmitter substances are associated with the sympathetic nervous system? Describe the effects of each.

13. A patient brought into the emergency room is experiencing severe hypotension. Blood pressure reads 90/50. What class of drugs is indicated for treatment? What would be the first indication that too much drug has been administered?

14. α and β blockers are both indicated for the treatment of hypertension. Explain the difference in the mechanism of action of these two drug classes to lower blood pressure.

APPLYING KNOWLEDGE ON THE JOB

Answer the following questions.

15. Following emergency administration of epinephrine (SQ) for an acute asthmatic attack, the physician prescribes terbutaline (Brethine) tablets three times daily. How is this drug classified? What is it supposed to do? What are its advantages over epinephrine in the treatment of chronic asthma?

16. One of your co-workers has been taking propranolol (Inderal) regularly for a fast heart rate (tachycardia). Recently, she has been complaining of tiredness

and a feeling that she might faint. Is this effect drug related, and if so, what is occurring? What advice might you give her?

17. Assume that your employer, a busy physician, has asked you to help screen patients for potential prescription drug problems. Patient X visited the doctor's office today complaining of "sinus"— sinus congestion, pressure, and headache. The doctor diagnosed an upper respiratory virus and prescribed phenylephrine for the sinus congestion and discomfort. You study Patient X's chart and note that he has a history of hypertension. What should you advise the doctor about the drug she has prescribed for Patient X?

18. Betty Parsons has asthma and diabetes. She has also developed high blood pressure, for which her doctor just prescribed the drug propranolol. One of your duties as a respiratory care practitioner is to make sure patients are not prescribed drugs that are contraindicated because of other health problems. What should you tell the doctor about Betty's prescription for propranolol?

Additional Reading

Albertson PC. Prostate disease in older men 1. Benign hyperplasia. *Hosp Pract* 1997;32(5):61.

Atenolol for high-risk patients undergoing noncardiac surgery. *Emerg Med* 1997;29(4):36.

Frishman WH. Beta-adrenergic blockers are cardioprotective agents. *Am J Cardiol* 1992;70:21.

Oral albuterol for acute cough. *Emerg Med* 1996;28(10):57.

Schatz IJ. Autonomic failure and orthostatic hypotension. *Hosp Pract* 1997;32(5):15.

Sohl LL, Applefeld MM. A new direction for dobutamine. *Nursing* 1990;20(10):42.

Teplitz L. Clinical close-up on epinephrine. *Nursing* 1989;19(10):50.

Teplitz L. Clinical close up on dopamine. *Nursing* 1989;19(12):50.

Wilde MI, Fitton A, Sorkin EM. Terazosin. A review of its pharmacodynamic and pharmacokinetic properties and therapeutic potential in benign prostatic hyperplasia. *Drugs Aging* 1993;3:258.

Internet Activities

Medicinenet (http://www.medicinenet.com) is a search engine that provides information on many diseases and drugs. After reaching the Web site, click "Diseases and Treatment" and then highlight the letter "R." Go down the list until you find Raynaud's disease; click on this heading and learn about this condition. What are some of the classes of drugs used to treat this condition? What adrenergic blocking drugs may be used? What other medications can aggravate this condition?

Another topic at this Web site under "Diseases and Treatment" at letter "B" is bee stings; click on this heading and determine the immediate treatment for a severe allergic reaction. What is the most serious type of reaction called?

Enter another Web site (**http://www.parsec.it/summit/pO.htm**) and read about prostatitis. Click on the headings "Anatomy and Physiology," "Diagnostic Approach," and "Treatment." What are the different drug classes used to treat prostatitis? Prepare a short presentation for your classmates about prostatitis and its treatment.

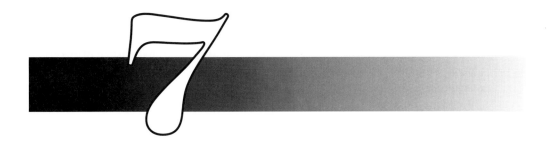

Drugs Affecting the Parasympathetic Nervous System

Henry Hitner, PhD
Barbara Nagle, PhD

Chapter Focus

This chapter describes the basic pharmacology of drugs that affect the parasympathetic nervous system. It also explains how cholinergic drugs increase parasympathetic activity and anticholinergic drugs increase parasympathetic activity and anticholinergic drugs decrease it.

Chapter Terminology

acetylcholinesterase: An enzyme that inactivates acetylcholine.

anticholinergic: Refers to drugs or effects that reduce the activity of the parasympathetic nervous system.

cholinergic: Refers to the nerves and receptors of the parasympathetic nervous system; also refers to the drugs that stimulate this system.

muscarinic receptor: An older but more specific term for the cholinergic receptor on smooth and cardiac muscle.

nicotinic-1 (NI) receptor: Cholinergic receptor located on both sympathetic and parasympathetic ganglia, also referred to as nicotinic$_{neural}$ (N_n).

nicotinic-2 (NII) receptor: Cholinergic receptor located at the neuromuscular junction of skeletal muscle, also referred to as nicotinic$_{muscle}$ (N_m).

parasympatholytic: Refers to drugs (anticholinergic) that decrease activity of the parasympathetic nervous system.

parasympathomimetic: Refers to drugs (cholinergic) that mimic stimulation of the parasympathetic nervous system.

Chapter Objectives

After studying this chapter, you should be able to:

- Describe the neuronal release and inactivation of acetylcholine.
- List the three types of cholinergic receptors and the tissues where they are located.
- Explain the effects of acetylcholine on the major internal organs and glands of the body.
- Name two direct- and two indirect-acting cholinergic drugs and the effects they produce.
- Name three anticholinergic drugs and the main effects they produce on the major body systems.
- List the most frequently observed adverse effects of both cholinergic and anticholinergic drug therapy.
- List two anticholinergic drugs used in the treatment of respiratory disorders.

The autonomic nervous system regulates the functions of the internal organs and glands. As previously discussed, the sympathetic division controls activity during physical exertion and stress (fight or flight). The parasympathetic division regulates body functions mainly during rest, digestion, and waste elimination. Parasympathetic stimulation increases the activity of the GI and genitourinary systems and decreases the activity of the cardiovascular system.

Parasympathetic System

The neurotransmitter of the parasympathetic system is acetylcholine (ACh). Nerves that release ACh are called cholinergic nerves; receptors that respond to cholinergic stimulation are called cholinergic receptors. Therefore, other drugs that bind to cholinergic receptors and produce effects similar to ACh are referred to as **cholinergic** drugs. Drugs that bind to cholinergic receptors and do not produce any effect (antagonism) are referred to as cholinergic blocking drugs. The cholinergic blocking drugs prevent ACh from acting on its receptors.

CHOLINERGIC NERVE ENDINGS

Acetylcholine is produced and stored within the cholinergic nerve endings. When a nerve is stimulated, ACh is released from its storage granules, travels to the smooth or cardiac muscle membrane, and binds to the cholinergic receptors. The binding of ACh to the receptors initiates the changes that result in parasympathetic stimulation. In the area of the cholinergic receptors is an enzyme called acetylcholinesterase.

Acetylcholinesterase inactivates ACh only when it is outside a nerve ending and not on the receptor. Inactivation of ACh occurs so quickly that the effects of ACh last for only a few seconds. A cholinergic nerve ending is shown in Figure 7-1.

CHOLINERGIC RECEPTORS

Three types of cholinergic receptors are found in the peripheral nervous system. ACh is the neurotransmitter for each receptor site. However, each of the cholinergic receptor types reacts differently to drugs that block the different cholinergic receptors. There are three distinct classes of cholinergic blocking drugs, one for each type of receptor. All three types of cholinergic blockers are required clinically to block all of the effects of ACh. Although the terminology used for the cholinergic receptors can be confusing to beginning students, learning the terminology is essential for understanding the mechanism of drug action.

Muscarinic Receptors   The cholinergic receptors at the parasympathetic postganglionic nerve endings *(as shown in Figure 7-2A)* are known as **muscarinic receptors.** The term *muscarinic* is derived from the drug muscarine, which is an alkaloid obtained from a particular type of mushroom. One of the first drugs used to establish the function of the autonomic nervous system (ANS), muscarine produces effects that are similar to those of ACh, but only at these particular receptor sites. Consequently, early pharmacologists referred to these receptors as muscarinic, and the terminology is still in use. Drugs that act like ACh or muscarine at these receptors are referred to as either cholinergic or muscarinic drugs. Drugs that block ACh at the muscarinic receptors are referred to as either anticholinergic or antimuscarinic drugs. Presently, the terms *cholinergic* and *anticholinergic* are preferred.

Nicotinic-I Receptors   The cholinergic receptors at the ganglionic sites of both sympathetic and parasympathetic nerves *(as seen in Figure 7-2B)* are known as

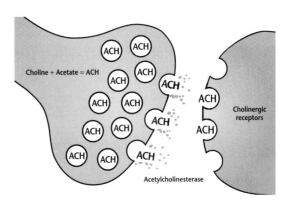

Figure 7-1
Characteristics of the cholinergic nerve ending. Presynaptic nerve releases acetylcholine (ACh). Postsynaptic membrane contains the cholinergic receptor. Acetylcholinesterase inactivates ACh.

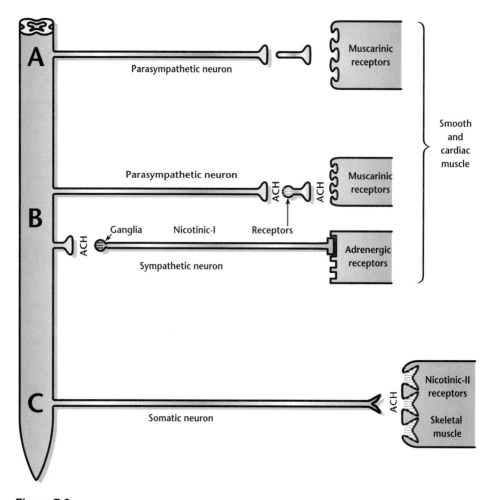

Figure 7-2

The three cholinergic sites of action and their specific receptors. **A:** A parasympathetic neuron with pre- and postganglionic fibers innervating smooth or cardiac muscle via the muscarinic receptor. **B:** The nicotinic-I receptor located on the ganglia of both parasympathetic and sympathetic neurons. **C:** A somatic neuron that innervates skeletal muscle via nicotinic-II receptors (ACh, acetylcholine).

nicotinic-I (NI) receptors. ACh is the neurotransmitter for these receptors. The term *nicotinic* is derived from the drug nicotine, which is an alkaloid obtained from the tobacco plant. Early pharmacologists also used nicotine to study the pharmacology of the ANS because nicotine stimulates the autonomic ganglia (sympathetic and parasympathetic) in low doses and blocks the autonomic ganglia in high doses. Drugs that act like ACh or low doses of nicotine at these receptors are known as ganglionic stimulants. Drugs that block ACh at these receptors or act like high doses of nicotine are referred to as ganglionic blockers. The ganglionic drugs are discussed in Chapter 8.

Nicotinic-II Receptors   The cholinergic receptors at the neuromuscular junction (NMJ) of skeletal muscle *(seen in Figure 7-2C)* are known as **nicotinic-II (NII) receptors.** Nicotine also stimulates or acts like ACh at the neuromuscular junction. Drugs that block the effects of ACh at the neuromuscular junction are neuromuscular blockers or skeletal muscle relaxants. The skeletal muscle relaxant drugs are discussed in Chapter 9.

Cholinergic Drugs

Cholinergic drugs mimic the actions of ACh at the muscarinic receptors. Another term with essentially the same meaning is **parasympathomimetic.** Cholinergic drugs are subdivided into two groups, the direct-acting and the indirect-acting drugs. The direct-acting drugs bind to the muscarinic receptors and produce effects similar to ACh. The indirect-acting drugs inhibit the enzyme acetylcholinesterase. By inhibiting acetylcholinesterase, these drugs allow ACh to accumulate at each of the cholinergic receptor sites (nicotinic and muscarinic). Consequently, a greater number of receptors become stimulated, and the effects of ACh are prolonged.

DIRECT-ACTING CHOLINERGIC DRUGS

Direct-acting cholinergic drugs bind to the muscarinic receptors. ACh is not useful as a drug because of its extremely short duration of action. Therefore, several derivatives of ACh were synthesized (methacholine and bethanechol) that produce effects like ACh but are more slowly inactivated by acetylcholinesterase. Consequently, the durations of action of these drugs are considerably longer than the duration of action for ACh. In all other respects, the derivatives of ACh stimulate the parasympathetic system similarly to ACh.

Pharmacologic Effects   The main effects are an increase in GI secretions and motility, an increase in genitourinary activity, bronchoconstriction, miosis, a decrease in blood pressure (vasodilation), and a decrease in heart rate. The cholinergic drugs are listed in Table 7-1.

In addition to the derivatives of ACh, there are a few alkaloids, such as muscarine and pilocarpine, that have parasympathomimetic effects. Muscarine has no clinical importance except in cases of accidental poisoning. Pilocarpine is another alkaloid that acts like ACh and is used only in the form of eye drops for the treatment of glaucoma.

Clinical Indications   Because of the short duration of ACh and some of its derivatives, the direct-acting cholinergic drugs are rarely used systemically. Bethanechol

Table 7-1

Cholinergic Drugs and Their Major Clinical Uses

Drug (Trade Name)	Main Use
Direct Acting	
Acetylcholine (Miochol)	Miotic in cataract surgery
Bethanechol (Urecholine)	Nonobstructive urinary retention
Carbachol (Miostat)	Treatment of glaucoma
Methacholine (Provocholine)	Diagnostic agent for asthma
Pilocarpine (Pilomiotin, Ocusert)	Treatment of glaucoma
Indirect Acting	
Ambenonium (Mytelase)	Treatment of myasthenia gravis
Demacarium (Humorsol)	Treatment of glaucoma
Edrophonium (Tensilon)	Diagnosis of myasthenia gravis, antidote for curare-type drugs
Isoflurophate (Floropryl)	Treatment of glaucoma
Neostigmine (Prostigmin)	Treatment of myasthenia gravis, antidote for curare-type drugs
Physostigmine (Antilirium, Eserine)	Antidote to anticholinergic drugs, treatment of glaucoma
Pyridostigmine (Mestinon)	Treatment of myasthenia gravis, antidote for curare-type drugs

is the exception; this drug is administered orally to stimulate the urinary and intestinal tracts. Certain drugs (general anesthetics) and conditions, especially in the elderly, cause urinary retention and intestinal stasis. Bethanechol may be administered several times a day to stimulate urination and defecation. The main adverse effects are the result of overstimulation of the bladder and intestines, resulting in increased urinary frequency and diarrhea.

Cholinergic drugs are used locally during ophthalmic examinations (miotic, to constrict pupil) and in the treatment of glaucoma. In glaucoma, there is increased intraocular pressure, which gradually destroys the retina of the eye and causes blindness. Topical application (eye drops) of cholinergic drugs produces miosis (pupillary constriction), which promotes better drainage of intraocular fluid from the eye. This lowers pressure and helps prevent retinal damage.

Methacholine has been used as part of bronchial provocation testing. This testing can be used as part of an evaluation of the efficacy of bronchodilators. By testing, we hope to simulate a real live challenge similar to allergens in the environment or cold air. Methacholine is prepared at a number of different concentrations and administered by inhalation. Asthmatics tend to be very sensitive to inhaled methacholine. Methacholine leads to bronchoconstriction and can be useful as part of confirming a diagnosis of asthma.

INDIRECT-ACTING CHOLINERGIC DRUGS

The indirect-acting drugs are known as the anticholinesterases. These drugs inhibit the enzyme acetylcholinesterase and allow the accumulation of acetylcholine at all cholinergic receptor sites. The anticholinesterase drugs are subdivided into reversible inhibitors and irreversible inhibitors of acetylcholinesterase.

Reversible Inhibitors   The reversible inhibitors are used in the diagnosis and treatment of myasthenia gravis. This is a disease in which there is severe muscle weakness caused by a lack of ACh. Reversible inhibitors are also used as antidotes to reverse the effects of drugs that block cholinergic and nicotinic receptors. Edrophonium has the shortest duration of action, about 30 minutes, and is used intravenously in order to diagnose myasthenia gravis. The durations of neostigmine (2–4 hours), pyridostigmine (3–6 hours), and ambenonium (4–8 hours) are longer. These drugs are administered orally for the treatment of myasthenia gravis and intravenously to reverse the effects of excessive cholinergic blockade. The previously mentioned drugs are all quaternary amines (charged compounds) that do not cross the blood–brain barrier and so produce effects only at peripheral receptor sites. Physostigmine is not a charged compound and does produce effects in the brain. It is used parenterally to reverse the CNS effects of excessive anticholinergic blockade and as eye drops in the treatment of glaucoma.

Irreversible Inhibitors   The irreversible inhibitors of acetylcholinesterase are derivatives of organophosphate compounds widely used as insecticides, pesticides, and as chemical warfare agents. These compounds have extremely long durations of action because they form irreversible bonds with the acetylcholinesterase enzyme. A few of these derivatives, for example, isoflurophate (Floropryl), are used in very small doses as drugs, primarily as eye drops in the treatment of glaucoma. In larger doses, these drugs produce severe toxicity, referred to as cholinergic crisis, that can quickly cause respiratory paralysis and death.

All of the anticholinesterase drugs, reversible and irreversible, produce effects that are similar to those of ACh and parasympathetic stimulation (parasympathomimetic).

ADVERSE AND TOXIC EFFECTS OF CHOLINERGIC DRUGS

The most common adverse effects of these drugs are caused by excessive stimulation of the parasympathetic nervous system. The symptoms include nausea, vomiting, diarrhea, blurred vision, excessive sweating, muscular tremors, salivation, increased frequency of urination, bronchoconstriction, bradycardia, and hypotension. In toxic overdosage, these drugs cause skeletal muscular paralysis, respiratory depression, and sudden death. The main antidote is the administration of anticholinergic drugs such as atropine, which compete with ACh for the muscarinic receptors and reverse the effects of excessive cholinergic stimulation.

Cholinergic Crisis   Cholinergic crisis is the term usually used to describe the effects of excessive drug dosage in patients with myasthenia gravis. At high concentrations, ACh causes excessive stimulation of cholinergic (muscarinic) receptors but blockade (paralysis) of nicotinic receptors. This may result in respiratory paralysis because respiratory muscles are skeletal (voluntary) in nature. In these situations, anticholinesterase drug administration must be stopped until the levels of ACh return to normal. Atropine can be administered to block the effects of excessive muscarinic stimulation.

Farmers who spray their fields with derivatives of the irreversible anticholinesterases (organophosphates) may also experience a cholinergic crisis. Unless protective masks or enclosed tractor cabs are used, the farmer may inhale too much of the insecticide or pesticide and develop signs of cholinergic crisis. With the irreversible drugs, the antidote is atropine to reverse the effects of excessive ACh and also an additional drug, pralidoxime (Protopam). Pralidoxime is a drug that can reactivate the acetylcholinesterase enzyme after it has been inhibited by an irreversible inhibitor. Pralidoxime is most effective immediately after organophosphate exposure. Pralidoxime is also the antidote to organophosphate chemical warfare agents.

CLINICAL INDICATIONS FOR ANTICHOLINESTERASE DRUGS

The anticholinesterase drugs are more widely used than the direct-acting cholinergic drugs. They are used in the treatment of glaucoma, myasthenia gravis, urinary retention, intestinal paralysis, and Alzheimer's disease, and as antidotes to the curare-type skeletal muscle blockers and the anticholinergic drugs.

Topical Use in Glaucoma   Several of these drugs (Table 7-1) are used topically as eye drops to lower intraocular pressure in glaucoma. By inhibiting the metabolism of ACh, they increase ACh levels in the eye to produce miosis, improved drainage of intraocular fluid, and lower intraocular pressure.

Treatment of Myasthenia Gravis   Myasthenia gravis is a disease of the skeletal muscle endplate where acetylcholine functions to stimulate muscle tone and contraction. The condition is believed to be the result of an autoimmune reaction in which the body produces antibodies that attack the nicotinic-II receptor. The result is loss of skeletal muscle tone and strength. The eyelids droop, and as the disease progresses, there is difficulty in physical movement. Eventually, patients may become bedridden and have difficulty breathing. The longer-acting reversible anticholinesterase drugs, pyridostigmine and ambenonium, are preferred and used orally to increase ACh levels and increase skeletal muscle tone and strength.

Treatment of Urinary Retention and Intestinal Stasis   Urinary retention (also referred to as atony of the bladder) and intestinal stasis or paralysis (also referred to as paralytic ileus) are usually treated with neostigmine. The increased levels of ACh stimulate bladder contraction and intestinal peristalsis.

Treatment of Alzheimer's Disease   Alzheimer's disease is a degenerative brain condition that occurs in some individuals with advanced age. There appears to be a loss of neuronal synapses and, in particular, a reduction of ACh levels in the brain. These changes cause memory loss, dementia, and general deterioration of mental function. There are very few drugs that have been discovered that are effective in this condition. Currently, two centrally acting reversible anticholinesterase drugs, tacrine (Cognex) and donepezil (Aricept), are used to increase ACh levels in the brain. Beneficial effects of the drugs are most notable in the early stages of the disease and lessen as the disease progresses. Lecithin (Phoschol) is a precursor of ACh, and it is often administered with the anticholinesterase drugs in an attempt to further increase ACh levels.

Antidotes to Skeletal Muscle Blockers   Skeletal muscle blockers (Chapter 9) are used in surgery to produce paralysis of skeletal muscles (nicotinic-II receptor). At high doses they may cause respiratory paralysis. In these situations, administration of neostigmine will increase ACh levels and antagonize the actions of the skeletal muscle blockers.

Antidotes to Anticholinergic Drug Poisoning   Anticholinergic drugs, such as atropine and scopolamine (next section), block the cholinergic receptors (muscarinic) and produce effects similar to decreasing the activity of the parasympathetic system (parasympatholytic). This includes urinary and intestinal inhibition, cardiac stimulation (tachycardia), and central effects in the brain that can cause a variety of stimulant (seizures) and depressant (coma) effects. The antidote is usually to administer physostigmine because this drug can pass the blood–brain barrier. The increased levels of ACh produced compete with the anticholinergic drug for the receptor. As the levels of ACh increase, the central effects of excessive anticholinergic blockade are reversed.

Anticholinergic Drugs

The cholinergic blocking drugs that bind to the muscarinic receptors are referred to as **anticholinergic,** or **parasympatholytic,** drugs. They act by competitive antagonism of ACh. In the presence of anticholinergic drugs, sufficient amounts of ACh are unable to bind to the cholinergic receptors to produce an effect. The oldest anticholinergic drugs, such as atropine and scopolamine, were obtained from the belladonna plant (deadly nightshade) and are commonly referred to as the belladonna alkaloids. Atropine, scopolamine, and the newer synthetic drugs are listed in Table 7-2.

PHARMACOLOGIC ACTIONS AND CLINICAL INDICATIONS

Cardiovascular System   By blocking the effects of ACh, anticholinergic drugs decrease the activity of the vagus nerve (parasympathetic nerve) on the heart. Consequently, an increase in heart rate occurs. In patients with excessively slow heart rates (bradycardia), anticholinergic drugs are used to increase heart rate and speed up atrioventricular conduction.

Respiratory System   Acetylcholine increases the secretions of the respiratory tract and may cause bronchoconstriction. Anticholinergic drugs are administered preoperatively to inhibit secretions that are increased by the administration of general anesthetics. Both atropine and scopolamine are used for this purpose.

Table 7-2

Anticholinergic Drugs and Their Main Uses

Drug (Trade Name)	Main Use	Usual Adult Daily Dose*
Belladonna Alkaloids		
Atropine	To increase heart rate, preop medication, enuresis, GI and biliary colic, antidote to cholinergic drugs	0.4–1.0 mg PO
	Mydriatic and cycloplegic	Topic eyedrops
Hyoscyamine (Cystospaz, Levsin)	Same as atropine	0.25–1.0 mg PO, IV
Scopolamine, transdermal	Same as atropine	1 patch every 3 days
Semisynthetic Drug		
Homatropine	Mydriatic	2–5% topical solution
Synthetic Drugs		
Dicyclomine (Bentyl)	Treatment of GI disorders such as ulcers, colitis	10–20 mg PO TID
Glycopyrrolate (Robinul)	Treatment of ulcers	1–2 mg PO TID
Propantheline (Pro-Banthine)	Treatment of GI disorders such as ulcers, colitis	15 mg PO QID

Abbreviations: BID, twice daily; IV, intravenously; PO, orally; QID, four times daily; TID, three times daily.

Anticholinergic drugs produce a moderate degree of bronchodilation and are administered by aerosol generators used in the treatment of asthma and chronic obstructive pulmonary disease (COPD). These medications have a unique mechanism of action by acting on the muscarinic receptors in the lungs. This results in bronchodilation. Ipratroprium bromide (Atrovent) is a derivative of atropine and is used in respiratory care, as a bronchodilator. However, because of its quaternary structure, it does not enter the brain and cause centralized anticholinergic effects.

Asthma, although not an emotional disease, can be triggered by emotional factors. Ipratroprium can be beneficial around times of increased anxiety, such as exam time for students, as an additional medication. Treatment a day or so before the exam as well as on the day of the exam can be very beneficial. More information can be found in Chapter 19.

In addition, ipratroprium is also used in a type of running nose called vasomotor rhinitis, which results from excess cholinergic activity in the nose. Ipratroprium can be very helpful in treating this condition.

Some patients produce an excessive amount of respiratory secretions and must be suctioned on a regular basis. These patients may benefit from the synthetic anticholinergic medication glycopyrrolate (Robinul). Care must be taken not to give too high a dose, or the secretions become very thick and difficult to remove. See Table 7-3 for anticholinergics used in respiratory care.

Table 7-3
Anticholinergic Drugs Used in Respiratory Care

Drug (Trade Name)	Main Use	Doses*
Atropine	Bronchospasm	0.03–0.05 mg/kg/dose 3–4 times daily via inhalation—children
		0.025–0.05 mg/kg/dose every 4–6 hours via inhalation—adult
Glycopyrrolate (Robinul)	Control respiratory secretions	40–100 μg/kg/dose 3–4 times daily PO—children
		4–10 μg/kg/dose every 3–4 hours IV, IM—children
Ipratropium bromide (Atrovent)	Bronchodilator	25 μg/kg/dose TID via inhalation—neonates
		125–250 μg TID via inhalation—infants and children
		1–2 puffs TID via MDI—children 3–12 years old
		500 μg 3–4 times daily via inhalation—children > 12 years old and adults
		2 puffs QID via MDI
	Seasonal rhinitis	2 sprays in each nostril 2–3 times daily—children > 5 years old and adults

* *Abbreviations:* IM, intramuscularly; IV, intravenously; MDI, metered dose inhaler; PO, orally; QID, four times daily; TID, three times daily.

GI System   Anticholinergic drugs reduce salivary and GI secretions. In addition, they decrease the motility of the GI tract. The anticholinergic drugs are used as antispasmodics in GI disorders such as irritable bowel syndrome. In the treatment of peptic ulcers, the anticholinergic drugs, which decrease gastric acid secretion, have been replaced by newer and more effective drugs.

Genitourinary System   Anticholinergic drugs inhibit urinary peristalsis and the voiding of urine. These drugs may be used in individuals suffering from enuresis (urinary incontinence) to promote urinary retention and in the treatment of various bladder disorders involving spasm and increased urinary urgency. However, anticholinergic drugs are contraindicated in men with hypertrophy of the prostate gland. These drugs increase urinary retention and further increase the difficulty of urination associated with this condition.

Central Nervous System   Most anticholinergic drugs that gain access to the brain produce a depressant effect, which generally results in drowsiness and sedation. Some over-the-counter preparations contain limited amounts of scopolamine and are used as sleep aids. At higher doses, there can be a mixture of both CNS stimulant and depressant effects. At toxic doses, both atropine and scopolamine may produce excitation, delirium, hallucinations, and a profound CNS depression that can lead to respiratory arrest and death. Anticholinergic actions are useful in the treatment of Parkinson's disease and as antiemetics in the treatment of motion sickness.

Ocular Effects   The anticholinergic drugs produce mydriasis (pupillary dilation) and cycloplegia (loss of accommodation). They are used in ophthalmology to facilitate examination of the retina and lens. Anticholinergic drugs increase intraocular pressure and should never be administered to patients with narrow-angle glaucoma.

ADVERSE AND TOXIC EFFECTS

The most frequently occurring adverse effects of the anticholinergic drugs are caused by excessive blockade of the parasympathetic nervous system. The symptoms include dry mouth, visual disturbances, urinary retention, constipation, flushing (redness) and dryness of the skin, fever (hyperpyrexia), tachycardia, and symptoms of both CNS stimulation and depression. The effects on the skin are the result of anticholinergic effects that inhibit the sweating mechanism and that vasodilate certain blood vessels to cause a flushing reaction. In toxic doses, hyperpyrexia and CNS depression can be severe and accompanied by depression of the vital centers in the brain. If untreated, this may result in respiratory paralysis and death.

The belladonna alkaloids are present in some over-the-counter preparations and in many common plant substances and inedible plant berries. Poisoning usually occurs in children who have mistakenly eaten the berries. Such children usually develop fever, tachycardia, dryness and flushing of the skin, and mydriasis. Emergency treatment is essential. If sufficient quantities have been ingested, respiratory paralysis, coma, and death may occur within a few hours.

Treatment involves inducing emesis or performing gastric lavage to limit absorption. Activated charcoal and saline cathartics are administered to inactivate the drug and accelerate its elimination. Physostigmine, given intravenously, antagonizes the actions of the anticholinergic drugs and is useful when CNS symptoms such as delirium and coma are present.

ADMINISTRATION AND PATIENT MONITORING

Observe the patient for signs of excessive anticholinergic effects, especially after parenteral administration: tachycardia, flushing of skin (redness), decreased urination, CNS stimulation or depression, and respiratory difficulties.

Explain to the patient the common anticholinergic side effects: dry mouth, blurred vision (pupillary dilation), sedation, or mental confusion.

Instruct the patient to report excessive blurred vision, rapid pulse rate, difficulty with urination, constipation, mental confusion, or hallucinations. Geriatric patients are particularly susceptible to anticholinergic effects and should be observed more closely, especially for mental confusion and disorientation.

Anticholinergic drugs are contraindicated in patients with narrow-angle glaucoma, men with prostate hypertrophy, and patients with urinary or intestinal obstruction.

The antidote to anticholinergic overdose is administration of anticholinesterase drugs, especially physostigmine when there are CNS symptoms.

Chapter 7 Review

UNDERSTANDING TERMINOLOGY

Match the drug effect or drug use in the left column with the appropriate drug in the right column. Answers can be used more than once.

1. Reactivates acetylcholinesterase.
2. Directly stimulates muscarinic receptor.
3. Increases ACh levels in the CNS.
4. Used to reverse CNS anticholinergic toxicity.
5. Used to decrease the volume of respiratory secretions.
6. Used to prevent motion sickness.
7. Used before surgery to dry respiratory secretions.
8. Blocks muscarinic receptors leading to bronchodilation.
9. Irreversibly inhibits acetylcholinesterase.
10. Used to treat nonobstructive urinary retention.

A. Bethanechol (Urecholine)
B. Glycopyrrolate (Robinul)
C. Scopolamine, transdermal
D. Isoflurophate (Floropryl)
E. Atropine
F. Physostigmine (Antilirium)
G. Pralidoxine (Protopam)
H. Ipratropium bromide (Atrovent)

Test your understanding of this chapter by discussing the following terms.

11. Differentiate between parasympatholytic and parasympathomimetic.
12. Explain the terms cholinergic and anticholinergic.

ACQUIRING KNOWLEDGE

Test your understanding of the material in this chapter by answering the following questions.

13. What is the function of the parasympathetic nervous system?
14. What is the function of acetylcholinesterase? Where is it found?
15. Where are the three different cholinergic receptors located? What class of drug is needed to block each receptor?
16. How do the direct-acting and indirect-acting cholinergic drugs produce their parasympathetic effects?
17. List the potential adverse effects of the cholinergic drugs.
18. List the potential adverse effects of the anticholinergic drugs.
19. Why are the side effects of the anticholinergic drugs similar to the side effects of the sympathetic drugs?

APPLYING KNOWLEDGE ON THE JOB

Answer the following questions.

20. Your next-door neighbor knows you are studying pharmacology, so she sometimes comes to you when she has questions about health problems. A few minutes ago, she came to your door in a state of panic. She said her 3-year-old had just swallowed some scopolamine tablets, which your neighbor takes for her irritable bowel syndrome. What should you do?

21. Your elderly patient, who was prescribed an antispasmodic drug for GI hyperactivity, is complaining of increased sensitivity to light and notices that she has difficulty urinating. What do you think is happening to this patient? What class of drugs do you think she was most likely prescribed? What drug class would be indicated if her condition worsened and treatment was required?

22. One of your patients is under good control of his asthma with his usual antiinflammatory medications. The only exception is around exam time in school, when his symptoms worsen. What could you suggest to help him?

Additional Reading

Bayer MJ, McKay C. Reversing the effects of pesticide poisoning, part 1: Insecticides and herbicides. *Emerg Med* 1997;29(4):72.

Bayer MJ, McKay C. Reversing the effects of pesticide poisoning, part 2: Rodenticides and miscellaneous agents. *Emerg Med* 1997;29(5):78.

Keeping an eye on vision: Primary care of age-related ocular disease. *Geriatrics* 1997;52(8):30.

Miller CA. What's new in treating and preventing Alzheimer's disease. *Geriatr Nurs* 1997;18(5):238.

Morris JC. Alzheimer's disease: A review of clinical assessment and management issues. *Geriatrics* 1997;52(Suppl 2):S22.

Ramsey F. Reversal of neuromuscular blockade. *Curr Rev Nurse Anesth* 1991;514(7):50.

Seybold ME. Update on myasthenia gravis. *Hosp Med* 1991;27(4):71.

Teplitz L. Clinical close-up on atropine. *Nursing* 1989;19(11):44

Internet Activities

Visit the **Medicinenet** Web site **(http://www.medicinenet.com);** under "Diseases and Treatments," click on letter "E" and look for Eye, Glaucoma. Organize a brief presentation that explains the causes, symptoms, detection, and treatments for glaucoma. Under "Diseases and Treatments," click on the letter "M" and find Myasthenia Gravis. Read about the prognosis and treatment of this condition in relation to the drugs presented in this chapter.

Drugs Affecting the Autonomic Ganglia

HENRY HITNER, PhD
BARBARA NAGEL, PhD

Chapter Focus

This chapter describes the drugs that affect autonomic ganglia and examines how ganglionic blocking drugs affect both sympathetic and parasympathetic activity.

Chapter Terminology

ganglionic blocker: Drug that blocks the nicotinic-I receptors and reduces the activity of the autonomic nervous system.

ganglionic stimulant: Drug that stimulates the nicotinic-I receptors to increase autonomic activity.

nicotine: Alkaloid drug in tobacco that stimulates ganglionic receptors.

nitotinic-I (NI) receptor: Cholinergic receptor at the ganglia.

Chapter Objectives

After studying this chapter, you should be able to:

- Describe the pharmacologic effects of both ganglionic stimulation and ganglionic blockade.
- List three ganglionic blocking drugs and describe their clinical uses.
- Discuss the adverse effects associated with the use of ganglionic blocking drugs.

The autonomic ganglia of both sympathetic and parasympathetic nerves are pharmacologically identical. Acetylcholine (ACh) is the neurotransmitter at the ganglionic synapses. Acetylcholinesterase is responsible for inactivation of ACh. Before the discovery of ACh, nicotine was found to stimulate the autonomic ganglia, and so the receptors at the ganglia were known as the **nicotinic-I (NI) receptors.** Drugs that stimulate the NI receptors are called **ganglionic stimulants.** There are no clinical conditions in which ganglionic stimulation is of significant clinical value. Therefore, as a drug class, the ganglionic stimulants are of little interest.

Individuals who smoke tobacco inhale **nicotine,** which produces ganglionic stimulation affecting both sympathetic and parasympathetic activity. Theoretically, if both systems are stimulated at the same time, the effects should cancel out. However, sympathetic stimulation appears to predominate in the cardiovascular system, whereas parasympathetic stimulation predominates in the GI tract. Consequently, after smoking, there is usually an increase in heart rate, blood pressure, and GI activity. Nicotine also stimulates the CNS to produce tremors and, most importantly, the pleasurable effects of smoking, whatever they are.

Ganglionic Stimulants

A chewing gum containing nicotine (Nicorette) is available for individuals who are trying to stop smoking. The gum releases nicotine that is meant to substitute for the nicotine supplied by smoking. In addition, transdermal skin patches (Habitrol, Nicoderm) slowly deliver nicotine into the bloodstream. The intention of these products is to prevent any withdrawal reactions caused by quitting the smoking habit. Later, the use of these products can be reduced and then eliminated altogether.

CAUTIONS AND CONTRAINDICATIONS

Pregnancy   Nicotine and tobacco smoke (contains nicotine) have been shown to be harmful to the fetus. Consequently, tobacco smoking and the use of nicotine substitutes should be avoided during pregnancy.

ADVERSE EFFECTS

Drugs that block the effects of ACh at the NI receptors are called **ganglionic blockers.** At toxic doses, ACh and nicotine act as ganglionic blockers and can block both ganglionic and neuromuscular transmission. This blockade can result in respiratory paralysis and death.

Ganglionic Blocking Drugs

The ganglionic blockers that are used clinically compete with ACh for the NI receptors. These drugs interfere with ganglionic transmission at both sympathetic and parasympathetic ganglia. Consequently, the effects are a combination of anticholinergic and sympathetic blocking effects. The main disadvantage of the ganglionic blockers is that there is no selectivity. As a result, many side effects are associated with their use. Newer drugs with greater selectivity have been discovered, and these have gradually replaced the ganglionic blockers.

MAIN EFFECTS OF GANGLIONIC BLOCKADE

Ganglionic blockade decreases the activity of the cardiovascular, GI, and genitourinary systems. The major effects are hypotension, bradycardia, decreased intestinal secretions and motility, and reduced urination. In men, impotence may occur. In addition, there are usually varying degrees of mydriasis and cycloplegia.

PHARMACOKINETICS

The first ganglionic blockers that were discovered (hexamethonium, pentolinium, and trimethaphan) possessed a quaternary ammonium ion. Quaternary ammonium ions are permanently charged molecules and are poorly absorbed from the GI tract. Therefore, parenteral administration (IM or IV) is usually required. On the other hand, one of the ganglionic blockers, mecamylamine, is not a quaternary ion and is almost completely absorbed after oral administration. Trimethaphan has an extremely short duration of action (10 to 20 minutes) and is administered by IV infusion. The ganglionic blocking drugs are listed in Table 8-1.

CLINICAL INDICATIONS

The most important therapeutic effect of the ganglionic blockers is the lowering of blood pressure. This effect results from ganglionic blockade of the sympathetic

Table 8-1
Ganglionic Blocking Drugs

Drug (Trade Name)	Main Use	Usual Dose*
Mecamylamine (Inversine)	Severe hypertension	2.5–10 mg PO BID, TID
Trimethaphan (Arfonad)	During surgery to lower blood pressure	1–4 mg/min IV (infusion)

Abbreviations: BID, twice a day; IV, intravenously; PO, orally; TID, three times a day.

ganglia, which results in vasodilation. Although the ganglionic blockers are very potent antihypertensive drugs, they produce numerous side effects that restrict their use. Therefore, the ganglionic blockers are reserved for the treatment of severe hypertension. In addition, they must also be used in combination with other antihypertensive drugs. Combination therapy allows a reduction of dosage of the ganglionic blocker, which reduces the frequency and severity of adverse effects.

The ganglionic blockers may also be used in the treatment of peripheral vascular disease, such as Raynaud's disease. The vasodilator effect increases peripheral blood flow.

ADVERSE EFFECTS

Almost all of the adverse effects of the ganglionic blockers are caused by excessive blockade of the autonomic ganglia. The result is a combination of anticholinergic and antiadrenergic effects, which usually include decreased GI activity (dry mouth and constipation), visual disturbances (mydriasis and cycloplegia), decreased cardiovascular function (hypotension and decreased cardiac output), and decreased genitourinary function (urinary retention and impotence). The ganglionic blockers are contraindicated in patients with glaucoma because the mydriatic effect increases intraocular pressure.

DRUG INTERACTIONS

Many drugs act on autonomic receptors, and the possibility of a drug interaction with ganglionic blockers is significant. Table 8-2 lists the potential drug interactions with ganglionic blockers.

Table 8-2

Drug Interactions with Ganglionic Blocking Drugs

Drug Class	Result
Adrenergic drugs	Antagonism of antiadrenergic effect of ganglionic blockade, especially on cardiovascular system
Adrenergic blocking drugs	Additive antiadrenergic effect to produce hypotension and possible cardiovascular collapse
Cholinergic drugs	Antagonism of anticholinergic effect of ganglionic blockade, especially on GI and urinary tract
Anticholinergic drugs	Additive anticholinergic effect
Vasodilator drugs	Additive vasodilating effect to produce hypotension and possible cardiovascular collapse

Chapter 8 Review

UNDERSTANDING TERMINOLOGY

Test your understanding of the material in this chapter by answering the following questions.

1. Differentiate between a ganglionic stimulant and a ganglionic blocker.
2. What is the name of the cholinergic receptors at the ganglia?

ACQUIRING KNOWLEDGE

Answer the following questions.

3. What neurotransmitter regulates ganglionic transmission?
4. List the main effects of ganglionic stimulation.
5. List the main effects of ganglionic blockade.
6. What are the main therapeutic uses of the ganglionic blocking drugs?
7. What is the major advantage of mecamylamine (Inversine)?
8. List the adverse effects of the ganglionic blocking drugs.
9. What other drugs may interact with the ganglionic blockers?

APPLYING KNOWLEDGE ON THE JOB

Answer the following questions.

10. Assume that you work in an HMO, where you act as patient liaison. Patients are encouraged to talk over problems with you if they feel that the problems have not been resolved by a doctor or if they feel uncomfortable discussing the problems with a doctor. One of the patients wants to talk to you about an "embarrassing problem." He says that ever since he started taking that "strong medicine" for his high blood pressure, he hasn't been able to make love to his wife. He also has a dry mouth, and he's constipated all of the time. What drug is the patient most likely taking? What other drugs might be tried to help control his hypertension without causing the side effects he's experiencing?
11. A patient has been brought by ambulance to the emergency room where you work. He's suffering from hypotension, and he's on the verge of cardiovascular collapse. The patient's wife, who accompanied him in the ambulance, says he was fine until he took some new medication for his high blood pressure. She has the bottle with her—the medication is mecamylamine. You ask her if he's taking any other medicine, and she replies that he takes something for his angina, but she doesn't remember what it is. What might the other medication be, and why is it producing these effects in this patient?

Additional Reading

The nicotine patch: A good deal? *Emerg Med* 1997;29(1):55.

Safety of the nicotine patch in cardiac patients. *Emerg Med* 1997;29(6):45.

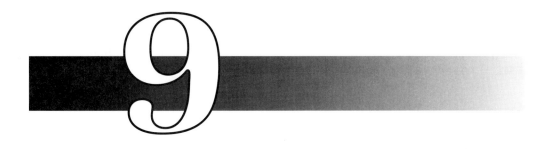

Skeletal Muscle Relaxants

Henry Hitner, PhD
Barbara Nagle, PhD

Chapter Focus

This chapter describes drugs that reduce the contraction of skeletal muscles, affecting posture and motor function. It also explains how surgery may be aided by removing the normal tone of skeletal muscles and how spastic muscle disorders are controlled.

Chapter Terminology

centrally acting skeletal muscle relaxant: Drug that inhibits skeletal muscle contraction by blocking conduction within the spinal cord.

depolarizing blocker: Produces paralysis by first causing nerve transmission, followed by inhibition of nerve transmission.

fasciculation: Twitchings of muscle fiber groups.

hyperthermia: Abnormally high body temperature.

incompatibility: Undesirable interaction of drugs not suitable for combination or administration together.

malignant hyperthermia: Condition in susceptible individuals resulting in a life-threatening elevation in body temperature.

neuromuscular junction (NMJ): Space (synapse) between a motor nerve ending and a skeletal muscle membrane; it contains acetylcholine receptors.

nondepolarizing blocker: Produces paralysis by inhibiting nerve transmission.

peripheral skeletal muscle relaxant: Drug that inhibits muscle contraction at the neuromuscular junction or within the contractile process.

potentiates: Produces an action that is greater than either of the components can produce alone.

vagolytic: Inhibition of the vagus nerve to the heart, causing the heart rate to increase (counteraction to vagal tone, which causes bradycardia).

vasodilator: Substance that relaxes the muscles (sphincters) controlling blood vessels, leading to increased blood flow.

Chapter Objectives

After studying this chapter, you should be able to:

- Describe at least two ways in which skeletal muscles may be relaxed.
- Explain why muscle relaxation is necessary during diagnostic and surgical procedures.
- Trace how these drugs may alter the ability to control respiration.
- Explain how tranquilizers relax skeletal muscles through a different mechanism of action than nondepolarizing blockers.
- Identify which drugs are used in the chronic treatment of spastic muscle disorders.
- List three potential adverse effects associated with muscle relaxants.

Contraction of skeletal muscles is voluntarily controlled by impulses that originate in the CNS. Impulses from the brain are conducted through the spinal cord to the somatic motor neurons *(Figure 9-1)*. Somatic motor neurons eventually connect with skeletal muscle fibers, forming a **neuromuscular junction (NMJ).** The neuronal endings of the somatic motor fibers contain neurotransmitter acetylcholine (ACh). When ACh is released into the neuromuscular synapses, it combines with cholinergic receptors known as nicotinic-II (NII) receptors. Although these receptors are cholinergic, they are not identical to the muscarinic (parasympathetic) and ganglionic receptors previously discussed (Chapters 8 and 9).

Depolarization of the muscle fibers occurs when ACh combines with NII receptors. Following depolarization, the contractile elements of the muscle fibers (actin and myosin) produce muscle contraction. Muscle relaxatation occurs after ACh is hydrolyzed by acetylcholinesterase; this terminates the action of ACh. Skeletal muscle function is essential to life because respiration depends on the rhythmic contraction of the diaphragm and chest muscles. In addition, skeletal muscle tone permits coordinated movement of the entire body to maintain posture. This muscle activity occurs continually without our conscious awareness.

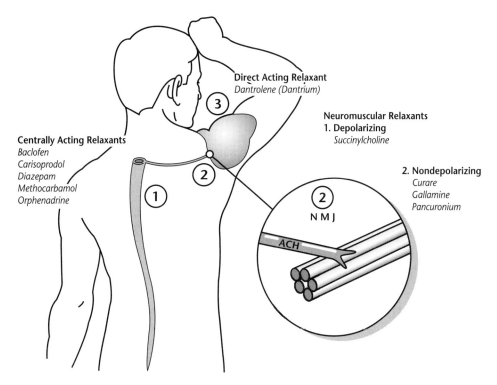

Figure 9-1
Innervation of skeletal muscle by somatic motor neurons. Site 1: impulse conduction from the CNS through the spinal cord. Site 2: neuromuscular junction (NMJ). Site 3: skeletal muscle fibers (ACh, acetylcholine).

Clinical Indications

Many drugs inhibit skeletal muscle contraction by interfering with neuromuscular function. Drugs that inhibit skeletal muscle contraction by blocking conduction within the spinal cord are known as **centrally acting skeletal muscle relaxants** *(Figure 9-1, site 1)*. In contrast, **peripheral skeletal muscle relaxants** inhibit muscle contraction at the neuromuscular junction *(Figure 9-1, site 2)* or within the contractile process *(Figure 9-1, site 3)*. Regardless of the site of action, drugs classified as skeletal muscle relaxants are clinically valuable because they selectively inhibit neuromuscular function. This inhibition then results in skeletal muscle relaxation.

Skeletal muscle relaxation is desirable in spastic diseases (multiple sclerosis and cerebral palsy), conditions in which the spinal cord has been damaged (trauma, paraplegia), and injuries in which pain accompanies overexertion of the muscles. In addition, surgical and orthopedic procedures and intubation (e.g., bronchoscopy) are often facilitated by the use of skeletal muscle relaxants. Without administering these agents before invasive diagnostic procedures, there is a greater possibility for the reacting muscles to tear or become strained.

Peripherally Acting Skeletal Muscle Relaxants

MECHANISM OF ACTION

Neuromuscular blockers inhibit skeletal muscle contraction by interfering with the NII receptors. There are two types of neuromuscular blockers: nondepolarizing (curare, gallamine, and pancuronium) and depolarizing (succinylcholine).

The **nondepolarizing blockers** combine with the NII receptors but do not stimulate the receptors. These agents occupy the NII sites so that ACh cannot combine with the receptors, and depolarization cannot occur (nondepolarizing, no depolarization).

The **depolarizing blockers** inhibit muscle contraction by a two-step process: (1) succinylcholine attaches to the NII receptors and induces depolarization, observed as muscle **fasciculations;** (2) then succinylcholine alters the NII receptors so that they cannot respond to endogenous ACh stimulation. This phase represents the neuromuscular blockade.

ROUTE OF ADMINISTRATION

The nondepolarizing neuromuscular blockers are usually administered intravenously because they are not well absorbed when taken by mouth. Following a single injection of a nondepolarizing blocker, neuromuscular blockade occurs within 3 to 5 minutes and lasts from 20 to 30 minutes. The muscles of the eyes and face are the first to become relaxed, followed by the limbs, trunk, and diaphragm. Recovery of muscle function occurs as the drug is metabolized and excreted. Curare and pancuronium are metabolized in the liver to some extent, whereas gallamine is excreted unchanged in the urine.

The depolarizing blocker succinylcholine is metabolized so rapidly that it is often administered by intravenous infusion to maintain skeletal muscle relaxation. Succinylcholine is rapidly hydrolyzed by the enzyme plasma cholinesterase, which is present in the blood. Some individuals do not have enough plasma cholinesterase or, because of a genetic abnormality, produce an abnormal (atypical) enzyme. These people metabolize succinylcholine very slowly, so its duration of action and potential toxicity increase. The intravenous doses of the peripheral neuromuscular blockers are given in Table 9-1.

EFFECTS ON CARDIOPULMONARY SYSTEMS

Although the primary site of action of the neuromuscular junction, neuromuscular blockers also produce cardiovascular changes at therapeutic doses through a different mechanism of action. Curare may cause hypotension because it releases histamine **(vasodilator)** and inhibits sympathetic tone on the blood vessels (ganglionic blockade). In contrast, gallamine may produce tachycardia by blocking the vagal tone on the SA (sinoatrial) node of the heart **(vagolytic).** Gallamine may also increase blood pressure.

Although pancuronium has no effect on the autonomic ganglia or histamine

Table 9-1

Peripheral Skeletal Muscle Relaxant Doses and Routes of Administration

Drug (Trade Name)	Type	Adult Dose
Atracurium besylate (Tracrium)	Nondepolarizing	0.4–0.5 mg/kg IV bolus
Cisatracurium besylate (Nimbex)	Nondepolarizing	0.15 or 0.2 mg/kg/IV
Dantrolene (Dantrium)	Direct-acting	1 mg/kg IV
Doxacurium (Nuromax)	Nondepolarizing	0.05 mg/kg IV
Metocurine (Metubine)	Nondepolarizing	0.1–0.3 mg/kg IV
Mivacurium (Mivacron)	Nondepolarizing	0.15 mg/kg IV
Pancuronium bromide (Pavulon)	Nondepolarizing	0.06–0.1 mg/kg IV
Pipecuronium (Arduan)	Nondepolarizing	70–85 mg/kg IV
Rapacuronium bromide (Raplon)	Nondepolarizing	1.5 mg/kg IV
Roncuronium bromide (Zemuron)	Nondepolarizing	0.6–1.2 mg/kg IV
Succinylcholine chloride (Anectine, Quelicin, Sucostrin)	Depolarizing	0.3–1.1 mg/kg IV 1–2 mg/mL at 2.5 mg/min continuous IV infusion
Tubocurarine (curare)	Nondepolarizing	6–9 mg followed by infusion
Vecuronium bromide (Norcuron)	Nondepolarizing	0.08–0.1 mg/kg IV

release, it may cause tachycardia by a vagolytic action. Succinylcholine has been reported to produce ventricular arrhythmias and changes in blood pressure, which vary with the amount of drug administered. Because succinylcholine causes potassium leakage from muscle cells, patients with electrolyte imbalances (burns or trauma) may develop arrhythmias more easily.

All of the blockers except pancuronium cause a release of histamine from mast cells, which leads to the production of bronchospasms and increased bronchial secretions in sensitive patients. Asthmatic patients are especially sensitive to the respiratory complications induced by histamine. Therefore, in asthmatic patients, pancuronium may be preferred to minimize bronchial (respiratory) complications.

ADVERSE AND TOXIC EFFECTS

The major toxicity associated with all neuromuscular blockers is paralysis of the respiratory muscles. This is life-threatening because the patient can no longer control breathing, consciously or unconsciously. Skeletal muscle paralysis caused by the nondepolarizing blockers may be reversed by the use of neostigmine or edrophonium, which inhibit acetylcholinesterase so that ACh accumulates within the junctions. The ACh displaces the blocker from the NII receptors and, because these receptors are not damaged or changed, initiates depolarization and muscle contraction. An added benefit of neostigmine and edrophonium is their ability to directly stimulate the NII receptors so that skeletal muscle paralysis is reversed.

Succinylcholine overdose presents a special problem because this drug alters the ability of NII receptors to become stimulated. There is no known antidote that reverses the neuromuscular blockade produced by succinylcholine. Administration of the acetylcholinesterase drugs may worsen the respiratory paralysis. Respiration must be supported artificially until the drug is metabolized and receptor responsiveness returns to normal. Skeletal muscle paralysis may be dangerously prolonged when succinylcholine is used in a patient who has atypical plasma cholinesterase.

Succinylcholine produces an unusual acute toxicity that is probably related to an existing genetic abnormality in 1 out of 20,000 individuals. Occasionally, a normal dose of succinylcholine in combination with an inhalation anesthetic produces a condition known as **malignant hyperthermia.** This condition is associated with a drastic increase in body temperature, acidosis, electrolyte imbalance, and shock. The mechanism by which hyperthermia occurs is believed to be related to the anesthetic-induced potentiation of calcium hyperreactivity leading to very rapid muscle contractions. These rapid contractions generate heat that raises the body temperature leading to very rapid muscle contractions. These rapid contractions generate heat that raises the body temperature. The hyperactive biochemical reactions progress so quickly that treatment must be started immediately to reduce the risk of death. Treatment of hyperthermia includes reducing body temperature with ice packs and controlling arrhythmias and acidosis with appropriate drugs. Unfortunately, the incidence of fatality in malignant hyperthermia is high. Prevention is primarily directed at obtaining a good family history about other episodes of difficulty during operative procedures. Muscle biopsy and elevated muscle enzyme levels may identify potentially sensitive patients. Such a workup before an operation allows the surgical team to avoid the use of sensitizing agents. Dantrolene is the drug of choice for malignant hyperthermia and will be discussed later in this chapter.

CAUTIONS AND DRUG INTERACTIONS

Neuromuscular blocking drugs should be used with extreme caution in patients with impaired neuromuscular function (myasthenia gravis and spinal cord lesions). Any medication that inhibits skeletal muscle function potentiates neuromuscular blockers. Antibiotics, antiarrhythmic drugs, and some general anesthetics directly inhibit neuromuscular function, causing skeletal muscle relaxation. Succinylcholine-induced neuromuscular blockade is potentiated by drugs that promote a loss of potassium, such as diuretics and digitalis. In contrast, drugs that stimulate the NII receptors or inhibit acetylcholinesterase antagonize nondepolarizing blockers. Drug interactions associated with skeletal muscle relaxants are given in Table 9-2. The only contraindication is their use in patients with a known hypersensitivity to any of these drugs.

CLINICAL INDICATIONS

The peripheral neuromuscular blockers are used primarily during surgical procedures to relax abdominal skeletal muscle. These agents are also used during electroconvulsive shock therapy and to reduce muscle spasms produced during tetanus. Because of its short action, succinylcholine may be used to aid intubations for surgical and diagnostic procedures (endoscopy).

Table 9-2

Drug Interactions of Skeletal Muscle Relaxants

Drug Class	Interaction
Acetylcholinesterase inhibitors Carbenazepine Corticosteroids Insecticides Ranitidine Theophylline	Antagonize the neuromuscular blockade of the nondepolarizing neuromuscular blockers

Alcohol
Antiarrhythmics
  Lidocaine
  Procainamide
  Quinidine
Antibiotics
  Clindamycin
  Kanamycin
  Lincomycin
  Neomycin
  Pipericillin
  Polymyxin B
  Streptomycin
  Tetracycline
Antiulcer
  Cimetidine
General anesthetics
  Cyclopropane
  Enflurane
  Ether
  Halothane
  Ketamine
  Methoxyflurane
Narcotic analgesics
Nitrates
Sedatives
Tranquilizers
Verapamil
	Potentiate the skeletal muscle relaxation produced by the neuromuscular blockers, dantrolene, and the centrally acting skeletal muscle relaxants including tizanidine

Digitalis Diuretics	Potentiate the skeletal muscle relaxation of succinylcholine

Curare can be used as a diagnostic test for myasthenia gravis. Myasthenic patients have impaired neuromuscular function and are five times more sensitive to drug-induced neuromuscular blockade. Administration of curare to a myasthenic patient produces a rapid loss of muscle tone.

Direct-Acting Skeletal Muscle Relaxants

Dantrolene is considered a direct-acting peripheral skeletal muscle relaxant because it inhibits the skeletal muscle fiber *(Figure 9-1, site 3)*.

MECHANISM OF ACTION

By interfering with biochemical pathways, dantrolene prevents actin and myosin contraction. The skeletal muscle contractile process cannot respond to stimulation, but conduction of impulses through the spinal cord and transmission across the neuromuscular junction are not affected.

CLINICAL INDICATIONS

Dantrolene is used in the treatment of malignant hyperthermia and spastic diseases. Muscle spasms associated with multiple sclerosis, cerebral palsy, and spinal cord injuries may reduce patients' ability to function. Dantrolene, taken orally, allows these individuals to use their residual motor function. In the prevention and treatment of malignant hyperthermia, dantrolene, given intravenously, interferes with the release of calcium in the sensitized muscles, reversing the biochemical crisis.

ADVERSE EFFECTS

The most frequent effects include dizziness, vomiting, fatigue, and weakness. Dantrolene has a potential for hepatotoxicity. As deaths have occurred from its hepatotoxicity, serum enzymes indicative of changes in liver function (AST, ALT) should be monitored frequently during dantrolene therapy. Contraindications to the use of dantrolene include hepatitis and cirrhosis, as well as other active hepatic diseases. The long-term safety of dantrolene is being evaluated through its continued use. Any drug that decreases muscle strength or depresses the CNS may potentiate the muscle weakness produced by dantrolene (Table 9-2).

Centrally Acting Skeletal Muscle Relaxants

Spastic contraction of skeletal muscles may occur in response to overexertion, trauma, or nervous tension. Usually, the muscles undergoing spasm are limited to the area of trauma (e.g., neck, back, or calf). Reflexes within the spinal cord repeatedly stimulate the motor neurons so that localized muscle fibers contract intermittently. This perpetuates a cycle of irritation or inflammation within localized muscle areas.

MECHANISM OF ACTION

Drugs that relax skeletal muscle by a central mechanism depress reflex impulse conduction within the spinal cord. This change in conduction reduces the number of impulses available to produce muscle contraction. Centrally acting skeletal muscle relaxants do not alter the function of the NII receptors or the skeletal muscle fibers. Some of these muscle relaxants interfere with select areas of the brain to interupt the spasticity. Although all of the drugs listed in Table 9-3 relieve muscle spasticity, chlordiazepoxide (Librium) and diazepam (Valium) are primarily used as tranquilizers (antianxiety). These agents are discussed in Chapter 12. Many people encounter muscle relaxants as outpatient therapy for muscle strain and overexertion during leisure activities; however, two relatively new drugs, baclofen and tizanidine, reduce the spasms that interfere with daily activities in patients with multiple sclerosis. Baclofen (Lioresal) is chemically related to a substance that naturally occurs in the brain (GABA, γ-aminobutyric acid). Like other centrally acting muscle relaxants, it inhibits reflexes at the spinal level. Baclofen is primarily used to relieve the symptoms of spasticity (flexor spasms, clonus, muscle rigidity) in patients with multiple sclerosis but may also be of value in patients with spinal cord injury resulting in severe spasticity.

Table 9-3

Centrally Acting Skeletal Muscle Relaxants

Drug (Trade Name)	Adult Dose
Baclofen (Lioresal)	10–20 mg PO QID
Carisoprodol (Rela, Soma)	350 mg PO TID, QID
Chlordiazepoxide* (Librium)	2–10 mg PO TID, QID
	2–20 mg IM,† IV; elderly, 2–2.5 mg daily, BID
Chlorphenesin carbamate (Maolate)	800 mg PO TID
Chlorzoxazone (Paraflex, Parafon Forte DSC, Remular-s)	250–750 mg PO TID, QID
Cyclobenzaprine (Flexeril)	10 mg PO TID
Diazepam* (Valium)	2–20 mg PO TID
(Valium, Zetran)	5–10 mg IM†
Metaxalone (Skelaxin)	800 mg PO TID, QID
Methocarbamol (Robaxin)	1.0–1.5 g PO QID
Orphenadrine citrate (Norflex)	100 mg PO BID
(Banflex, Flexon, Myolin)	60 mg IV, IM (every 12 hours as needed)†
Tizanidine (Zanaflex)	8 mg PO every 6–8 hours

*These drugs are used primarily as antianxiety agents rather than skeletal muscle relaxants.
†Should be changed to tablets as soon as the symptoms are relieved.

Through a different mechanism of action, tizanidine (Zanaflex) reduces spasticity by interacting with α_2-adrenergic receptors in the central nervous system. Neither of these drugs reverses the pathology of multiple sclerosis. They are adjunct medications that improve the quality of life for many patients with spastic muscle conditions.

ROUTE OF ADMINISTRATION AND ADVERSE EFFECTS

The centrally acting skeletal muscle relaxants may be administered orally or parenterally. To some degree, these drugs are metabolized in the liver and excreted in the urine. The most frequently reported adverse effects include blurred vision, dizziness, lethargy, and decreased mental alertness. The intensity of these effects may require patients to avoid driving or operating mechanical equipment. With large doses, skeletal muscle tone decreases, resulting in ataxia and hypotension. Tizanidine has the potential to decrease blood pressure because of its action on the sympathetic and α_2 receptors. This may result in orthostatic hypotension in patients with multiple sclerosis.

Prolonged use of diazepam or chlordiazepoxide may lead to dependency. Discontinuation of therapy in patients who have received any of these drugs for long periods (chronically) must be gradual to avoid precipitating withdrawal symptoms. Usually, the dose is decreased over a 4- to 8-week period. Baclofen may cause nausea, headache, insomnia, and frequent or painful urination, which should be reported to the physician for further evaluation. Special precautions must be taken in reducing the dose of baclofen during chronic therapy. If an adverse reaction occurs that prompts termination of baclofen therapy, the dose must be reduced gradually. Although this drug is not associated with dependence, hallucinations and/or seizures have been reported to occur when the drug was abruptly stopped. Any of the muscle relaxants should be discontinued under medical supervision if a hypersensitivity reaction develops.

Overdose of centrally acting skeletal muscle relaxants will produce symptoms of confusion, somnolence, and depression of vital functions including respiration, heart, and pulse rates. Coma may precede death if the patient does not receive adequate evaluation and treatment in time. The patient must be monitored for respiratory and cardiovascular activity while a clear airway is maintained and ventilation is supported. In the event that hypotension develops, an IV infusion should be available for parenteral fluid therapy. There is a specific benzodiazepine antagonist, flumazenil, which may be of value in the treatment of overdose. Benzodiazepines include Valium, Lebrium and will be discussed in Chapter 12. This antagonist has no ability to reverse the depression associated with other centrally acting muscle relaxants.

DRUG INTERACTIONS

Drugs that depress the CNS (alcohol, sedatives, and tranquilizers) or impair neuromuscular function potentiate the actions and adverse effects of all skeletal muscle relaxants.

Note to the Respiratory Care Practitioner

Skin rash, nasal congestion, persistent fever, or yellowish discoloration of the skin or eyes should be reported to the physician immediately for further evaluation.

Considerations for the Respiratory Care Practitioner

When skeletal muscle relaxants are used in surgical settings, the potential for adverse effects may be minimized through close observation of the patient during the recovery period. With diagnostic procedures or intubations performed under outpatient conditions, or in chronic therapy for spastic muscle conditions, there is a greater likelihood that patients may experience adverse effects, putting them at risk for injury. Because the respiratory care practitioner can be immediately involved in postoperative patient care, he or she should be clear about which adverse effects are worthy of physician notification and which may interfere with successful respiratory care.

The respiratory care practitioner must be aware of the end-organ action of these drugs because it directly affects the ability of the patient to comply with respiratory care treatments. Patient sensitivity to the neuromuscular muscle relaxants could result in a sustained muscle blockade. Partial blockade or paralysis of the diaphragm and intercostal muscles will result in apnea. Even though the patient may be receiving mechanical ventilation, the recovering patient must be monitored very closely to avoid hypoxemia from hypoventilation. During the postoperative recovery period, patients may have residual muscle relaxation. Patients with chronic respiratory problems may require respiratory support through mechanical ventilation and/or chest physical therapy. For these patients, when skeletal muscle function is less than optimal, there may be inadequate muscle response to support good ventilation and bronchial hygiene during the recovery period.

On the other hand, neuromuscular blocking drugs may be warranted when the patient is receiving mechanical ventilation in order to eliminate inconsistent spontaneous (asynchronous) breathing. Asynchronous breathing increases the patient's work of breathing because the patient is, in effect, fighting the ventilator. By removing the reflex respiratory muscle action, the neuromuscular blocking drugs allow the patient to make a smooth transition to ventilator control, thus facilitating more efficient oxygenation. Remember that all of the blockers except pancuronium cause a release of histamine from mast cells, which leads to bronchospasms and the production of increased bronchial secretions. Depending on the postprocedure status of the patient, whether ICU patient, elderly, or with a chronic respiratory condition, the histamine release contributes additional residual secretion during the patient's recovery period.

In the outpatient setting, the respiratory care practitioner also needs to be aware of medications the patient may be taking that interfere with patient compliance with instructions or respiratory care techniques. The centrally acting skeletal muscle relaxants may cause persistent drowsiness that interferes with mental alertness and concentration. For chronic spastic conditions, this effect is usually tolerable, so the treatment schedule does not need to be interrupted. It should be noted that dose adjustment does not always mitigate the drowsy effect. Therefore, with short-term therapy of muscle strain, the patient may need to incorporate other solutions to circumvent the difficulties associated with drowsiness.

Alcohol and other CNS depressant drugs should be avoided. This includes OTC medications that contain alcohol as a significant active ingredient. These drugs may potentiate poor coordination, drowsiness, and dizziness (postural hypotension). In general, the lack of concentration, drowsiness, or poor coordination may not permit the patient to follow through with proper self-administered respiratory care.

USE IN PREGNANCY

Drugs in this class have been designated Pregnancy Category B or C. Safety for use during pregnancy has not been established. The recommendation is that no drug should be administered during pregnancy unless it is clearly needed and the potential benefits to the patient outweigh the potential risks to the fetus.

Female patients who become pregnant or who expect to become pregnant during therapy should discuss the potential risks of therapy to the fetus with the physician.

Chapter 9 Review

UNDERSTANDING TERMINOLOGY

Test your understanding of the material in this chapter by answering the following questions.

1. Differentiate between depolarizing blockers and nondepolarizing blockers.

2. Explain the difference between peripheral skeletal muscle relaxants and centrally acting skeletal muscle relaxants.

3. Use the following terms in a short paragraph: *fasciculation, hyperthermia, vagolytic,* and *vasodilator.*

ACQUIRING KNOWLEDGE

Answer the following questions.

4. What are the physiological events that precede skeletal muscle contraction?
5. What is a neuromuscular junction (NMJ)?
6. What sites are involved in the production of skeletal muscle relaxation?
7. What are the two types of neuromuscular blockers? How do they differ in their mechanism of action?
8. Why are neuromuscular blockers administered IV?
9. What adverse effects are produced by the neuromuscular blockers as a result of histamine release?
10. Describe the major toxicity associated with neuromuscular blockers and the antidote used.
11. How does dantrolene differ from neuromuscular blockers?
12. What is the mechanism of action of centrally acting skeletal muscle relaxants?
13. When are centrally acting skeletal muscle relaxants used?

APPLYING KNOWLEDGE ON THE JOB

Answer the following questions.

14. Assume that you work in a busy HMO. You work with dozens of patients each day. You've noticed that each of the following three patients who were treated today has been prescribed a drug that could cause problems. For each patient, identify and explain the potential drug problem.

    a. Patient A came to the HMO this morning complaining of muscle pain following a back injury. He was prescribed the muscle relaxant cyclobenzaprine. Patient A is always joking with the nurses about how much he drinks. It's clear that he takes several drinks of whiskey every day.

    b. Patient B came into the HMO last week with strep throat, for which he was prescribed streptomycin. Today, he's complaining of neck and shoulder pain, which he attributes to driving his car for a total of 20 hours over the past 2 days. Patient B was prescribed metaxalone for the muscle pain.

15. Assume that you work in a surgical unit where you coordinate patient medications. For each of the following patients, identify a potential drug problem and how it might be avoided.

    a. Jeri Curran is about to have a type of orthopedic surgery that requires a muscle relaxant for best results. Jeri's medical history indicates that she has asthma but is otherwise in good health.

    b. Linda Petersen is scheduled for surgery on her back. Her surgeon is planning to give her succinylcholine to relax her muscles during the procedure. As far as the surgeon is aware, Linda is in great health other than the vertebrae that require surgery. Linda has confided in you, however, that she has bulimia, which you know can lead to electrolyte imbalance.

   c. Susan Willis has knee surgery scheduled. A note on her chart indicates that she will be given succinylcholine during the operation to relax the muscles in her leg. Her chart also indicates that she takes digitalis for a heart problem.

Additional Reading

Biddle C. Use and abuse of muscle relaxants. *Curr Rev Nurse Anesth* 1996;15(16):131.

Gianino J. Intrathecal baclofen for spinal spasticity: Implication for nursing practice. *J Neurosci Nurs* 1993;2:254–263.

New Drugs. Roncuronium (Zemuron): A safer, faster muscle relaxant? *Am J Nurs* 1995;95(3):56.

Porter B. Surgical nursing: A review of intrathecal baclofen in the management of spasticity. *Br J Nurs* 1997;6(5):253.

Waldman HJ. Centrally acting skeletal muscle relaxants and associated drugs. *J Pain Symptom Manage* 1994;9(7):434.

Internet Activities

Web pages that present information on adjuncts to anesthesia, malignant hyperthermia, and the management of malignant hyperthermia discuss the use of skeletal muscle relaxants. This material is designed to be read by medical associates and the general public and therefore is user friendly to access and comprehend. Go on the internet and select Yahoo (search engine) by entering **www.Yahoo.com.** You will be presented a list of topics; click on "health, medicine, drugs." When the next screen appears, do one of the following:

a. Select "medicine" to access the next menu of medical conditions and diseases. Then select "anesthesiology" and subsequently, select "malignant hyperthermia." You will have entered the Malignant Hyperthermia home page. The Malignant Hyperthermia Associations of America (MHAUS) and Japan maintain the categories of information identified on the home page, including a North American Registry of patients who are susceptible to malignant hyperthermia plus a quarterly newsletter, *The Communicator.* This on-line service provides the most current information on malignant hyperthermia and its management. Conditions that trigger muscle spasticity are described on the home page, with a simple color schematic explaining the action at the neuromuscular junction.

b. Remain on the malignant hyperthermia web page. Select the category "FAQ," frequently asked questions. At the next screen, scroll down to the end of the document to review a list of drugs that can be safety used in patients with malignant hyperthermia.

Another source of drug information is the education service provided by Yale University. Enter the URL (Universal Resource Locator) **www.groucho.med.yale.edu.** At the new web page, click on SEARCH, gasnet. Then type "valium" into the query box and hit search. You will be provided with a list of topics and articles that describe the use of Valium. Select "Valium versus Versed" and review the information provided by anesthesiologists who are using these agents. When you are ready, click the right mouse button to return to the home page or the previous page. Enter any term or drug of interest into the query box and hit SEARCH to continue gathering information.

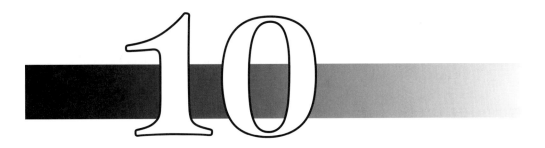

Local Anesthetics

HENRY HITNER, PhD
BARBARA NAGLE, PhD

Chapter Focus

This chapter describes the drugs that influence patients' responses to pain and how painful stimuli can be inhibited without affecting consciousness (without depressing higher centers of the brain).

Chapter Terminology

amide local anesthetic: Anesthetic that has a long duration of action.

cardiac arrhythmia: Variation in the normal rhythm (motion) of the heart.

caudal anesthesia: Injection of a local anesthetic into the caudal or subcaudal spinal canal.

epidural anesthesia: Injection of a local anesthetic into the extradural space.

ester local anesthetic: Anesthetic that has a short or moderate duration of action.

general anesthetic: Drug that abolishes the response to pain by depressing the CNS and producing loss of consciousness.

hypersensitivity: Exaggerated response such as rash, edema, or anaphylaxis.

infiltration anesthesia: Injection of a local anesthetic directly into the tissue.

intradermal anesthesia: Injection of a local anesthetic under the skin.

local anesthetic: Drug that reduces response to pain by affecting nerve conduction. The action can be limited to an area of the body according to the site of administration.

nerve conduction: Transfer of impulses along a nerve by the movement of sodium and potassium ions.

spinal anesthesia: Injection of a local anesthetic into the subarachnoid space.

topical application: Placing a drug on the surface of the skin or a mucous membrane (e.g., mouth, rectum).

vasoconstriction: Tightening or contraction of muscles (sphincters) in the blood vessels, which decreases blood flow through the vessels.

vasodilation: Relaxation of the muscles (sphincters) controlling blood vessel tone, which increases blood flow through the vessels.

Chapter Objectives

After studying this chapter, you should be able to:

- Describe how a local anesthetic works (mechanism of action).
- Explain how a local anesthetic can reduce pain without affecting the muscles that control posture and breathing.
- Identify which local anesthetics must be administered by injection.
- Describe the adverse effects associated with local anesthetic use.
- Identify two local anesthetic drugs that are important in the treatment of cardiac dysfunction because of their action on the heart (antiarrhythmic).
- Identify local anesthetic use in respiratory patients.

Drugs may be used in many different ways to control pain. **General anesthetics,** which are discussed in Chapter 13, abolish the response to pain by depressing the CNS and producing loss of consciousness. It may be desirable, however, to relieve pain without altering the alertness or mental function of the patient. To accomplish this, analgesics (narcotic and nonnarcotic) or local anesthetics may be used. The source and intensity of the pain determine which of these pharmacologic agents is most useful to decrease the response to the painful stimuli. **Local anesthetics,** as their name suggests, produce a temporary loss of sensation or feeling in a confined area of the body.

Mechanism of Action

The most common clinical use of local anesthetics is to abolish painful stimulation before surgical, dental (tooth extraction), or obstetric (delivery) procedures. In addition, local anesthetics are ingredients in many over-the-counter products for sunburn, insect bites, and hemorrhoids. Local anesthetics abolish the response to pain because they inhibit sensory nerves that carry painful stimuli to the CNS. In particular, local anesthetics block nerve fiber conduction by acting directly on nerve membranes to inhibit sodium ions from crossing the membranes. If sodium ion movement is inhibited, nerves cannot depolarize, and conduction of impulses along the nerves is blocked *(Figure 10-1)*. This blockade of **nerve conduction** is reversible, which means that when the local anesthetic is carried away from the nerve by the circulation, the action of the local anesthetic ends. The local anesthetic is then metabolized.

Sensory nerves carry impulses for pain, touch, warmth, and cold to the brain. The sensory and autonomic nerves are the first fibers to become blocked by local anesthetics because these fibers are relatively small in diameter and unprotected by myelin sheaths. Therefore, local anesthetics can easily penetrate the membranes and inhibit nerve conduction. In contrast, the motor nerves that supply skeletal muscle are the last fibers to be inhibited because motor nerves are large fibers with thick myelin coverings. The importance of this varying degree of nerve

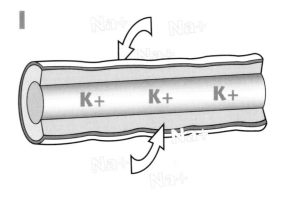

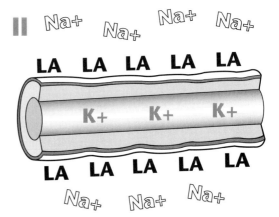

Figure 10-1

The action of local anesthetics on nerve conduction. **I:** Normal conduction along a nerve membrane. **II:** Local anesthetics (LA) inhibit nerve conduction by blocking sodium (Na^+) movement.

Table 10-1

Order of Depression of Nerve Fibers by Local Anesthetics

Order of Depression	Type of Nerve Fibers
Earliest	A. Small-diameter unmyelinated nerves: postganglionic autonomic,
	sensory — pain / temperature: warmth, cold / itch / tickle
Intermediate	B. Intermediate-diameter myelinated nerves, preganglionic autonomic
Last	C. Large-diameter myelinated nerves
	somatic motor ⟶ skeletal muscle
	sensory (visceral) ⟶ proprioception / sharp pain

depression, presented in Table 10-1, is that pain fibers can be blocked without altering skeletal muscle function, such as muscles critical to respiration (diaphragm) or maintaining posture. Another benefit is that recovery occurs in the direction that favors pain relief; that is, the pain fibers are the last to recover from local anesthetic blockade.

Pharmacology

The most commonly used local anesthetics are listed in Table 10-2. These agents produce adequate nerve block by inhibiting nerve conduction. They differ in their duration of action, site of metabolism, and potency. There are two classes of local anesthetics: ester local anesthetics and amide local anesthetics.

In general, the **ester local anesthetics** have a short or moderate duration of action because they are metabolized by enzymes (cholinesterases) that are present in the blood and skin. Examples of ester local anesthetics are benzocaine, cocaine, procaine, and tetracaine. However, tetracaine is the only ester derivative that has a very long duration of action. It is too large a molecule to be rapidly metabolized by the liver.

The **amide local anesthetics** are usually the longer-acting drugs because these agents must be metabolized in the liver. The amide group includes dibucaine, lidocaine, mepivacaine, and procainamide.

Table 10-2
Characteristics of Commonly Employed Local Anesthetics

Drug (Trade Name)	Duration	Route	Preparations
Esters			
Benzocaine (Boil-ease, Dermoplast, Lanacane, Solarcaine)[†]	0.5–0.75 hour	Topical	5% cream, ointment 2–20% spray
Cocaine[‡]	0.25–0.75 hour	Topical	1–4% solution
Chloroprocaine (Nesacaine)	0.25–0.50 hour	Injection	1–3% solution
Procaine (Novocain) infiltration	0.25–1.0 hour	Injection	1–2% and 10% solutions
Tetracaine (Pontocaine)	2–3 hours	Injection	0.2%, 0.3%, and 1% solutions
(Pontocaine cream/ ointment)[†]	—	Topical	1% cream, 5% ointment
Amides:			
Bupivacaine (Marcaine)	2–4 hours	Injection	0.25–0.75% solution
Dibucaine (Nupercaine)	3–4 hours	Injection	0.25% solution
(Nupercainal)[†]		Topical	0.5% cream, 1% ointment
Etidocaine (Duranest)	5–10 hours	Injection	1% solution
Lidocaine (Xylocaine, Solarcaine Aloe Extra)	0.5–1 hour	Injection	2% and 4% solution
(Bactine spray, Unguentine Plus)[†]		Topical	2% jelly, 2.5% and 5% ointment
Mepivacaine (Carbocaine)	0.75–1.5 hours	Injection	1% and 2% solutions
Prilocaine (Citanest)	0.5–1.5 hours	Injection	1–4% solutions
Other			
Ethyl chloride	Minutes	Topical*	Spray
Fluroethylchloride			
Fluori-methane aerofreeze			
Prez-Pak			

* Decreases surface temperature.
† Over-the-counter preparations.
‡ Federally restricted drug, Schedule II.

Routes of Administration

The duration of action and potency of local anesthetics determine which route of administration to employ. Local anesthetics are administered topically or by injection. Ester anesthetics, particularly those found in over-the-counter preparations, are applied topically to the skin or mucous membranes in the form of ointments, salves, drops, and lozenges. Injection of local anesthetics may involve several differ-ent sites, including under the skin (**intradermal**) and into the spaces around the spinal cord (**spinal, epidural,** or **caudal anesthesia**). The long-acting, potent amide anesthetics are administered primarily by injection.

Infiltration anesthesia is achieved by injecting a local anesthetic directly into the tissue. The extent of anesthesia is determined by the depth of tissue pene-trated, that is, the tissue infiltrated. The duration of action following infiltration anesthesia for several injectable local anesthetics is presented in Table 10-2. When those local anesthetics are administered in combination with epinephrine (usually 1:200,000 dilution), the duration of anesthesia may be doubled. For example, prilocaine, mepivacaine, dibucaine, and bupivacaine administered with epineph-rine may have their duration of action extended up to 6 hours. The addition of epi-nephrine retards absorption of the local anesthetic from the site of injection.

Adverse Effects

Local anesthetics are administered to produce a pharmacologic response in a well-defined area of the body. However, local anesthetics can be absorbed into the blood from the site of administration and pass through the circulation, affecting tissues and organs along the way. The most frequent and serious side effects from systemic absorption of a local anesthetic involve the blood vessels, heart, and brain.

VASCULAR EFFECTS

Cocaine was the first local anesthetic to be discovered. Although it has potent local anesthetic activity, cocaine cannot be used by injection because it produces intense **vasoconstriction.** Cocaine interferes with the sympathetic nervous system and the blood vessels. Today, cocaine is used topically in surgical procedures on the eyes and nasal mucosa because its vasoconstrictor action decreases operative bleeding and improves surgical visualization.

All of the other local anesthetics used today produce **vasodilation;** procaine, in particular, produces a marked dilation of blood vessels, which may lead to hy-potension. Except for cocaine, toxic levels of the local anesthetics relax vascular smooth muscle and produce significant hypotension. Depending on the concen-tration of the local anesthetic in the blood and the sensitivity of the patient (i.e., compromised, elderly, debilitated patients), these effects may lead to cardiovascu-lar collapse.

CARDIAC EFFECTS

Local anesthetics depress the function of the cardiac conduction system and the myocardium. Usually, these drugs produce a negative chronotropic (bradycardia) and a negative ionotropic response in the heart. In toxic doses, local anesthetics produce **cardiac arrhythmias.** It must be pointed out that in therapeutic (subtoxic) doses, two of the local anesthetics can be administered intravenously to correct certain cardiac arrhythmias. Lidocaine and procainamide are unique drugs because at very low doses they can protect cardiac function, whereas at toxic doses they inhibit normal cardiac function. Lidocaine is one of the standard drugs on the "crash cart" or emergency drug cart. During resuscitation, lidocaine may be required because it protects the patient from developing fibrillation during episodes of the ventricular tachycardia or premature ventricular contractions (PVCs).

CENTRAL NERVOUS SYSTEM EFFECTS

All of the local anesthetics can affect the CNS. In large or toxic doses, the local anesthetics can cross the blood–brain barrier and initially stimulate the cerebral cortex. The symptoms of cortical stimulation are nervousness, excitation, tremors, and convulsions. In general, the more potent the anesthetic, the more readily convulsions occur. As the concentration of local anesthetic increases in the brain, all areas of the CNS become depressed. Finally, at toxic levels, local anesthetics produce coma and death through total depression of the CNS.

Treatment of a local anesthetic overdose when CNS excitation is present includes barbiturates and diazepam (Valium). Once total CNS depression has occurred, the only available treatment is supportive restoration of breathing and blood pressure. In particular, artificial respiration is the essential feature of treatment in the late phase of anesthetic intoxication.

TOPICAL EFFECTS

The use of topical lidocaine with prilocaine (EMLA) has some unique dermatologic reactions. In about one third of patients the skin blanches, which makes it difficult to find the vein. In another third of patients there is redness (erythema) around the area.

Clinical Application

Topical application of local anesthetics relieves pain and itching associated with sunburn, skin abrasions, insect bites, and other allergic reactions, and skin eruptions from chickenpox. Occasionally, a topical anesthetic, such as the lidocaine/prilocaine combination EMLA, can be used before blood is drawn for a lab test. This will reduce the pain associated with the needle stick. If it is used, it must be placed on the skin 1 hour before the needle stick and covered with an occlusive dressing. Rectal suppositories relieve the pain produced by hemorrhoids. Injection of local anesthetics, especially the long-acting amides, is used for surgical, suturing, and obstetric procedures (epidural, caudal, spinal anesthesia) where the patients remain conscious. Dentistry is one of the most frequent clinical applications of local anesthetics.

> **Note to the Respiratory Care Practitioner**
>
> *Local anesthetic solutions occasionally contain epinephrine to counteract the vasodilation that occurs with use. Always read the contents of the bottle before administering a local anesthetic. Local anesthetic preparations that contain epinephrine should not be used for nerve block in the areas of the fingers, toes, ears, nose, or penis. In such areas, epinephrine may produce intense vasoconstriction, leading to ischemia and gangrene. Epinephrine also is contraindicated in conjunction with general anesthetics that increase cardiac excitability (arrhythmogenic).*

CAUTIONS AND CONTRAINDICATIONS

Local anesthetics may release histamine from mast cells located at the site of injection, producing a rash and local itching typical of a histaminic response of Lewis (see Chapter 18). Occasionally, a patient is hypersensitive to local anesthetics. If a rash or edema occurs, the drug should be stopped immediately. **Hypersensitivity** may develop to ester local anesthetics when they are used frequently. For this reason, topical preparations (creams, ointments, and sprays) should never be used continually for prolonged periods. If hypersensitivity develops and a local anesthetic is required, amide derivatives may be substituted, usually without fear of enhancing the allergic response.

Topical application of local anesthetics for sunburn, skin abrasions, and corneal wounds may result in systemic drug levels and toxic responses. When the skin is damaged or opened, local anesthetics can easily reach the blood vessels, and when the pain is intense, patients usually apply local anesthetics several times a day. It is not unusual for a patient to develop hypotension, tremors, and convulsions from overdose of a local anesthetic.

SPECIAL CONSIDERATIONS

When a local anesthetic is administered parenterally, the cardiovascular and respiratory vital signs must be monitored after each injection. Restlessness, dizziness, blurred vision, and slurred speech may be early signs of CNS toxicity. The local anesthetic should always be injected slowly to avoid systemic reactions. Debilitated patients, as well as elderly and pediatric patients, may require reduced doses because these patients are often more susceptible to the actions of local anesthetics. Local anesthetic solutions that contain a vasoconstrictor must be used with extreme caution in patients who have a medical history of hypertension, cerebral vascular insufficiency, heart block, thyrotoxicosis, or diabetes. (Review the effects of sympathomimetic drugs on the cardiovascular and metabolic systems, Chapter 6.)

Overdose of topical anesthetics may result in the same life-threatening response as from parentally administered drugs. If convulsions occur, it is an acute emergency. There is no specific antidote. Supportive treatment includes maintaining a clear airway and assisting ventilation with oxygen. If convulsions persist, an ultrashort-acting barbiturate or benzodiazepine may be given parenterally. Intravenous fluids and vasopressors are used when the circulation and organ perfusion are compromised.

DRUG INTERACTIONS

Local anesthetics are not involved in many drug interactions. However, they may enhance hypotension that occurs with antihypertensive drugs and muscle relaxants. Drugs that directly relax skeletal muscle are enhanced by the use of local anesthetics introduced into the spinal cord. Local anesthetics may increase the release of histamine even when they are being used to relieve an allergic reaction, and this histamine release will only worsen the clinical condition.

Procaine has been shown to inhibit the action of sulfonamide antibiotics. Procaine is metabolized to *p*-aminobenzoic acid, which competes with the sulfonamide for the bacterial site of action. Table 10-3 describes the interactions associated with the use of local anesthetics.

Patients who have experienced a hypersensitivity reaction to an ester local anesthetic are more likely to experience a similar reaction if exposed to other ester local anesthetics. Generally, it is advisable to use an amide local anesthetic as an alternative; rarely cross-sensitivity with lidocaine has been reported.

When local anesthetics are used in operating and emergency rooms, adverse effects may be minimized if the patient is closely monitored during the procedure. Local anesthetics are often used before endotracheal intubation to facilitate intubation by reducing potential muscle spasm and minimize the pain from irritation

Table 10-3
Drug Interactions Involving Local Anesthetics

Drug	Interacts with	Response
Sulfonamide antibiotics	Procaine, chloroprocaine, tetracaine	Reduce antibiotic efficacy by antagonizing sulfonamide action on bacteria
Benzocaine, chloroprocaine, procaine, tetracaine	Previous hypersensitivity to ester drug	Hypersensitivity, release of histamine
Injectable local anesthetics with epinephrine	Tricyclic antidepressants, MAO* inhibitors	Increased sympathetic response, sustained hypertension
	General anesthetics of chloroform, cyclopropane, halothane, trichloroethylene	Potential for arrhythmias to occur
Sedatives	Local anesthetics	Potentiate CNS depression
Muscle relaxants of curare, diazepam, succinylcholine, tubocurarine	Local anesthetics (spinal)	Increased hypotension, increased muscle relaxation

Abbreviation: MAO, monoamine oxidase.

and muscle strain. The use of anesthetics in dental procedures as well as available products for self-medication exposes the general population to a greater risk of experiencing certain adverse effects. The respiratory care practitioner should be aware of predictable local anesthetic actions that could cause the patient problems, namely loss of sensory perception and motor function.

PATIENT INSTRUCTIONS

The patient should be advised that loss of sensory perception and motor function may persist for a short time. This means the anesthetized region cannot respond to hot or cold stimuli, to deep scratching, or, in the case of oral anesthesia, provide a good seal around mouth pieces of nebulizers, aeosolizers, or breathing exercisers. The patient should avoid such activity for at least 1 hour or until full sensation and motor function have returned.

Following topical application to relieve a sore throat, the patient should not eat for 1 hour. Because sensation is impaired, there is always the danger that the patient may aspirate food particles.

NOTIFY THE PHYSICIAN

Patients routinely use OTC products containing local anesthetics for a multitude of conditions from sore throat to vaginal and/or rectal itch. Although the patient may have ten preparations for use on different body parts, they all probably contain a local anesthetic. Moreover, these are the types of products used by the more sensitive patients such as the elderly and children. The patient should be reminded that any time the skin or mucous membrane is broken, as in sunburn, minor scratches, or irritated mucosa, the local anesthetic may be more easily absorbed. Development of mental confusion and changes in pulse or respiration should be reported to the physician for further evaluation.

A small percentage of people are allergic (hypersensitive) to the *para*-aminobenzoic acid metabolites of procaine and tetracaine. Local swelling, edema, itching, difficulty breathing, or bronchospasm may indicate hypersensitivity to the anesthetic. If such symptoms occur while using any local anesthetic, the patient should be reminded to notify the doctor immediately and discontinue the anesthetic. The respiratory care practitioner, who may have frequent contact with the patient, should be alert for indications or signs of patient reaction to medication.

Note to the Respiratory Care Practitioner

In the respiratory care setting, it is not unusual to encounter lidocaine as a cough suppressant. On physician's orders, the pharmacist prepares a solution of 1% to 2% lidocaine mixed with saline administered through a hand-held nebulizer. In the presence of intractable nonproductive coughing, where the patient cannot achieve a normal breathing pattern, nebulized lidocaine reduces the reaction to the source of the cough.

USE IN PREGNANCY

Drugs in this class have been designated Pregnancy Category B and C. The safety of local anesthetic use in pregnancy has not been established through research in humans; however, the short-term exposure during labor and delivery limits the potential risk to the patient and newborn. Adverse effects observed in the newborn, primarily depression of the CNS and cardiovascular tone, quickly reverse once exposure is terminated. The degree of depression is related to the type and amount of local anesthetic administered to the mother.

Chapter 10 Review

UNDERSTANDING TERMINOLOGY

Test your understanding of the material in this chapter by answering the following questions.

1. Differentiate between local and general anesthetics.

2. Explain the difference between vasodilation and vasoconstriction.

Match the definition in the left column with the appropriate term in the right column.

3. An exaggerated response (such as rash or edema) to a local anesthetic.

4. Placing a drug on the surface of the skin or a mucous membrane.

5. Injection of a local anesthetic into the subarachnoid space.

6. Injection of a local anesthetic into the extradural space.

7. Injection of a local anesthetic into the caudal or subcaudal canal.

8. Injection of a local anesthetic directly into the tissue.

9. Injection of a local anesthetic under the skin.

a. caudal anesthesia

b. epidural anesthesia

c. hypersensitivity

d. infiltration anesthesia

e. intradermal anesthesia

f. spinal anesthesia

g. topical application

ACQUIRING KNOWLEDGE

Answer the following questions.

10. Explain how local anesthetics block the response to pain.

11. Which nerves are first affected when a local anesthetic is applied? What is the order of depression?

12. What are two classes of local anesthetics? How do they differ?

13. What body systems are mainly affected by systemic absorption of local anesthetics?

14. What are the adverse effects of local anesthetics on the heart?

15. What are the adverse effects of local anesthetics on the CNS?

16. Compare the effects of cocaine and procaine on blood pressure.

17. Why is epinephrine added to some local anesthetic preparations?

18. What precautions are associated with the use of local anesthetics and vasoconstrictors?

19. What drugs may interact with local anesthetics to produce undesirable effects?

APPLYING KNOWLEDGE ON THE JOB

Answer the following question.

20. Mrs. Brown was rushed to the emergency room by ambulance after her husband found her lying on the kitchen floor having convulsions. She had no previous history of convulsions and appeared to be in good health earlier in the day. You notice that Mrs. Brown has abrasions on her lower right arm, which her husband says she received when she fell to the pavement when bicycling yesterday. He says that she has been self-medicating with an over-the-counter ointment for pain ever since. What do you think caused Mrs. Brown's convulsions?

Additional Reading

Edlick RF. Repair of lacerations: Sedation and anesthesia. *Hosp Med* 1994;30(10):39.

Hersch EV. Analgesic efficacy and safety of an intraoral lidocaine patch. *JAMA* 1996;127(11):1626.

Hussey VP. Perioperative pharmacology: Effectiveness of lidocaine HCl on venipuncture sites. *Assoc Oper Room Nurs* 1997;66(3):472.

Johansson A. Nerve blocks with local anesthetics and corticosteroids in chronic pain: A clinical follow-up study. *J Pain Symptom Management* 1996;11(3):181–187.

Yaster M. Local anesthetics in the management of acute pain in infants and children. *J Pediatr* 1994;124:165.

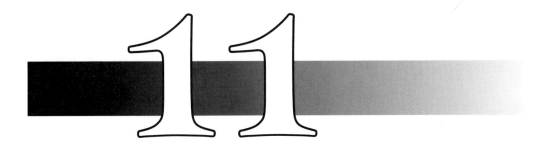

Introduction to the Central Nervous System

HENRY HITNER, PhD
BARBARA NAGLE, PhD

Chapter Focus

This chapter describes the major structural and functional features of the brain. It also describes how different parts of the brain regulate specific body functions.

Chapter Terminology

basal ganglia: Extrapyramidal system; part of the brain that regulates motor activity.

cerebellum: Part of the brain that coordinates body movements and posture and helps maintain body equilibrium

cerebral cortex: Part of the brain that controls the body's voluntary activities.

cerebral medulla: Part of the brain that conducts nerve impulses to and from different areas of the brain.

cerebrum: Uppermost part of the brain that controls higher intellectual abilities.

electroencephalogram (EEG): A recording of the electrical activity of the cortex.

hypothalamus: Part of the brain that controls many body functions.

limbic system: Neural pathway connecting different brain areas involved in regulation of behavior and emotion.

medulla oblongata: Part of the brain that controls cardiac, vasomotor, and respiratory functions.

pons: Part of the brain that serves as a relay station for nerve fibers traveling to other brain areas.

reticular formation: Network of nerve fibers that travel throughout the brainstem and cerebrum; regulates level of wakefulness.

thalamus: Part of the brain that regulates sensory impulses traveling to the cortex.

Chapter Objectives

After studying this chapter, you should be able to:

- Describe the three major parts of the brain.
- List the main parts of the brainstem and discuss the functions associated with each part.
- Describe the reticular formation and the limbic system and discuss the importance of each.

The central nervous system (CNS) is composed of the brain and spinal cord. The primary functions of the CNS are to coordinate and control the activity of other body systems. Distinct nerve pathways in the CNS interconnect different areas of the brain that serve the same function. Neurons in these pathways are linked together by synapses. These neurons release neurotransmitters, which regulate transmission across the synapses. In this way, nerve impulses are conducted to different areas of the brain to influence the levels of activity.

There are a significant number of neurotransmitters, including acetylcholine (ACh), norepinephrine (NE), dopamine, and serotonin, that have been identified in the brain. Some mental illnesses and pathologic conditions are associated with abnormal changes in the amount or activity of a specific neurotransmitter. Many of the drugs that act on the CNS do so by affecting neurotransmitter concentrations and activity. Although there are a large number of different neurotransmitters in the brain, the function and activity of each are similar to the function of the neurons and nerve endings (adrenergic, cholinergic) previously discussed with the autonomic nervous system.

Generally, a neuron releases one specific type of neurotransmitter that crosses the synapse and binds to its receptor located on the dendrites of the next adjoining neuron. Neurotransmitters can be either excitatory or inhibitory. Excitatory receptor stimulation generates action potentials that flow along the nerve axon to stimulate release of the neurotransmitter from the nerve endings of that neuron, and so on. Inhibitory neurotransmitters produce actions on the next adjoining neuron that inhibit the generation of action potentials. In this manner, neurotransmitters function to either generate nerve impulses that transmit information among the different brain centers or function to inhibit the flow of action potentials, which reduces neural activity. The

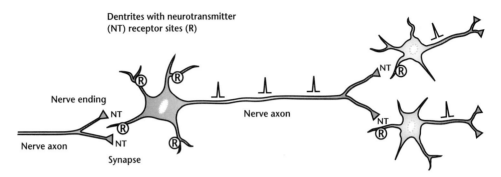

Dentrites with neurotransmitter
(NT) receptor sites (R)

Nerve ending

NT

Nerve axon

NT

Nerve axon

Synapse

Nerve axon

NT

Figure 11-1
Illustration of the synaptic connections between brain neurons. Nerve ending from one neuron releases neurotransmitter (NT), which crosses synapse to bind to NT receptor (R) on dendrites of next neuron. Receptor stimulation generates an action potential (⊥) that travels down the nerve axon to stimulate the release of NT from nerve endings.

released neurotransmitters are inactivated by metabolism or reuptake into their respective nerve endings. Figure 11-1 illustrates the synaptic connections of a typical brain neuron.

In the CNS, neurons having the same functions are generally grouped together. The cell bodies of these neurons form control centers for the various body functions. Consequently, the CNS is anatomically divided into different parts. In order to understand how drugs affect the CNS, the main structures and functions of the CNS are reviewed.

Parts of the Brain

The brain may be divided into three main parts: the cerebrum, brainstem, and cerebellum. Each of these parts is described in the following sections. The main structures of the CNS are illustrated in Figure 11-2.

CEREBRUM

The **cerebrum** is the largest and uppermost part of the brain. All of the higher intellectual abilities of human beings are controlled by the cerebrum. Anatomically, the cerebrum is divided into right and left cerebral hemispheres. Each hemisphere is composed of an outer cerebral cortex and an inner cerebral medulla.

Cerebral Cortex   The **cerebral cortex** contains the cell bodies of neurons (gray matter) that control voluntary activities of the body. The cortex is subdivided into four main lobes. The cortical lobes are named after the skull bones and include

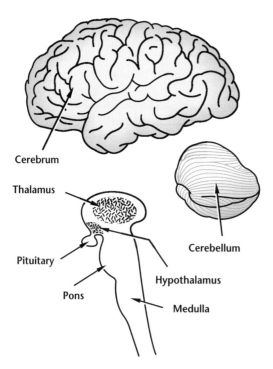

Cerebrum

Thalamus

Pituitary

Pons

Cerebellum

Hypothalamus

Medulla

Figure 11-2
The main structures of the brain.

the frontal, parietal, temporal, and occipital lobes. The frontal lobe is responsible for control of muscle movement, the motor components of speech, abstract thinking, and problem-solving activity. The parietal lobe is responsible for the sensory sensations of touch, pressure, pain, temperature, and vibration. The temporal lobes are involved in memory and language functions. The occipital lobes function in vision. There are neural connections between the lobes and each area of integration of neural function. An **electroencephalogram (EEG)** is a recording of the electrical activity of the cortex. The EEG is useful in diagnosing various brain disorders.

Cerebral Medulla   The inner **cerebral medulla** is composed of the myelinated axons (white matter) of the neurons. The axons conduct nerve impulses to and from different areas of the nervous system. Also, there is a group of cell bodies (gray matter) in the medulla known as the basal ganglia.

BASAL GANGLIA

The **basal ganglia** are involved in the regulation of motor activity. The basal ganglia are sometimes referred to as the extrapyramidal system. Degeneration of certain neurons within the basal ganglia is responsible for Parkinson's disease and Huntington's chorea.

BRAINSTEM

The brainstem is continuous with the spinal cord and extends up to the cerebrum. The brainstem controls many body functions that are not under conscious control. The main parts of the brainstem include the thalamus, hypothalamus, pons, and medulla oblongata.

Thalamus Located at the top of the brainstem, the **thalamus** regulates sensory impulses (pain, temperature, and touch) traveling to the cortex. The thalamus evaluates sensory information and directs it to the appropriate centers in the cortex. Some tranquilizers and analgesic drugs affect sensory information by interfering with the function of the thalamus.

Hypothalamus Located below the thalamus, the **hypothalamus** controls many body functions including temperature, water balance, appetite, sleep, the autonomic nervous system, and certain emotional or behavioral responses. The pituitary gland is attached to the hypothalamus. Referred to as the master gland of the body, the pituitary gland regulates the function of many other endocrine glands.

Pons Located below the hypothalamus, the **pons** is involved in the regulation of respiration and serves as a relay station for nerve fibers traveling to other brain areas.

Medulla Oblongata The **medulla oblongata** lies just above the spinal cord. Within the medulla oblongata are the three vital centers: cardiac (heart), vasomotor (blood pressure), and respiratory (breathing). Normal functioning of the vital centers is essential for life support. Injury to the medulla oblongata frequently results in death. Overdose with drugs, such as alcohol or barbiturates, causes death by depressing the function of the vital centers. Several important reflexes are also regulated by the medulla oblongata, including swallowing, coughing, vomiting, and gagging.

CEREBELLUM

The **cerebellum** lies behind the brainstem and below the cerebrum. The major functions of the cerebellum, which is divided into right and left cerebellar hemispheres, are to coordinate body movements and posture and to help maintain body equilibrium. Drugs that depress the cerebellum, such as alcohol, usually decrease body coordination and increase reaction time.

SPINAL CORD

The spinal cord is a collection of nerve axons that travel to and from the brain. Nerve axons traveling from the peripheral parts of the body (skin, muscle, visceral organs) to the brain carry sensory information (touch, pain, hot and cold sensations, etc.). Nerve axons traveling from the brain to the peripheral organs and skeletal muscle carry motor impulses that direct organ activity and muscle movement. Drugs that act on the spinal cord, mainly anesthetics, analgesics, and muscle relaxants, are primarily used to alter pain sensation and reduce the tone and activity of skeletal muscle.

FUNCTIONAL COMPONENTS

In addition to the main anatomic parts of the brain just described, several other functional neuronal pathways are located within the brain. These components form diffuse nerve networks that connect many different areas of the brain together. The reticular formation and the limbic system are two such components.

Reticular Formation   The **reticular formation** is a network of nerve fibers that travel throughout the brainstem and cerebrum. It is composed of two types of fibers: excitatory and inhibitory.

When the excitatory fibers are stimulated by various external stimuli (noise, bright light, or danger), the degree of alertness increases, preparing the body for a situation that requires action. The excitatory fibers are usually referred to as the reticular activating system.

When there is a lack of external stimuli, the inhibitory fibers become more active, decreasing the activity of this system and, consequently, the degree of arousal or alertness. This decrease normally occurs during periods of rest or sleep. Consequently, the reticular formation helps regulate the degree of alertness or wakefulness of the nervous system.

The reticular formation is sensitive to the effects of many drugs. Alcohol, barbiturates, and other depressant drugs decrease its activity and may induce sleep or unconsciousness. Stimulants, such as amphetamines and caffeine, increase the activity of the reticular formation and are usually used or abused to maintain wakefulness.

Limbic System   The **limbic system** refers to a collection of neurons and brain areas that form a specific neural pathway. Most of the structures of the limbic system are located around the hypothalamus and lower portions of the cerebrum. The limbic system appears to be involved with the emotional and behavioral responses of the body associated with reward and punishment, sexual behavior, anger or rage, fear, and anxiety; therefore, the limbic system appears to be important to mental health. The functions of the limbic system are not completely understood. However, certain drugs, such as the antianxiety agents, exert a selective effect on the limbic system and are useful for the treatment of certain behavioral and emotional disorders.

The area of pharmacology that deals with drugs affecting the CNS is known as neuropharmacology. In the following chapters, the major classes of drugs that affect the CNS are considered.

Chapter 11 Review

UNDERSTANDING TERMINOLOGY

Match the description in the left column with the appropriate part of the brain in the right column.

1. Coordinates body movements and posture, helps maintain equilibrium.
2. Regulates motor activity.
3. Conducts nerve impulses to and from different areas of the nervous system.
4. Uppermost part of brain that controls higher intellectual abilities.
5. Regulates sensory impulses traveling to cortex.
6. Controls cardiac, vasomotor, and respiratory functions.
7. Controls body's voluntary activities.

a. basal ganglia
b. cerebellum
c. cerebral cortex
d. cerebral medulla
e. cerebrum
f. medulla oblongata
g. thalamus

ACQUIRING KNOWLEDGE

Test your understanding of the material in this chapter by answering the following questions.

8. What are the main functions of the central nervous system?
9. List some of the neurotransmitters found in the brain. What is the function of a neurotransmitter?
10. Where are the basal ganglia located, and what function is associated with them?
11. List the main structures in the brainstem.
12. List the main functions of the hypothalamus and the medulla oblongata.
13. Why are the vital centers important? What are the consequences of injury to the medulla oblongata?
14. What is the reticular formation? How does it function to regulate the level of wakefulness or arousal?
15. What is the limbic system? What functions are associated with this system?

APPLYING KNOWLEDGE ON THE JOB

Answer the following questions.

16. As patient liaison in a large metropolitan hospital, one of your duties is to educate patients and their families about their illnesses and treatments. For the following cases, explain why the patients present with the signs and symptoms that they do.

    a. Patient A, a 16-year-old girl, took an overdose of Amytal and was brought to the emergency room by her parents. She presents in the ER with a heart rate of 45, blood pressure of 85 over 55, and slow, irregular breathing.

    b. Patient B took an accidental overdose of Biphetamine and presents at the ER in a state of excitability, with rapid breathing, heart palpitations, excessive perspiration, anxiety, and irritability.

    c. Patient C is an 18-year-old man who has had a few beers once or twice a month since he turned 18. He has never consumed hard liquor until tonight, when he attended a party where he participated in a drinking contest. At that time, he drank several ounces of whiskey in a few minutes. He passed out and could not be awakened. A sober friend brought him to the ER, still unconscious. His heart rate is slow, his blood pressure down, and he has irregular breathing.

17. Assume a patient of the doctor you assist has Parkinson's disease. He and his wife think his problem is in his muscles. Explain to them what is really affected and why he has the symptoms he does.

Additional Reading

Hanson HR. Clinical evaluation of cranial nerves I through VII. *Hosp Med* 1995;31(10):37.

Pellegrin TR. A faster, focused neurologic exam. *Emerg Med* 1997;29(6):68.

Sedative-Hypnotic Drugs and Alcohol

HENRY HITNER, PhD
BARBARA NAGLE, PhD

Chapter Focus

This chapter describes the pharmacology of drugs used to produce sedation and hypnosis (sleep). It also describes the sleep cycle, how hypnotic drugs affect the stages of the sleep cycle, and the pharmacology of alcohol, a CNS depressant drug.

Chapter Terminology

automatism: Drug-induced confusion that can cause increased drug consumption.

barbiturate: CNS depressant drug possessing the barbituric acid ring structure.

benzodiazepine: Class of drugs used to treat anxiety and sleep disorders.

GABA: γ-aminobutyric acid, an inhibitory neurotransmitter in the CNS.

hypnotic: Drug used to induce and maintain sleep.

induction: An increase in the amount of drug-metabolizing enzymes in the liver.

nonbarbiturate: Refers to hypnotic drugs that do not possess the barbituric acid structure, such as benzodiazepines.

NREM sleep: States of sleep not characterized by rapid eye movement.

REM sleep: Stage of sleep characterized by rapid eye movement (REM) and dreaming.

sedative: Drug used to produce mental relaxation and to reduce the desire for physical activity.

Chapter Objectives

After studying this chapter, you should be able to:

- Name three barbiturate hypnotic drugs and describe their mechanism of action and effect on the sleep cycle.
- Describe the adverse effects of barbiturates, the addiction liability, and treatment of barbiturate overdose.
- Name three benzodiazepine hypnotic drugs and explain the mechanism by which they produce hypnotic effects.
- List four advantages of using benzodiazepines over barbiturate drugs.
- Explain the major pharmacologic effects and adverse reactions of ethyl alcohol.

The central nervous system (CNS) coordinates and controls the activity of all other body systems. As a result, anything that directly affects the CNS ultimately influences the overall function of the body. With increased CNS stimulation, a person responds by becoming more alert, anxious, and occasionally more irritable. Excessive CNS stimulation can cause convulsions or various forms of abnormal behavior. Abuse of amphetamines or cocaine can cause these effects. In contrast, depression of the CNS reduces both physical and mental activity. Excessive CNS depression can produce unconsciousness, coma, and death. CNS depression is frequently related to abuse of barbiturates and alcohol.

Sedatives and hypnotics (drugs to induce sleep) are used therapeutically to decrease CNS activity. **Sedatives** are used to reduce the desire for physical activity. Usually a sedative will be prescribed after a heart attack or some other condition, when overexertion may be harmful. Various emotional or medical situations can cause enough anxiety and tension to interfere with sleep. When an individual is unable to sleep (insomnia), excessive tiredness can contribute to greater anxiety and make any situation worse. In this instance, **hypnotic** drugs may be prescribed to induce and maintain sleep (Table 12-1). Use of hypnotics should be intermittent and only when medically judged to be needed. Regular use should be limited to 2 to 4 weeks at any one time. Tolerance develops to the hypnotics, and effectiveness decreases after several weeks of continuous use.

Several different drug classes are used as sedatives and hypnotics. These drugs are generally classified as the barbiturates and the nonbarbiturates. The **nonbarbiturates** include several miscellaneous drugs and the class of drugs known as the **benzodiazepines**.

The benzodiazepines have important advantages over the other drugs and are currently considered to be the drugs of choice for both sedation and hypnosis.

Table 12-1
Doses for Sedation and Hypnosis of the Most Frequently Employed Sedative-Hypnotic Drugs

		Oral Adult Dose	
Drug (Trade Name)	Duration	Sedation	Hypnosis
Barbiturates			
Amobarbital (Amytal)	Intermediate	50–300 mg	100–200 mg
Butabarbital (Butisol)	Intermediate	50–120 mg	50–100 mg
Pentobarbital (Nembutal)	Intermediate	30 mg TID, QID	100 mg
Phenobarbital (Luminal)	Long	30–120 mg	50–100 mg
Secobarbital (Seconal)	Short	—	100 mg
Nonbarbiturates			
Chloral hydrate (Noctec)	Short	250 mg	500–1000 mg
Ethchlorvynol (Placidyl)	Short	100–200 mg	500–1000 mg
Zolpidem (Ambien)	Short	—	5–10 mg
Zaleplon (Sonata)	Short	—	5–10 mg
Benzodiazepines			
Estazolam (ProSom)	Intermediate	—	0.5–1.0 mg
Flurazepam (Dalmane)	Long	—	15–30 mg
Quazepam (Doral)	Long	—	7.5–15 mg
Temazepam (Restoril)	Intermediate	—	15–30 mg
Triazolam (Halcion)	Short	—	0.125–0.5 mg

Table 12-1 lists the most frequently prescribed sedative-hypnotic drugs. Before we discuss the pharmacology of the sedatives and hypnotics, we present a brief review of the sleep cycle.

Sleep Cycle

Although sedative-hypnotic drugs are primarily used to induce and maintain sleep, many of these drugs alter the normal sleep cycle. The normal sleep cycle is divided into two different states: non–rapid eye movement (**NREM**) and rapid eye movement (**REM**) sleep. NREM has been divided into four stages. Progression from Stage 1 to Stage 4 is characterized by deepening levels of sleep and usually takes between 60 and 90 minutes to occur. After Stage 4, individuals normally enter REM sleep for approximately 20 minutes. Dreaming usually occurs during REM sleep. After a period of REM sleep, individuals return to NREM sleep and repeat the cycle. Depending on the length of sleep, most individuals usually go through four to six sleep cycles per night.

STAGE 1 NREM

Individuals are somewhat aware of surroundings but relaxed. Stage 1 normally lasts a few minutes and occupies 4% to 5% of total sleep time.

STAGE 2 NREM

Individuals become unaware of surroundings but can be easily awakened. Stage 2 occupies about 50% of total sleep time.

STAGES 3 AND 4 NREM

Stages 3 and 4 are referred to as "slow-wave sleep" because of the high-amplitude, low-frequency δ waves observed on the electroencephalogram (EEG). These deep stages of sleep are believed to be particularly important for physical rest and restoration. They occupy approximately 20% to 25% of total sleep time.

REM

The REM stage is characterized by bursts of rapid eye movement, increased autonomic activity, and dreaming. It is believed to be essential for mental restoration. During REM sleep, daily events are reviewed, and information is integrated into memory. Like Stages 3 and 4, REM is a deep state of sleep and occupies about 20% to 25% of total sleep time.

Barbiturate Sedatives and Hypnotics

The barbiturates are among the oldest drugs in the sedative-hypnotic class. These drugs have a number of disadvantages in use and have in large part been replaced by newer drugs. All of the **barbiturates** are structurally similar to the parent compound, barbituric acid. The barbiturates produce a dose-dependent depression of the CNS. At higher doses, all barbiturates can produce general anesthesia. The barbiturates discussed in this chapter are used primarily for sedation and hypnosis. Barbiturates that are used as general anesthetics are discussed in Chapter 13.

MECHANISM OF ACTION

Barbiturates are believed to have two mechanisms of action. At lower doses, barbiturates increase the inhibitory actions of **γ-aminobutyric acid (GABA).** GABA is an inhibitory neurotransmitter in the CNS that reduces neuronal excitability, especially in the reticular activating system. Increasing the effects of GABA reduces brain activity and promotes sleep. At higher doses, barbiturates also cause a general depression of the entire CNS that is similar to the actions of the general anesthetics. This action of the barbiturates is not well understood but may be related to the ability of the barbiturates to dissolve in neuronal membranes, where they interfere with the normal function and movement of ions that regulate neuronal excitability and the release of excitatory neurotransmitters.

The main sites of action of the barbiturates for sedation and hypnosis are the reticular formation and the cerebral cortex. Inhibition of the reticular activating system reduces excitatory stimulation of the cerebral cortex. As a result, individuals become sedated and, with further CNS depression, become sleepy. The dose of barbiturate required to produce hypnosis is usually three to five times greater than the dose required to produce sedation.

Barbiturates usually increase Stage 2 sleep but decrease slow-wave sleep (Stages 3 and 4). In addition, barbiturates suppress REM sleep. When barbiturates are discontinued, patients often spend excess time in REM sleep during the next night or two as if to make up for the lost REM sleep (REM rebound effect). During the rebound period, there is increased dreaming, which may cause restlessness, anxiety, and nightmares.

PHARMACOKINETICS

The barbiturates are well absorbed following oral administration. Once in the circulation, these drugs are readily distributed to all tissues. Symptoms of CNS depression occur within 30 to 60 minutes following oral administration. The drug microsomal metabolizing system (DMMS) in the liver is responsible for inactivation of the barbiturates.

When taken regularly for more than several days, barbiturates begin to induce the microsomal enzymes. **Induction** refers to an increase in the amount of drug-metabolizing enzymes in the liver. Induction results in faster metabolism of the barbiturate. Consequently, the duration of action is decreased, and patients must take larger doses of the drug to attain the same pharmacologic effect as before. When this occurs, patients are said to have developed tolerance.

When induction of the metabolizing enzymes occurs, all of the drug-metabolizing enzymes are increased. Therefore, any other drugs taken at the same time are also metabolized faster. This effect is responsible for a number of drug interactions. Barbiturates are eliminated mostly by the urinary system.

BARBITURATE DRUGS

Phenobarbital (Luminal)   Phenobarbital is classified as a long-acting barbiturate, with a duration of 6 to 12 hours. When used as a hypnotic, phenobarbital may produce a "hangover effect," during which individuals feel drugged the next morning as a result of the prolonged duration of action. For this reason, phenobarbital is used primarily as a sedative, where one dose is to produce sedation for most of the day. Phenobarbital is also used in the treatment of epilepsy.

Pentobarbital (Nembutal)   Pentobarbital is classified as an intermediate-acting sedative-hypnotic with a duration of 4 to 6 hours.

Amobarbital (Amytal)   Amobarbital is similar to pentobarbital. In addition, both of these barbiturates can be used parenterally to stop convulsions.

Secobarbital (Seconal)   Secobarbital is a short-acting hypnotic with a duration of 2 to 4 hours. It is particularly useful in individuals who have difficulty falling asleep but not staying asleep.

ADVERSE EFFECTS

The side effects associated with the sedative-hypnotic drugs are an extension of their therapeutic action (CNS depression). Drowsiness, dry mouth, lethargy, and incoordination occur most frequently. These adverse effects are more annoying than harmful. However, depressed reflexes and impaired judgment may contribute to serious accidents if patients operate motor vehicles or heavy machinery while taking these drugs.

Elderly patients are particularly sensitive to CNS side effects, especially mental confusion and memory difficulties. When memory is impaired as a result of CNS depression, patients may not remember when the drug was last taken. As a result, more drug may be consumed within a short time. This phenomenon, known as **automatism,** may lead to drug intoxication and death. Mild overdosage of the sedative-hypnotic drugs resembles alcohol intoxication (inebriation). Slurred speech, ataxia, impaired judgment, irritability, and psychological disturbances are characteristic of intoxication.

ADDICTION LIABILITY

Prolonged and excessive use of barbiturates results in tolerance and physical dependence. In addition, cross-tolerance (resistance) develops to the depressant effects of other CNS depressants such as alcohol and benzodiazepines.

The mechanism for the production of tolerance and dependence has not yet been clearly determined. Physical dependence usually develops when greater therapeutic dosages are taken on a regular basis for more than 1 to 2 months. Once physical dependence develops, the drug must be used continuously to avoid the onset of withdrawal symptoms. Withdrawal symptoms include anxiety, insomnia, cramping, tremors, paranoid behavior, delirium, and convulsions. The abstinence syndrome (withdrawal) associated with sedative-hypnotics is especially dangerous. If withdrawal is not conducted within an adequately supervised medical center, death may occur.

BARBITURATE POISONING

Overdose with the barbiturates results in extensive cardiovascular and CNS depression. In large doses, these drugs depress all brain activity, including that of the vital centers in the medulla oblongata. Inhibition of vasomotor centers in the medulla oblongata removes sympathetic control of the blood vessels, and dilation of the blood vessels contributes to the production of hypotension and shock.

In the presence of hypotension, kidney function decreases. There is little or no production of urine (oliguria or anuria) to remove the toxic products from the body. Medullary respiratory centers are also depressed, leading to irregular breathing and hypoxia (cyanosis). **Severe intoxication with the barbiturates usually leads to coma, respiratory depression, and death, most commonly from respiratory arrest.**

There is no antidote for barbiturate overdose. Treatment of comatose patients includes supportive therapy to maintain respiration and blood pressure. Endotracheal intubation and artificial respiration may be employed. Also, sympathomimetic (α-adrenergic) drugs and IV fluids may be administered to elevate blood pressure. Osmotic diuretics administered intravenously may stimulate urine production so that renal excretion of the drug can occur. In addition, alkalinization of the urine (pH 7.0 or above) will increase the excretion of the more acidic barbiturates such as phenobarbital. Hemodialysis or peritoneal dialysis may be required when kidney function is depressed.

CAUTIONS AND CONTRAINDICATIONS

The barbiturates are the drugs most frequently used for attempted suicide. Because of their rapid action, the short-acting drugs are particularly dangerous. Many patients die before medical treatment can be administered. To prevent hospitalized patients from hoarding medication, precautions must be taken to ensure that each dose has been swallowed at the scheduled time. The pills must never be left on the nightstand to be taken at a patient's discretion.

Most of the barbiturates are contraindicated in patients who have acute intermittent porphyria. In this condition, an overproduction of hemoglobin (porphyrin) precursors accumulates in the liver. Sedative-hypnotics such as the barbiturates stimulate and increase the production of porphyrins, which can precipitate an attack (may cause nerve damage, pain, paralysis) in patients prone to this condition.

PREGNANCY

The barbiturates are designated as FDA Pregnancy Category D, which indicates that they can cause harmful effects to the fetus. Consequently, these drugs should be avoided during pregnancy.

DRUG INTERACTIONS

Sedative-hypnotic drugs undergo extensive interactions with other drugs. Sedative-hypnotic agents will potentiate the actions of other CNS depressant drugs, leading to greater CNS and respiratory depression. Sedative-hypnotics and alcohol can be a deadly combination and should never be taken together.

Because barbiturates cause enzyme induction, other drugs may be metabolized more rapidly in their presence. This rapid metabolism results in a decreased pharmacologic effect of drugs, such as the oral anticoagulants and oral contraceptives. Most of the sedative-hypnotic drugs are bound to plasma proteins; therefore, they compete with other drugs for protein-binding sites. Protein-binding displacement usually leads to a potentiation of the pharmacologic effect of the drug displaced.

Miscellaneous Nonbarbiturates

The nonbarbiturate sedative-hypnotics (Table 12-1) are a diverse group of drugs that produce effects similar to those of barbiturates. Some of these agents were developed with the hope that they would not produce tolerance or physical addiction as the barbiturates do. Unfortunately, this has not been true. Prolonged abuse of these drugs usually results in the development of tolerance and physical addiction. Only chloral hydrate and two newer drugs, zolpidem and zaleplon, are discussed here.

CHLORAL HYDRATE (NOCTEC, SK-CHLORAL)

Choral hydrate is related in a general way to alcohol. In the liver, it is metabolized by alcohol dehydrogenase to trichloroethanol, which also produces hypnotic effects (active metabolite). The main use of chloral hydrate is as a hypnotic, particularly in the elderly. Chloral hydrate produces less suppression of REM sleep than do the barbiturates. Side effects usually involve excessive CNS depression and gastric irritation. Although capable of producing tolerance and addiction, chloral hydrate is not particularly popular with drug abusers.

ZOLPIDEM (AMBIEN)

Zolpidem is not a benzodiazepine but acts on GABA in a manner that is similar to the barbiturates and benzodiazepines. The drug is used only as a hypnotic and does not have useful anticonvulsant or skeletal muscle-relaxing properties. Zolpidem does not appear to disrupt the normal stages of the sleep cycle, nor is it associated with the development of drug dependence and withdrawal reactions. The drug has a short half-life (2–3 hours) and is excreted in the urine. Adverse effects are infrequent and usually limited to dizziness, headache, nausea, and diarrhea. Zolpidem is designated FDA Pregnancy Category B.

ZALEPLON (SONATA)

Zaleplon is classified as a nonbenzodiazepine hypnotic that acts on GABA in a manner similar to zolpidem. The drug has a short half-life (1 hour), does not accumulate with repeated use, and is not associated with rebound insomnia after discontinuation or drug dependence when used for long periods of time. Adverse effects usually involve headache, GI disturbances, rash, minor CNS disturbances, tremor, and myalgia. Zaleplon is designated Pregnancy Category C.

Benzodiazepines

The **benzodiazepines** are a class of drugs widely used in the treatment of anxiety. They are commonly referred to as the antianxiety drugs. The general pharmacology of the benzodiazepines is presented more fully in Chapter 8. However, in addition to producing antianxiety effects, benzodiazepines also depress the reticular activating system to produce sedation and hypnosis. Several benzodiazepines are marketed specifically as sedatives and hypnotics, and these drugs are included in this chapter (Table 12-1).

MECHANISM OF ACTION

The benzodiazepines produce sedative and hypnotic effects by increasing the inhibitory activity of γ-aminobutyric acid (**GABA**), a neurotransmitter in the CNS. When GABA is released by certain neurons, it binds to GABA receptors and leads to a reduction in neuronal excitability. The benzodiazepines bind to receptor sites (named benzodiazepine receptors) that are in close relationship to the GABA receptors. When benzodiazepines bind to their receptors, there appears to be an additional increase in the inhibitory activity of GABA, which further decreases neuronal excitability. In the reticular activating system, this depression produces sedation or hypnosis, depending on the dose of drug administered.

PHARMACOKINETICS

Benzodiazepines are lipid-soluble drugs that readily enter the CNS. They are well absorbed after oral administration. The benzodiazepines are metabolized by the drug microsomal enzymes. Some of the benzodiazepines are metabolized to active metabolites, which also produce sedation and hypnosis and thereby prolong the duration of action. Unlike the barbiturates, the benzodiazepines do not cause induction of the microsomal metabolizing enzymes at therapeutic doses. Elimination is mainly by way of the urinary tract.

Flurazepam (Dalmane)   Flurazepam is classified as a long-acting benzodiazepine. It forms several active metabolites, some of which have long half-lives. For this reason, the sedative and antianxiety effects of flurazepam are usually evident the day following a hypnotic dose. This prolonged action can be useful in anxious patients when sedating drug effects are desired on the following day. On the other hand, daytime sedation and drowsiness may interfere with employment or other activities.

Temazepam (Restoril)   Temazepam is an intermediate-acting hypnotic that does not form any important active metabolites. The duration of hypnotic action is 8 to 10 hours, and there are usually few or no drug effects evident the following day. One preparation of temazepam is marketed in a hard gelatin capsule that produces a delayed onset of action. This drug dosage form should be taken 1 to 2 hours before sleep is desired.

Triazolam (Halcion)   Triazolam is a short-acting hypnotic with no active metabolites. This hypnotic does not usually cause residual effects the day following a hypnotic dose. However, the short duration of action may cause early morning awakenings.

EFFECTS ON SLEEP CYCLE

All benzodiazepines produce similar effects on the sleep cycle. NREM Stage 2 is increased, but NREM Stage 4 is usually decreased. The benzodiazepines do not significantly suppress REM sleep and, therefore, do not usually cause REM rebound when discontinued.

ADVANTAGES OF BENZODIAZEPINE HYPNOTICS

The benzodiazepines generally do not interfere with REM sleep. They produce less tolerance and, therefore, are effective for a few weeks longer than are the barbiturates. They also do not induce microsomal metabolizing enzymes significantly. When abused, the benzodiazepines generally cause less physical dependence than barbiturates. These factors, along with the low incidence of adverse effects, give the benzodiazepines a number of advantages over the barbiturates for both sedation and hypnosis.

ADVERSE EFFECTS

The benzodiazepine hypnotics are well tolerated and produce few adverse effects when used properly. Flurazepam, because of its longer half-life, may cause sedation or a "hangover effect" the following day. Triazolam, which has a very short duration of action, has been associated with rebound insomnia. This involves insomnia occurring over several days following abrupt discontinuance of the drug. In addition, triazolam has been associated with increased daytime anxiety. The adverse effects of the benzodiazepines are further discussed in Chapter 8.

CAUTIONS AND CONTRAINDICATIONS

Pregnancy   Benzodiazepine hypnotic drugs have been shown to cause harmful effects during pregnancy. They are designated as FDA Pregnancy Category X and, therefore, should not be used during pregnancy.

DRUG INTERACTIONS

The benzodiazepines potentiate the actions of other CNS depressant drugs such as alcohol and barbiturates. Such drugs should never be taken together unless specifically ordered by a physician.

The metabolism of the benzodiazepines has been shown to be inhibited by cimetidine (Tagamet), a drug used in the treatment of intestinal ulcers. Consequently, using these drugs together may increase the duration of action of the benzodiazepines.

Alcohol

Alcohol (ethanol, whiskey, ethyl alcohol, or grain alcohol) is probably the most widely used (self-prescribed) nonprescription sedative-hypnotic and antianxiety agent.

PHARMACOLOGIC EFFECTS

Alcohol has many pharmacologic effects that are seen throughout the body, including the CNS, heart, gastrointestinal tract, and kidneys.

CNS Effects   The CNS is extremely senstive to the depressant action of alcohol. As with other sedative-hypnotic drugs, alcohol produces a dose-dependent depression of the CNS. After drinking alcoholic beverages, people usually feel "stimulated," uninhibited, and less self-conscious. However, this stimulation is actually caused by an initial depression of inhibitory areas within the brain. As the level of alcohol in the brain increases, excitatory and inhibitory fibers are progressively depressed, leading to sedation, hypnosis, and possibly coma. Unlike the other sedative-hypnotic drugs, alcohol produces some analgesia and antipyresis (reduces fever). The mechanisms of alcohol's action in the CNS have not been fully established, but alcohol also appears to increase the inhibitory effects of GABA.

Vascular Effects   In low to moderate amounts, alcohol does not produce any direct deleterious effects on the heart. However, alcohol may induce dilation of the blood vessels in the skin (cutaneous), producing a warmed, flushed sensation. The dilation of blood vessels may lead to a rapid loss of body heat, so that body temperature begins to fall. Depression of vasomotor centers in the CNS is most likely responsible for producing the peripheral vasodilation.

GI Effects   Alcohol stimulates the secretion of saliva and gastric juices (acid and pepsin). Overall, this action usually results in an increased appetite. However, ingestion of strong concentrations of alcohol may irritate the gastric mucosa, causing a local inflammation (gastritis). Increased acid secretion coupled with gastritis may lead to GI ulceration in sensitive patients.

Renal Effects   Alcohol promotes an increased excretion of urine (diuresis) that is partly caused by the increased fluid intake that accompanies the ingestion of alcoholic beverages. In addition, alcohol blocks the pituitary secretion of ADH (antidiuretic hormone), which decreases the renal reabsorption of water. Therefore, the water is excreted into the urine. Alcohol inhibits the renal secretion of uric acid by an unknown mechanism, which allows uric acid to build up in the blood. In susceptible patients (with gout or gouty arthritis), this elevation in uric acid levels may lead to attacks of joint inflammation.

NUTRITIONAL EFFECTS

In addition to its direct effects on the various organs, alcohol exerts a profound influence on the nutritional state of individuals. Alcohol is a natural product that possesses calories. For this reason, many people often substitute alcohol for nutritionally rich foods such as protein. Over a period of time, individuals who consume moderate to large amounts of alcohol in conjunction with a poorly balanced diet may suffer from vitamin and amino acid deficiencies. In particular, deficiency of the B vitamins leads to abnormal growth and function of nervous tissue. Therefore, multiple nutritional deficiencies associated with alcohol consumption produce various conditions such as neuropathies, dermatitis (pellagra), anemia, and psychosis.

METABOLISM OF ALCOHOL

Alcohol is readily absorbed throughout the entire GI tract following ingestion. Subsequently, alcohol is distributed to all tissues. However, the CNS receives a significant concentration of alcohol because of its rich blood supply. The concentration of alcohol in the brain is proportional to the concentration of alcohol in the blood.

Unlike other drugs, alcohol is metabolized at a constant rate in the liver. No matter how much alcohol is consumed, only 10 to 15 mL of pure alcohol per hour is metabolized, which is the amount of alcohol in one beer, a glass of wine, or an average-size cocktail. This limits the amount of alcohol that can be consumed without producing intoxication. Alcohol is metabolized primarily to acetaldehyde, which the body can use in the synthesis of cholesterol and fatty acids. Overall, alcohol is efficiently metabolized (about 95%) to useful biochemical products and water.

Enzyme induction develops during chronic use of alcohol. Therefore, habitual drinkers often experience shorter durations of action of other drugs metabolized by the microsomal system of the liver (oral anticoagulants and many others).

ADVERSE EFFECTS

The adverse effects associated with the use of alcohol are separated into acute and chronic effects. Acute intoxication (inebriation) produces extensive CNS depression. Individuals may exhibit ataxia, impaired speech, blurred vision, and loss of memory, similar to the symptoms of intoxication caused by other sedative-hypnotic drugs.

When CNS depression is severe, stupor and coma may result. The skin is cold and clammy, the body temperature falls, and the heart rate may increase. Treatment is usually directed at supporting respiration so that the brain remains well oxygenated. Even while patients are unconscious, their body tissues can metabolize alcohol until the blood level is safely reduced.

Chronic consumption of alcohol is associated with progressive changes in cell function. Elevated blood alcohol levels for long periods result ultimately in drug tolerance and physical dependence. The abstinence syndrome associated with alcohol addiction is similar to that described for the other sedative-hypnotic drugs. In addition, chronic use of alcohol produces alterations in body metabolism, some of which may be the result of the development of malnutrition. Alcohol-induced malnutrition and vitamin deficiency can cause a number of neurologic disorders, such as Wernicke encephalopathy and Korsakoff psychosis. In addition, malnutrition and alcohol contribute to the production of fatty liver and cirrhosis of the liver.

CAUTIONS AND CONTRAINDICATIONS

The symptoms of alcohol intoxication often resemble those associated with diabetic coma, head injuries, and drug overdose (other sedative-hypnotics). Patients who appear intoxicated should always be kept for observation until an accurate diagnosis is made. If possible, the blood alcohol level should be determined to confirm the suspected diagnosis.

Alcohol should never be combined with other CNS-depressant medications. Potentiation occurs with any central-acting depressant, including muscle relaxants, anesthetics, analgesics, and antianxiety drugs. Alcohol is absolutely contraindicated in patients who have hepatic or renal disease, ulcers, hyperacidity, or epilepsy.

Pregnancy   The consumption of alcohol has been associated with harmful fetal effects and should be avoided during pregnancy. Alcohol readily crosses the placenta and distributes to all tissues of the fetus. Infants who were exposed to circulating levels of alcohol in utero have shown depressed respiration and reflexes at birth. Babies born to alcoholic mothers are unusually small, are frequently premature, and may be mentally retarded. It is not unusual for a newborn of an alcoholic mother to undergo withdrawal symptoms after birth. Fetal alcohol syndrome is the term used to describe the fetal abnormalities, which may include low IQ, microcephaly, and a variety of facial abnormalities.

CLINICAL INDICATIONS

When applied to the skin, alcohol produces a cooling effect as a result of rapid evaporation from the skin surface. For this reason, it is used as a sponge bath to reduce elevated body temperature. Also, 70% alcohol applied to the skin acts as a bactericidal agent (disinfectant). There is very little medicinal value associated with the consumption of alcohol. However, many over-the-counter (nonprescription) cold remedies and cough syrups contain a significant amount of alcohol; the alcohol present in these preparations is sufficient to produce sedation and hypnosis. Therefore, exposure of patients to alcohol may occur without their knowledge.

DISULFIRAM (ANTABUSE)

Disulfiram is a drug used to treat chronic alcoholism. It interferes with the metabolism of alcohol. Alcohol is metabolized through a series of steps to acetyl coenzyme A:

- alcohol
- acetaldehyde
- acetate
- acetyl coenzyme A

Disulfiram slows the conversion of acetaldehyde to acetate. Therefore, acetaldehyde accumulates in the blood, producing nausea, vomiting, headache, and hypotension. This is known as a disulfiram reaction. Any drug that is metabolized through a similar biochemical pathway, such as paraldehyde, also produces a disulfiram reaction in the presence of disulfiram. Patients taking disulfiram are instructed not to ingest any alcoholic beverages, including cough syrups, special wine sauces, and fermented beverages (cider). As long as a patient is taking disulfiram, even a small amount of alcohol (1 ounce) will produce the unpleasant effects. In this manner, the disulfiram therapy acts as a reinforcing deterrent to alcohol consumption.

Chapter 12 Review

UNDERSTANDING TERMINOLOGY

Test your understanding of the material in this chapter by answering the following questions.

1. Differentiate between REM sleep and NREM sleep.
2. What is the difference between a sedative and a hypnotic?
3. Explain the meaning of automatism.
4. Differentiate between barbiturates and nonbarbiturates.
5. What is GABA an abbreviation for?

ACQUIRING KNOWLEDGE

Answer the following questions.

6. What is the major indication for the use of sedatives and hypnotics?
7. Explain the mechanism of action of barbiturate hypnotics. What are the main sites of action to produce this effect?
8. List the different stages of sleep and the characteristics of each.
9. How do barbiturates alter the normal sleep cycle?
10. What is the importance of enzyme induction caused by sedative-hypnotic drugs?
11. What adverse effects are caused by barbiturates?
12. How does GABA normally function?
13. Explain the mechanism of action of the benzodiazepine hypnotics.
14. How do benzodiazepine hypnotics alter the sleep cycle?
15. What is the main difference between flurazepam (Dalmane) and triazolam (Halcion)?
16. What are the advantages of the benzodiazepines over the barbiturate hypnotics?
17. List some of the effects that alcohol produces on the different body systems.
18. Explain how disulfiram (Antabuse) is used in the treatment of alcoholism and describe the disulfiram reaction.

Additional Reading

Ancoli-Israel S. Sleep problems in older adults: Putting myths to bed. *Geriatrics* 1997;52(1):20.

Kuhn W. Shift work: Circadian rhythm and survival in the ER. *Emerg Med* 1996;29(3):80.

Lewis DC. Alcoholism in the elderly. *Hosp Pract* 1997;32(3):211.

Mahowald MW. Initial evaluation of the patient with insomnia. *Hosp Med* 1995;31(2):50.

Mahowald MW. Update on treating insomnia. *Hosp Med* 1995;31(3):31.

Warmer TM. New strategies for treating alcohol withdrawal syndrome. *Hosp Med* 1995;31(3):54.

Internet Activities

Visit the **MedicineNet** Web site **(http://www.medicinenet.com)**. Under "Diseases and Treatments," click on the letter "A" and find the topic Alcohol, Pregnancy. Under this heading click on "Fetal Alcohol Syndrome." How is this condition diagnosed? What are the main problems, causes, and features of this syndrome?

Another search engine is the **National Clearinghouse for Alcohol and Drug Information (http://www.health.org)**. Click on "Alcohol and Drug Facts" and familiarize yourself with the topics and information available. This information may be useful for preparing reports on alcohol abuse and prevention.

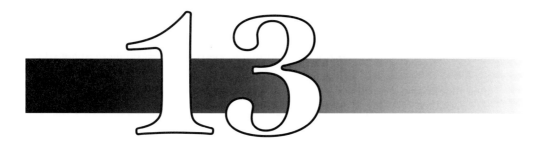

General Anesthetics

Henry Hitner, PhD
Barbara Nagle, PhD

Chapter Focus

This chapter describes drugs that reduce patient response to painful stimuli by altering patient consciousness.

Chapter Terminology

adipose tissue: Tissue containing fat cells.

analgesia: Decreased response to pain; condition in which painful stimuli are not consciously interpreted (perceived) as hurting.

dissociative anesthesia: Form of general anesthesia in which patients do not appear to be unconscious.

euphoria: Feeling of well-being or elation; feeling good.

general anesthesia: Deep state of unconsciousness in which there is no response to stimuli, including painful stimuli.

halogenated hydrocarbon: Compound that contains halogen (chlorine, fluorine, bromine, iodine) combined with hydrogen and carbon.

hypothalamus: Center of the brain that influences mood, motivation, and the perception of pain.

hypoxia: Reduction of oxygen supply to tissues below the amount required for normal physiological function.

induction of general anesthesia: Time required to take a patient from consciousness to Stage III of anesthesia.

maintenance of general anesthesia: Ability to keep a patient safely in Stage III of anesthesia.

medullary depression: Inhibition of automatic responses controlled by the medulla, such as breathing or cardiac function.

medullary paralysis: Condition in which overdose of anesthetic shuts down cardiovascular and respiratory centers in the medulla, causing death.

neuroleptanalgesia: Condition in which a patient is quiet, calm, and has no response to pain after the combined administration of a narcotic analgesic, fentanyl, and a tranquilizer, droperidol.

neuroleptanesthesia: State of unconsciousness plus neuroleptanalgesia produced by the combined administration of nitrous oxide, fentanyl, and droperidol.

synergistic: When the action resulting from a combination of drugs is greater than the sum of their individual drug effects.

Chapter Objectives

After studying this chapter, you should be able to:

- Identify the various stages of general anesthesia and describe the physical responses as the CNS functions are depressed.
- Name two classes of general anesthetics by their routes of drug administration.
- Explain why ketamine would be used in a patient with asthma.
- Explain the use of general anesthetic agents in the treatment of resistant asthmatic attacks.
- Explain what an adjunct to anesthesia is and cite two examples of drug adjuncts used with general anesthetics.
- List three side effects that may be associated with anesthetic use.
- Explain how postanesthesia residual effects can interfere with respiratory care.

Mild inhibition of cortical activity reduces anxiety, whereas more intense depression of the limbic and reticular systems produces sleep. Sleep is a state of unconsciousness in which stimulation such as yelling or shaking will arouse an individual. **General anesthesia** is a deeper state of unconsciousness (sleep) in which an individual cannot respond to stimulation.

General Anesthesia

Drugs discussed in the previous chapters selectively depress the CNS. During general anesthesia, all sensations are inhibited. Because sensations are suppressed, general anesthesia is used primarily to prevent the reactions to painful stimuli associated with surgery. General anesthesia agents are CNS depressants that abolish pain by inhibiting the function of the CNS through an unknown mechanism.

The extent of CNS depression under general anesthesia is much greater than that produced by other CNS depressant drugs (tranquilizers, sedatives, and hypnotics) at therapeutic doses. All of the major areas of the CNS are suppressed except for the medullary centers that regulate the vital organs (heart and lungs). An anesthesiologist controls the delicate balance between the beneficial effects of anesthesia and **medullary depression,** which can result in medullary paralysis and death.

SIGNS AND STAGES OF ANESTHESIA

General anesthesia is produced by gradually depressing the CNS. The sequence of depression is divided into four stages, as illustrated in Figure 13-1. During Stage I, the cerebral cortex is gradually inhibited. This stage is characterized by a decreased response to pain **(analgesia),** a feeling of **euphoria** (well-being or elation), and a loss of consciousness (sleep). Once the cerebral cortex is fully depressed, the **hypothalamus** assumes control of body functions (Stage II). Stage II is known as the "excitement phase" because there is an overall increase in sympathetic tone. Blood pressure, heart rate, respiration, and muscle tone increase during this stage. During Stage II, cardiac arrhythmias may occur. Eventually, however, the hypothalamus is depressed, and patients enter Stage III.

Stage III is usually referred to as surgical anesthesia because surgery is most ef-

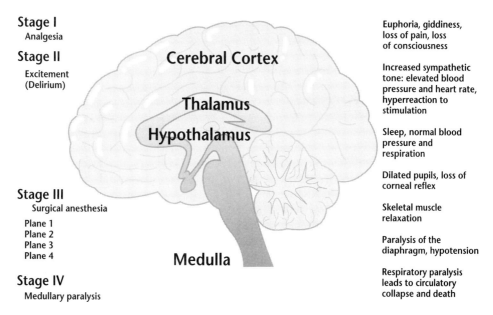

Stage I
Analgesia

Stage II
Excitement
(Delirium)

Stage III
Surgical anesthesia
Plane 1
Plane 2
Plane 3
Plane 4

Stage IV
Medullary paralysis

Cerebral Cortex

Thalamus

Hypothalamus

Medulla

Euphoria, giddiness, loss of pain, loss of consciousness

Increased sympathetic tone: elevated blood pressure and heart rate, hyperreaction to stimulation

Sleep, normal blood pressure and respiration

Dilated pupils, loss of corneal reflex

Skeletal muscle relaxation

Paralysis of the diaphragm, hypotension

Respiratory paralysis leads to circulatory collapse and death

Figure 13-1
Signs and stages of anesthesia associated with CNS depression.

ficiently performed at this level of general anesthesia. Stage III is divided into four planes (1–4) that reflect the progressive depth of CNS depression. During this stage, cardiovascular and respiratory functions return to normal, spinal reflexes are inhibited, and skeletal muscles are relaxed. Surgical incisions can be made throughout Stage III without producing pain or skeletal muscle contraction.

Stage IV is the phase of **medullary paralysis.** This stage represents an overdose of general anesthetic in which cardiovascular and respiratory centers in the medulla are inhibited, and death occurs.

The clinical signs associated with each stage of general anesthesia vary with the general anesthetic being used. Some anesthetics produce excellent analgesia at Stage I, whereas others do not produce any analgesia until Stage III. However, most anesthetics used today are capable of producing Stage III and IV anesthesia as just described. An anesthetic that produces all stages of general anesthesia (I, II, III, and IV) is a *complete* anesthetic.

INDUCTION AND MAINTENANCE

Induction of general anesthesia is the time required to take a patient from consciousness to Stage III. **Maintenance of general anesthesia** is the ability to keep a patient safely in Stage III. The ideal general anesthetic would produce rapid induction and slow maintenance without entering Stage IV anesthesia. In addition, recovery from the ideal general anesthesia would occur rapidly and without side effects.

Unfortunately, there is no ideal general anesthetic. Some anesthetics are excellent for induction (nitrous oxide, thiopental, and a combination of fentanyl citrate and droperidol), whereas others are better for maintenance of general anesthesia. Also, all anesthetics are associated with side effects. Today, anesthesiologists usually employ a combination of anesthetics to meet the needs of surgeons and to minimize patient reaction. Rapid, smooth induction with well-controlled maintenance is the key to good general anesthesia.

ROUTE OF ADMINISTRATION

General anesthetics are administered by inhalation or intravenous injection. These routes provide rapid delivery of the drug into the blood, which facilitates smooth induction of general anesthesia. Unlike other drugs, most of the general anesthetics do not bind to plasma proteins. General anesthetics dissolve in the blood before they are distributed to other tissues. Eventually, general anesthetics are carried to the CNS, where the primary pharmacologic effect is produced. The degree of CNS depression is related to the concentration of the anesthetic in the brain. However, the level of drug necessary to produce general anesthesia varies with each anesthetic. Induction and duration of general anesthesia also vary with each anesthetic and are related to the physical properties of the drug.

PHYSIOLOGICAL EFFECTS

Although the primary action of anesthetics is on the CNS, anesthetics also influence a variety of other tissues. Selection of the proper anesthetic may depend on the drug's alteration of cardiac, bronchial, or hepatic function.

CNS In general, all nervous tissue is depressed by general anesthetics. Voluntary (motor) and involuntary (autonomic) systems are inhibited. Respiratory function is depressed through a central action. However, oxygen deprivation does not occur because ventilation is controlled by the anesthesiologist. Some anesthetics cause pituitary secretion of ADH (antidiuretic hormone), resulting in postoperative urinary retention, especially in elderly patients.

Cardiovascular System The myocardium (heart muscle) and blood pressure may be depressed by general anesthetics. However, the degree of depression varies with the anesthetic used. Blood pressure may decrease because sympathetic tone is inhibited, whereas heart rate may increase as a result of vagal inhibition. Occasionally, catecholamines are secreted from the adrenal medulla, and these circulating catecholamines may counteract the myocardial depression. On the other hand, some anesthetics sensitize the heart to the catecholamine stimulation, and ventricular arrhythmias may occur.

Salivary and Bronchial Secretions Inhalation anesthetics irritate the mucosal lining of the respiratory tract and salivary glands. This irritation leads to the secretion of mucus, coughing, and spasms of the larynx in unconscious patients.

Skeletal Muscle Depression of pyramidal systems and spinal reflexes causes skeletal muscle relaxation in Stage III (Plane 3) anesthesia. However, certain anesthetics produce additional skeletal muscle relaxation by inhibiting neuromuscular function. Usually, acetylcholine is blocked from interacting with the skeletal muscle membrane in these situations.

GI Tract Nausea and vomiting are the most common side effects associated with the use of general anesthetics. These effects frequently occur during recovery, making patients uncomfortable. Decreased intestinal motility may lead to postoperative constipation.

Liver Halothane, enflurane, and chloroform, in particular, are suspected of producing liver damage (hepatotoxicity). Repeated exposure to these agents may cause altered enzyme production, jaundice, or hepatic necrosis. Patients with liver damage, jaundice, or known sensitivity to these anesthetics should not be exposed to them.

Use of General Anesthetics

General anesthetics include inhalation anesthetics and injectable anesthetics. In addition, there are adjuncts to general anesthesia.

INHALATION ANESTHETICS

Inhalation anesthetics include volatile liquids such as ether and **halogenated hydrocarbons** and gases such as nitrous oxide (see Table 13-1). These anesthetics are

Table 13-1

Side Effects and Uses of General Anesthetics

Anesthetic (Trade Name)	Use	Effect on Respiratory System	Nausea and Vomiting	Potentially Hepatotoxic
Inhalation Anesthetics—Volatile Liquids				
Chloroform	Obsolete	Seldom	Moderate	Yes
Ether	Maintenance	Frequently, increases secretions	High	—
Enflurane (Ethrane)	Maintenance	Seldom	—	Yes
Isoflurane (Forane)	Maintenance	Seldom	Low	Yes
Halothane (Fluothane)	Maintenance	Seldom	Low	Yes
Methoxyflurane (Penthrane)	Maintenance	Seldom	Low	Yes
Sevoflurane (Ultane)	Maintenance	Seldom	Low	No
Inhalation Anesthetic—Gas				
Nitrous oxide	Induction	—	Low	Yes
Injectable Anesthetics				
Etomidate (Amidate)	Induction	Bronchospasm	Low–moderate	—
Fentanyl citrate and droperidol	Induction	Seldom secretions, laryngospasms	Low	—
Ketamine (Ketalar)†	Induction and maintenance	Salivation and laryngospasm	High	—
Methohexital (Methohexital)‡	Induction and maintenance	Bronchial secretions	Moderate	—
Midazolam (Versed)‡	Preoperative sedation and induction	Salivation and bronchospasm	—	—
Propofol (Diprivan)	Induction and maintenance	Salivation	Low–moderate	—
Thiamylal (Surital)†	Induction	Bronchial secretions	Moderate	—
Thiopental (Pentothal)†	Induction	Seldom	Low–moderate	—

* Schedule II drug.
† Schedule III drug.
‡ Schedule IV drug.

usually inhaled through the nose and mouth by means of a face mask. Air (oxygen) must be included in the anesthetic mixture, or patients will rapidly develop **hypoxia** (reduction of oxygen supply to tissues below the amount required for normal physiological function). Anesthesiologists control the mixture and rate of delivery of anesthetic throughout the surgical procedure. When the face mask is removed, patients quickly exhale inhalation anesthetics. As a result of exhalation, the blood drug level falls, and the patients begin to recover from general anesthesia.

Most general anesthetics are excreted through the lungs. However, a small percentage of the halogenated hydrocarbons (halothane, enflurane, isoflurane, and methoxyflurane) are metabolized in the liver. All of the inhalation anesthetics except nitrous oxide (it is not potent enough to maintain Stage III, Plane 3 anesthesia) produce all stages of general anesthesia; therefore, they can be used for induction and maintenance of general anesthesia. Nitrous oxide ("laughing gas") can be used only for induction of general anesthesia. However, nitrous oxide produces such good analgesia that it is frequently used alone for dental procedures or in combination with other anesthetics.

Some of the anesthetic gases are potent bronchodilators and have been used in the treatment of asthmatic attacks that are resistant to other treatments. The primary gas had been halothane, but because of concerns over effects on the heart's ability to contract and the likelihood of electrical disturbances, it has been replaced with isoflurane. Isoflurane is equal to halothane in its bronchodilating effect without some of the toxicities. Its mechanism of action is not known but may be through release of endogenous catecholamines, interference with β-agonist receptors, or direct relaxation of airway smooth muscles.

There are some limitations of its use:

- Isoflurane, and the equipment to administer it, are expensive.
- Special equipment is needed to monitor its inspired and expired concentrations.
- It alters the metabolism of other drugs.
- Prolonged use leads to tolerance.

In most cases it is discontinued within 12 hours.

INJECTABLE ANESTHETICS

Injectable anesthetics include the barbiturates (methohexital, thiamylal, and thiopental), etomidate (Amidate), ketamine (Ketalar), midazolam (Versed), propofol (Diprivan), and a combination of fentanyl citrate and droperidol (see Table 13-1 for a display of injectable anesthetic effects). The barbiturate anesthetics can be used for induction or maintenance of general anesthesia. These drugs are usually administered intravenously because extravascular injections cause pain, swelling, and ulceration.

Thiopental, an ultrashort-acting barbiturate, induces general anesthesia within 30 seconds, but the tissue levels fall slowly. Barbiturate anesthetics are highly fat soluble and thus are redistributed to fatty tissues. The drug accumulates in **adipose** (fat) **tissue** and leaves the tissue so slowly that it takes a long time for these anesthetics to become metabolized and excreted into the urine. As the anesthetic leaves the adipose tissue, it is redistributed to other organs. Redistribution of the drug leads to residual CNS depression (hangover), mental disorientation, and nausea during the recovery period.

Barbiturate anesthetics are associated with the same effects and contraindications as other barbiturates (their adverse effects are discussed in Chapter 12). Barbiturate anesthetics may cause laryngospasm or bronchospasm during the postoperative recovery period. It is important to observe patients carefully because they may choke or aspirate fluid into the lungs. An absolute contraindication to the use of thiopental or methohexital as anesthetics is a history or predisposing evidence of status asthmaticus.

Etomidate (Amidate) and propofol (Diprivan) are hypnotic drugs used for intravenous induction of general anesthesia. Neither etomidate nor propofol has analgesic activity. These anesthetics depress the heart and respiratory centers less than the barbiturates. Because of their cardiorespiratory profile, these drugs may be advantageous for use in high-risk surgical patients who cannot tolerate tissue depression. Both have a rapid onset of action and, in the absence of repeated administration, are short-acting CNS depressants. Propofol is used in combination with other anesthetics for induction or maintenance of general anesthesia.

Midazolam (Versed) is a short-acting CNS depressant related to the benzodiazepines [diazepam (Valium) and chlordiazepoxide (Librium)] but more potent. Midazolam is frequently administered intravenously, orally, or intranasally before short diagnostic or endoscopic procedures (e.g., bronchoscopy) to produce conscious sedation. Patients are awake but do not fight against the intubation procedures. Midazolam is also used for induction of general anesthesia before administration of other anesthetics or to supplement nitrous oxide. Because of the significant CNS depressant action of midazolam, preanesthetic narcotic medications will potentiate its hypnotic effect. Elderly patients and patients with chronic obstructive pulmonary disease are often more sensitive to midazolam, experiencing a deeper depression of ventilatory mechanisms.

Ketamine (Ketalar) is a short-acting nonbarbiturate **dissociative anesthetic** that produces good analgesia and loss of memory but does not relax skeletal muscles. Therefore, patients appear to be awake although not responding to stimulation. Ketamine is thought to act primarily on the limbic system so that very little respiratory and cardiovascular depression is produced. In fact, blood pressure and heart rate may be elevated during the anesthesia. Ketamine is not the drug of choice in patients in whom a significant increase in blood pressure would be hazardous. However, it is the drug of choice when a bronchodilator is needed. Ketamine is a bronchodilator and has been used in the prevention of bronchospasm during general anesthesia and in the treatment of an acute asthmatic attack (status asthmaticus). It works by releasing endogenous catecholamines that relax airway smooth muscle.

This short-acting anesthetic is rapidly metabolized in the liver. It can be given intramuscularly or intravenously to induce anesthesia. Vivid dreams and hallucinations usually occur during the recovery period. In a small percentage of patients, delirium occurs. Severe reactions are treated with short-acting barbiturates. Ketamine is a restricted drug and is chemically related to phencyclidine, a hallucinogen of high abuse potential.

When a mixture of a narcotic analgesic (fentanyl) and a tranquilizer (droperidol), is administered, **neuroleptanalgesia** is produced. This type of anesthesia provides excellent analgesia while patients remain conscious. This combination cannot produce unconsciousness (**neuroleptanesthesia**) unless a third anesthetic (nitrous oxide) is added. Fentanyl and droperidol are eventually metabolized by the liver. Droperidol has an antiemetic effect that is advantageous as a surgical premedication. Droperidol reduces patient anxiety, nausea, and vomiting during diagnostic procedures. Unusual side effects that occur with the use of droperidol are extrapyramidal symptoms. Occasionally, a parkinsonian syndrome—uncontrolled movements of the tongue and head—occurs. The fentanyl–droperidol product may be administered intramuscularly or by slow intravenous injection. If a narcotic analgesic is prescribed following this kind of anesthesia, the dose of the narcotic may be significantly reduced to one-fourth of the recommended dose because these drugs have a **synergistic** action on the CNS.

ADJUNCTS TO GENERAL ANESTHESIA

In addition to the anesthetic agents, a variety of different drugs are routinely used before and after surgical procedures, as outlined in Table 13-2. Preanesthetic and postanesthetic medications are administered to aid induction of general anesthesia, counteract the side effects of anesthetics, or make recovery more comfortable for patients. Many people approach surgery with fear and apprehension; usually, there is intense anxiety about the existing medical problem and concern about the outcome of the operation. Some individuals also experience severe pain as a result of their medical condition. Anxiety and CNS stimulation tend to counteract a smooth induction into anesthesia. Therefore, CNS depressants such as narcotic analgesics, tranquilizers, or sedative-hypnotics may be administered before surgery. Often, these adjunct medications are given the evening before so that patients are groggy and unaware of the preparations being carried out before surgery.

Table 13-2
Adjunct Medications Used with Anesthetics

Pharmacologic Class	Administration	Reason for Use
Analgesics (narcotic)	Preanesthesia, postanesthesia	Relieve pain and produce sedation
Antianxiety agents	Preanesthesia	Decrease apprehension
Antiarrhythmic drugs	During surgery	Control arrhythmias
Antibiotics	Preanesthesia	Decrease infection
Anticholinergics	Preanesthesia	Decrease salivary and bronchial secretions
	During surgery	Prevent bradycardia
Cholinergic drugs	Postanesthesia	Relieve urinary retention
Sedative-hypnotic drugs (short-acting agents)	Preanesthesia	Decrease apprehension
Skeletal muscle relaxants	During surgery	Sustain skeletal muscle relaxation
Tranquilizers	Preanesthesia, postanesthesia	Sedate, control nausea and vomiting

Most general anesthetics that take patients into Stage III, Plane 3 anesthesia produce skeletal muscle relaxation. However, it may be advantageous in certain operations (abdominal and thoracic) to have skeletal muscle relaxation for a long time with minimal CNS depression. For this purpose, neuromuscular blocking drugs, such as tubocurarine or succinylcholine, may be administered during surgery. These drugs produce adequate skeletal muscle relaxation while patients are maintained in early Stage III anesthesia.

Anticholinergic drugs may be used as preanesthetic medications to prevent the salivary and bronchial secretions induced by some anesthetics. Bronchial secretions of mucus usually line the respiratory tract and may impair the transfer of oxygen and anesthetic across the lungs. If the secretions are not controlled, hypoxia may develop.

CAUTIONS AND DRUG INTERACTIONS

Many patients are not aware of possible drug reactions, allergies, or hypersensitivities that they have. This lack of awareness is especially likely if patients have not previously encountered surgery or preanesthetic medications. Therefore, patients should be carefully observed for any unusual reactions to medications before and after general anesthesia. Most of the problems that arise following general anesthesia result from residual depression of the CNS. Patients frequently feel "hung over," dizzy, or nauseous and should be assisted because mental disorientation may lead to impaired judgment and incoordination. Postanesthetic medications such as analgesics, muscle relaxants, and tranquilizers will potentiate the residual CNS depression of general anesthetics. Antibiotics such as streptomycin, kanamycin, and erythromycin will potentiate the skeletal muscle relaxation to produce muscle weakness and fatigue.

Several of the inhalation anesthetics and surgical adjuncts (skeletal muscle relaxants) produce malignant hyperthermia in certain individuals. This acute toxicity is associated with a genetic defect.

Special Considerations   With the use of any complete anesthetic, patient vital signs should be monitored frequently before, during, and after anesthesia. During the postoperatve recovery period, patients' airways must be kept unobstructed. It is important to check patients for signs of hypoxia (cyanosis), laryngospasm, or gagging, which can precipitate aspiration of fluid into a patient's lungs. Patients should be positioned so that the potential for aspiration of secretions is minimized. Intravenous fluids and vasopressor drugs should be kept available for the treatment of hypotensive episodes. Patients should be monitored and positioned to avoid redistribution of anesthetic to the CNS, which may precipitate severe hypotension and respiratory arrest during the recovery period.

Overdose occurs most often as a result of too much anesthetic administered or an excessively fast rate of administration. With supportive therapy, fluid replacement, and mechanical support of respiration, the effects usually reverse once the anesthetic is stopped. The patient is continually monitored until the vital signs return to an acceptable stable level.

Postoperative nausea often associated with the barbiturate anesthetics may be lessened or avoided by having patients fast before receiving the drug. Patients have experienced mental confusion following ketamine anesthesia. Because drugs such as ketamine may be used as adjuncts in diagnostic procedures, patients should be cautioned not to drive or operate hazardous machinery for 24 to 36 hours after recovering from general anesthesia.

Considerations for the Respiratory Care Practitioner

Patients are usually exposed to these drugs in the operating room environment. For all procedures it is expected that the patient will be closely monitored during and after surgery to ensure that adverse reactions are minimized. Even for diagnostic procedures, the patient is kept for observation until it is clear there is no immediate risk. An opportunity for adverse effects is more likely to occur because information was inadequate before the selection of the anesthetics and premedication regimen. Patient history is extremely important to ascertain which drugs are most appropriate. The patient interview provides information that is critical to minimizing adverse reactions to anesthetics. Alcohol consumption, blood pressure medication, antibiotics, and OTC product use should be thoroughly reviewed. For example, Midazolam (Versed) will be potentiated by CNS depressants, including the alcohol in any cough/cold preparations the patient may be taking.

The respiratory care practitioner plays an important role in postoperative recuperative therapy. This is especially true for patients who have a chronic respiratory condition in addition to the condition for which surgery was performed. The respiratory care practitioner may encounter residual effects in the patient postanesthesia that increase the difficulty of returning the patient to a state of good bronchial hygiene. The length of the procedure, the duration of exposure to anesthetics, and the respiratory condition of the patient before surgery all affect the amount of retained secretions the patient must mobilize during the postoperative recovery period. In addition, the duration of endotracheal intubation contributes to localized secretions through direct irritation of the tissue.

If the patient experiences residual recirculation of anesthetic in the blood (i.e., leaching from adipose tissue), the patient may not be able to control certain skeletal muscles to produce good, deep breaths during respiratory care treatment. This is further complicated when patients have had surgery on abdominal organs because the abdominal muscles may not be able to contract in a concerted efficient manner for several days. On the other hand, where secretions have been minimized by the combined effect of tissue dehydration in the bronchial tree during surgical procedures and antisecretory premedication, the patient may be "dry as a bone" during the postoperative recovery period. As a result, spontaneous coughing is usually nonproductive, and it requires the efforts of the respiratory care practitioner to educate and assist the patient in mobilizing bronchial secretions.

Hypersensitivity to anesthetics and/or premedications from previous exposure, or knowledge of a family member experiencing difficulty during surgery, may provide evidence of a contraindication to specific anesthetics. This is especially valuable as an indication of predisposition to malignant hyperthermia.

Chapter 13 Review

UNDERSTANDING TERMINOLOGY

Test your understanding of the material in this chapter by answering the following questions.

1. Name the brain center that influences mood, motivation, and the perception of pain.
2. Differentiate among analgesia, general anesthesia, dissociative anesthesia, medullary depression, and medullary paralysis.
3. Explain the difference between induction of anesthesia and maintenance of anesthesia.

ACQUIRING KNOWLEDGE

Answer the following questions.

4. How does general anesthesia differ from sleep?
5. How is general anesthesia produced?
6. Why is ketamine used for asthmatics?
7. What do the various stages of anesthesia represent?
8. What effects do general anesthetics have on the cardiovascular and respiratory systems?
9. How may the general anesthetics produce skeletal muscle relaxation?
10. How do the inhalation anesthetics differ from the injectable anesthetics?
11. How are general anesthetics used in the treatment of resistant asthmatic attacks?
12. For what purpose are the various adjunct medications administered?
13. What types of drug interactions may occur in postsurgical patients?

Additional Reading

Hazen SE. Elder care—general anesthesia and elderly surgical patients. *Assoc Oper Room Nurs J* 1997;65(4):815.

Humphries Y. Superiority of oral ketamine as an analgesic and sedative for wound care procedures in the pediatric patient with burns. *J Burn Care Rehabil* 1997;18(1):34.

McAuliffe MS. Anesthetic drug interactions. *CRNA Clin Forum Nurse Anesth* 1997;8(2):84.

Moore JL. Malignant hyperthermia. *Am Fam Physician* 1992;45(5):2245.

Strazis KP. Malignant hyperthermia: A review of published cases. *Anesth Analg* 1993;77(2):297.

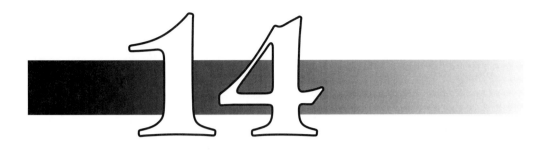

Narcotic (Opioid) Analgesics and Antitussives

Henry Hitner, PhD
Barbara Nagle, PhD

Chapter Focus

This chapter describes drugs that minimize the response (reaction or perception) to intense pain without altering consciousness. Narcotic analgesics are not general or local anesthetics, although they can be used in conjunction with general anesthetics to provide analgesia and reduce preoperative anxiety. The chronic use of narcotic analgesics at any dose for any indication can lead to tolerance and physical dependence. The potential for addiction is extremely rare when narcotic analgesics are prescribed for medical treatment. Patients should be aggressively managed for the treatment of pain.

Chapter Terminology

analgesic: Substance (synthetic or naturally occurring) that inhibits the body's reaction to painful stimuli or the perception of pain.

antidiuretic hormone (ADH):   Substance produced in the pituitary gland that decreases urine production by allowing the kidneys to reabsorb water.

antitussive: Able to suppress coughing.

anuria: No formation of urine.

dysphoria: Feeling of discomfort or unpleasantness.

emesis: Vomiting.

endogenous: Naturally occurring within the body.

expectorant: Substance that causes the removal (expulsion) of mucous secretions from the respiratory system.

narcotic: Substance extracted or derived from opium, or a synthetic substance that acts on the brain as do opiate drugs to relieve pain and induce sleep.

narcotic antagonist: Drug that attaches to opioid receptors and displaces the narcotic analgesic.

oliguria: Smaller than normal amount of urine produced.

opiate: Drug derived from opium and producing the same pharmacologic effects as opium.

opioid: Synthetic drug that produces the same pharmacologic effects as opium or a narcotic-like substance produced by the body.

peripheral nerve: Part of the nervous system that is outside the central nervous system (the brain or spinal cord), usually near the surface of the tissue fibers or skin.

physical dependency: Condition in which the body requires a substance (drug) not normally found in the body in order to avoid symptoms associated with withdrawal or the abstinence syndrome.

spasmogenic: Causing a muscle to contract intermittently, resulting in a state of spasms.

synthetic drug: Drug produced by a chemical process outside of the body.

tolerance: Ability of the body to alter its response (to adapt) to side effects so that the effects are minimized.

Chapter Objectives

After studying this chapter, you should be able to:

- Describe the sources of narcotic analgesics.
- Discuss the pharmacologic effects of these drugs.
- Discuss absorption and metabolism of these drugs.
- List the adverse effects of these drugs.
- Explain acute narcotic poisoning.
- Discuss the clinical actions of narcotic antagonists.
- Discuss narcotic effects that impact respiratory function encountered by the respiratory care practitioner.
- List the commonly prescribed antitussives.

Pain functions primarily as a protective signal. Pain may warn of imminent danger (fire) or the presence of internal disease (appendicitis or tumors). On the other hand, pain may be part of the normal healing process (inflammation). Relief from pain is necessary when the duration and intensity of pain alter the ability of an individual to function efficiently. In such situations, **analgesic** drugs are useful because these agents relieve pain without producing a loss of consciousness. There are two major classes of analgesics: the narcotic analgesics and the nonnarcotic analgesics. Narcotic analgesics are usually referred to as strong analgesics, whereas nonnarcotic drugs are considered mild analgesics. Such classification suggests the type of pain that can be alleviated by each group. Narcotic analgesics are capable of inhibiting pain of *any* origin. However, these drugs are used primarily to relieve the moderate to severe pain of trauma, pain associated with myocardial infarction, pain associated with terminal illness, and pre- and postoperative pain.

Narcotic Analgesics

SOURCE

Narcotic analgesics are derivatives of opium or synthetic chemicals that produce the same pharmacologic effects as opium. The naturally occurring narcotic analgesics, **opiates,** include morphine and codeine. Many of the other narcotic analgesics used today are **synthetic drugs** referred to as **opioids** (see Table 14-1). Morphine is considered the prototype, or standard, narcotic analgesic.

All narcotic analgesics relieve severe pain; however, they vary in potency, onset of action, and incidence of side effects, as shown in Table 14-2. Certain narcotics, such as fentanyl or sufentanil citrate, are selectively used as adjuncts to anesthesia. Because of their ability to provide excellent analgesia, the patient becomes more manageable and less anxious, and lower concentrations of general anesthetic are required to reach the surgical stage of anesthesia.

Regardless of the therapeutic indication for narcotic analgesics, all drugs in this class produce tolerance and physical dependence with chronic use. Narcotic analgesics are federally restricted drugs (Schedule II) because of their potential for abuse. Schedule II drugs can be obtained only by prescription (see Table 14-3).

Certain narcotic analgesics (codeine and dextromethorphan) are **antitussive** (suppress coughing) at doses that do not alter consciousness. In general, the antitussive narcotics are much less potent analgesics than morphine and possess a lower potential for abuse. Therefore, codeine and dextromethorphan are considered relatively safe and are frequently found in over-the-counter cough remedies (see Table 14-4).

In contrast, heroin is a derivative of morphine considered in the United States to have *no medicinal value* (it is used to treat terminal cancer patients in England). Heroin is one of the most potent and rapidly addicting narcotic analgesics and is absolutely restricted (Federal Comprehensve Drug Abuse Prevention and Control Act) from any clinical use (Schedule I).

Table 14-1

Analgesic Doses of Narcotic Analgesics

Drug (Trade Name)	Schedule	Adult Dose Analgesia	Intramuscular Administration	
			Onset (min)	Duration (h)
Opiates				
Codeine	II	15–60 mg PO, SC, IM, IV*	15–30	4–6
Heroin	I	No recognized medicinal value in the United States		
Hydromorphone (Dilaudid)	II	2 mg PO, 1–2 mg SC, IM, IV*	15–30	4–5
Morphine	II	5–20 mg IM, SC†	15–20	3–7
Opium tincture	II	0.6 mL QID	—	—
Oxycodone (Roxicodone)	II	5 mg PO*	15–30	4–6
Oxymorphone (Numorphan)	II	1–1.5 mg IM, SC*; 0.5 mg IV	5–10	3–6
Paregoric	III	5–10 mL PO (0.25–0.5 mg/kg for child) QD–QID	—	—
Opioids				
Alfentanil (Alfenta)	II	8–75 µg/kg IV	—	60
Buprenorphine (Buprenex)	V	0.3 mg IM, IV*	—	—
Butorphanol (Stadol)‡		0.5–2 mg IM,† IV	10	3–4
Butorphanol nasal spray (Stadol NS)‡		1 mg (one spray in one nostril); repeat if needed in 90 min	—	—
Dezocine (Dalgan)	II	5–20 mg IM, IV†	30	2–4
Fentanyl (Sublimaze)	II	0.05–0.1 mg/kg IM	5–15	1–2
Fentanyl transdermal (Duragesic)	II	Individualized dose		
Levorphanol (Levo-Dromoran)	II	2–3 mg PO, SC	30–90	6–8
Meperidine (Demerol)	II	50–150 mg PO, SC, IM†	10–15	2–4
Methadone (Dolophine, Methadone)	II	2.5–10 mg PO, IM, SC†	10–15	4–6
Nalbuphine (Nubain)‡	IV	10 mg/70 kg SC, IM, IV*	15	3–6
Pentazocine (Talwin)‡	IV	50–100 mg PO; 30 mg IM, SC†	20	3

Table 14-1 *(continued)*

Analgesic Doses of Narcotic Analgesics

Drug (Trade Name)	Schedule	Adult Dose Analgesia	Intramuscular Administration	
			Onset (min)	Duration (h)
Opioids (continued)				
Propoxyphene (Darvon, Dolene)	IV	65 mg PO†	15–30	4–6
Remifentanil (Ultiva)	II	Continuous infusion		
Sufentanil (Sufenta)	II	8–30 µg/kg IV	—	—
Central Analgesic (Nonopioid Receptor Active)				
Tramadol (Ultram)		50–100 mg PO*	15–30	2–4

* Dose repeated every 6 hours.
† Dose repeated every 3–4 hours.
‡ These drugs are partial antagonist analgesics.

SITE AND MECHANISM OF ACTION

The sensation of pain is composed of at least two elements: the local irritation (stimulation of **peripheral nerves**) and the recognition of pain (within the CNS). Recognition of pain involves a psychological component that intensifies the response to pain because the CNS anticipates how painful the irritation will be. This recognition leads to anxiety and apprehension (CNS stimulation), which heighten the patient's reaction to pain. Narcotic analgesics relieve severe pain by selectively acting within the CNS to decrease anxiety and reduce the reaction to pain. Narcotic analgesics do not impair the function of peripheral nerves. The pain is still present, but patients either can tolerate the pain or "don't care." In order to obtain the full analgesic effect, narcotic analgesics should always be given before intense pain is present. This technique is the basis for patient analgesic administration known as patient-controlled analgesia (PCA).

Morphine and other narcotic analgesic drugs are believed to act by mimicking the effects of narcotic-like substances that are produced in the body. The **endogenous** opioids, called endorphins, are present in the brain and spinal cord, where they bind to specific opioid receptors. An important function of endorphins is regulation of pain transmission from the periphery to the CNS. When administered intravenously, endorphins have been shown to be three to four times more potent than morphine. In addition to effects on pain perception, endorphins appear to play a role in mood control and in regulation of the cardiovascular, respiratory, and endocrine systems. The narcotic analgesic drugs interact with specific endogenous opioid receptors within the CNS. Narcotic analgesics reduce the awareness and perception of pain by stimulating the µ, κ, and σ receptors within the brain. The µ receptors mediate morphine-like analgesia, euphoria, and respiratory depression. The κ receptors mediate pentazocine-like analgesia and sedation. The σ receptors mediate dysphoria, hallucinations, and respiratory and vasomotor stimulation. By interacting with these three receptors, each narcotic analgesic expresses

Table 14-2
Pharmacologic Effects of Narcotic Analgesics

Drug	Risk of Physical Dependence	Analgesic Potency	Antitussive Activity*	Incidence of Nausea and Vomiting*	Respiratory Depression*
Alfentanil	NR	Same as morphine	Not rated	Not rated	Not rated
Codeine	Low	Less than morphine	3	1	1
Heroin	Highest	Greater than morphine	?	1	2
Hydrocodone	Low	Less than morphine	3	?	1
Hydromorphone	High	Greater than morphine	3	1	2
Levorphanol	High	Same as morphine	2	1	2
Meperidine	High	Same as morphine	1	2	2
Methadone	Low	Same as morphine	2	1	2
Morphine	High	Good	3	2	2
Oxycodone	High	Same as morphine	3	2	2
Oxymorphone	Highest	Greater than morphine	1	3	3
Pentazocine	Moderate	Less than morphine	Not rated	2	2
Propoxyphene	Low	Less than morphine	Not rated	2	1
Sufentanil	NR	Greater than morphine	Not rated	Not rated	Not rated

* 3, high; 2, moderate; 1, low; NR, not rated.

different degrees of pain control, respiratory depression, and liability for physical dependence.

Many of the narcotic analgesics such as morphine, codeine, oxycodone, hydromorphone, methadone, and fentanyl have predominately μ receptor activity. The μ agonists produce analgesia, which can be continually increased as the dose of the drug increases (no ceiling for analgesic effect). These analgesics are relatively short acting (3 to 6 hours); however, continuous-release preparations provide up to 12 hours of pain relief. Although tramadol is a κ agonist, it also inhibits serotonin and norepinephrine reuptake, which confers analgesia through a different mechanism.

Table 14-3
Drug Schedules Defined in the Federal Comprehensive Drug Abuse Prevention and Control Act

Schedule	Definition	Controlled Drugs
Schedule I (CI)	Drugs with high abuse potential and no accepted medical use	Heroin, hallucinogens; these drugs are not to be prescribed
Schedule II (CII)	Drugs with high abuse potential, severe dependence liability, and accepted medical use	Narcotics (morphine and pure codeine), cocaine, amphetamines, short-acting barbiturates; no refills without a new written prescription from the physician
Schedule III (CIII)	Drugs with less abuse potential than Schedule II, moderate dependence liability, and accepted medical use	Moderate- and intermediate-acting barbiturates, glutethimide, preparations containing codeine plus another drug; prescription required, may be refilled five times in 6 months when authorized by the physician
Schedule IV (CIV)	Drugs with low abuse and dependency potential and accepted medical use	Phenobarbital, chloral hydrate, antianxiety drugs (Librium, Valium); prescription required, may be refilled five times in 6 months when authorized by the physician
Schedule V (CV)	Drugs with *limited* abuse potential and accepted medical use	Narcotic drugs used in limited quantities for antitussive and antidiarrheal purposes; preparations containing 12.5 mg codeine plus another drug

Certain narcotics (nalbuphine, butorphanol, pentazocine) are partial antagonists. These drugs stimulate κ receptors (agonists) while blocking μ receptors (antagonists); hence the classification as partial antagonists. This group provides relatively less analgesia with lower abuse potential than pure narcotic agonists (morphine). Because of the dual receptor action, this group may produce dysphoria, reverse analgesia, and precipitate withdrawal in patients who are physically dependent on μ opioids.

PHARMACOLOGIC EFFECTS

Like the endogenous opioids, narcotic analgesics produce effects on a variety of tissues.

Effects on CNS   Narcotic analgesics may influence CNS function by increasing or decreasing certain CNS activities. For example, narcotic analgesics do not cause a loss of consciousness at therapeutic doses. However, these drugs do alter mental behavior. In particular, narcotic analgesics produce changes in mood and decrease mental alertness. Some individuals experience a feeling of well-being—a warm

Table 14-4
Combination Cold Preparations Containing Narcotic Antitussive Drugs*

Product Name	Antitussive	Liquid Concentration	Other Ingredients	Amount of Alcohol
Benylin Cough	10 mg dextromethorphan	2.0 mg/mL	Ammonium chloride, sodium citrate	5%
Children's Nyquil	5 mg dextromethorphan†	1.0 mg/mL	Pseudoephedrine, chlorpheniramine	—
Cheracol D	10 mg dextromethorphan	2.0 mg/mL	Guaifenesin	4.8%
Dimacol Caplets	10 mg dextromethorphan	—	Guaifenesin, pseudoephedrine	—
Multisymptom Tylenol Cold	15 mg dextromethorphan	1.0 mg/mL	Chlorpheniramine, pseudoephedrine	—
Novahistine DH Liquid	10 mg codeine‡	0.4 mg/mL	Pseudoephedrine, chlorpheniramine, guaifenesin	5%
Novahistine DMX Syrup	10 mg dextromethorphan	2.0 mg/mL	Pseudoephedrine	10%
Nyquil Nighttime Cold Medicine	5 mg dextromethorphan†	1.5 mg/mL	Pseudoephedrine, doxylamine, acetaminophen	25%
Robitussin A-C	10 mg codeine†	2.0 mg/mL	Guaifenesin	3.5%
Tylenol Cold Medication, Non-Drowsy	15 mg dextromethorphan	—	Pseudoephedrine, acetaminophen	—
Vicks Formula 44D	10 mg dextromethorphan†	2.0 mg/mL	Pseudoephedrine	10%
Vicks Formula 44M	10 mg dextromethorphan†	1.5 mg/mL	Pseudoephedrine, chlorpheniramine, acetaminophen	—

* Not an all-inclusive list of available products.
† Dose of dextromethorphan reduced from earlier formulation.
‡ Dose of codeine increased from earlier formulation.

glow—known as euphoria. This pleasant experience may entice the individuals to use the narcotic continually, thus contributing to the development of drug dependence. In contrast, other individuals may experience **dysphoria,** an unpleasant reaction, which enhances anxiety and fear. Dysphoric individuals are less likely to abuse these drugs.

In low doses, most narcotic analgesics produce nausea and vomiting. **Emesis** (vomiting) is a direct result of CNS stimulation of the chemoreceptor trigger zone, which in turn leads to direct stimulation of the vomiting center in the medulla. In some individuals, the frequency of vomiting increases when the patient is standing. (If gastrointestinal upset occurs after oral administration, the patient can be advised to take the medication with meals or milk.) As the dose of the narcotic is increased, the drug depresses the vomiting center. Therefore, at large doses, narcotic analgesics counteract their emetic response by inhibiting the vomiting center *(Figure 14-1)*.

One of the most important CNS effects produced by the narcotic analgesics is respiratory depression. All dose levels of narcotic analgesics depress respiratory activity by directly inhibiting the respiratory centers in the medulla and the pons. Respiratory rate and volume are reduced so that carbon dioxide (CO_2) is retained in the blood. Mild retention of CO_2 may produce headaches because CO_2 increases cerebral fluid pressure and intracranial pressure. As respiratory depression increases, so does CO_2 retention. However, the suppressed medulla cannot respond to CO_2 stimulation, and hypoventilation persists. The depth of respiratory depression increases as the dose of the drug increases. Death from narcotic poisoning is usually attributed to respiratory arrest.

Although only a few narcotic analgesics are used as antitussives, most narcotic analgesics suppress the coughing reflex at therapeutic doses. The antitussive effect is produced by direct inhibition of the coughing center in the medulla. These drugs do not cure the underlying cause of the irritation; they merely decrease the intensity and frequency of the cough. Once the cough reflex has been suppressed, patients become less irritable, less anxious, and are usually able to sleep comfortably.

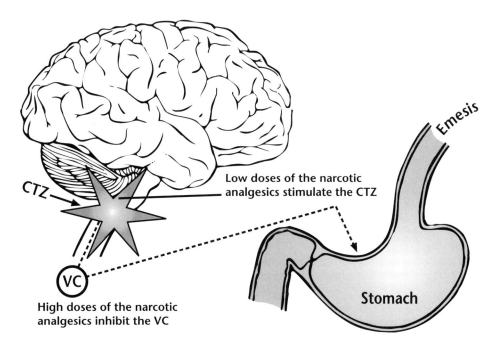

Figure 14-1
Vomiting reflex: Pathway between the chemoreceptor trigger zone (CTZ), the vomiting center (VC), and the stomach.

Effects on Smooth Muscle   Most of the other pharmacologic effects produced by the narcotic analgesics are a result of their **spasmogenic** activity. Narcotic analgesics increase smooth muscle tone, resulting in periodic muscle contractions or spasms. When spasms occur within the intestinal smooth muscle, peristalsis is inhibited. In addition, narcotic analgesics inhibit parasympathetic stimulation of the intestines by blocking the release of acetylcholine. Both of these effects can result in constipation, which frequently occurs with the use of narcotic analgesics. Only one narcotic analgesic derivative, diphenoxylate, is used in the treatment of persistent diarrhea. Constipation, a common problem with older patients, may be potentiated by the opioid analgesics, including over-the-counter preparations. Patients should be evaluated to assess bowel function so that appropriate stool softeners or laxatives may be recommended to maintain bowel function.

Many narcotic analgesics, especially morphine, produce spasm of the common bile duct, which causes pressure to increase in the gallbladder. Usually, this effect is accompanied by intense pain. In the presence of a narcotic analgesic, however, the painful signal may be eliminated, even though the pressure continues to increase. For this reason, narcotics such as morphine should be used with caution in patients with possible biliary obstruction. Urine formation and urination are both decreased by narcotic analgesics because these drugs stimulate the secretion of **antidiuretic hormone (ADH),** which allows the kidneys to reabsorb water. This decreases the volume of urine produced. In addition, spasmogenic activity of the ureters and sphincter muscles inhibits urine from passing out of the bladder. The combination of these effects usually produces **oliguria** (a smaller than normal amount of urine) rather than **anuria** (no formation of urine).

Narcotic analgesics affect bronchial smooth muscle by two actions. In addition to their spasmogenic action, narcotic analgesics cause the release of histamine, which directly constricts the bronchioles (see Chapter 18, Antiallergic and Antihistaminic Drugs). Constriction of the bronchioles narrows the airways, increasing the work of breathing. This response is dangerous in individuals who already have respiratory disease, including chronic bronchitis, obstructive lung disease, and asthma. Asthmatic patients may be unusually sensitive to histamine release, to the point that narcotic analgesics may induce an asthmatic attack.

Effects on Cardiovascular System   Narcotic analgesics do not depress cardiac function in therapeutic doses. This lack of effect is important because it allows these drugs to relieve the pain accompanying myocardial infarction without worsening the condition. Although the cardiac muscle is not affected, hypotension may occur as a result of histamine release and medullary vasomotor depression. Hypotension is frequently encountered on changing from a sitting position to a standing position (orthostatic hypotension).

Effects on Eyes   Most narcotic analgesics produce miosis (constriction of the pupil). This effect is caused by stimulation of the cholinergic center in the brain.

Most narcotic analgesics produce pinpoint pupils in toxic doses. However, meperidine produces mydriasis (dilation). Therefore, the pupil size cannot be used to determine what drug was used by unconscious (overdose) patients.

ABSORPTION AND METABOLISM

Because the narcotic analgesics are weak bases, these drugs are not well absorbed in the acid environment of the stomach. They are absorbed in the intestines, where the pH is more alkaline. However, certain narcotics, such as morphine, may be given by the oral route if the dose is adjusted. Three to six times the parenteral dose is required orally to produce comparable analgesic effects. Regardless of the route of administration, metabolic inactivation of the narcotics eventually occurs in the hepatic drug microsomal metabolizing system. Heroin is a particularly unusual drug because it is not metabolized to an inactive product. Heroin is rapidly changed into morphine, which then produces several pharmacologic responses.

Eventually, the kidneys excrete the metabolic products of the narcotic analgesics. Anything that causes the urine to become alkaline, such as alkalosis and diuretics, increases tubular reabsorption of the narcotics. This action elevates the concentration of drug in the blood and increases the risk of developing drug toxicity.

CLINICAL INDICATIONS OF ANALGESICS

Narcotic analgesics are approved for relief of severe acute and chronic pain that responds to opioids. Such pain is often associated with myocardial infarction, posttrauma back, head, or neck injury, or cancer. Occasionally, the root cause remains undefined. This is not the pain associated with chronic inflammatory conditions such as osteoarthritis. Recently, there has been a significant change in the attitude and methods regarding the treatment of chronic severe pain. Specialists in pain and symptom management use aggressive drug treatment schedules in which dosing is often under the control of the patient. This patient-controlled analgesia, known as PCA, allows the patient to use the lowest effective dose of opioid before the pain becomes unbearable. In effect, the patient minimizes the opportunity for dependence through lower dose exposure and a customized administration schedule. Drug delivery systems have also improved. Once available only through parenteral administration, certain opioids are now available in a transdermal patch so effective drug blood levels can be consistently achieved without invasive catheterization. For those patients requiring catheterization, implantable pumps have been developed that provide drug through intrathecal administration.

Another approved indication is opioid analgesic use as preoperative medication to facilitate sedation and reduce patient apprehension. By making the patient less apprehensive, physiological mechanisms are no longer poised to fight the anesthesia. As a result, premedication with narcotics often reduces the amount of anesthetic required and facilitates induction of anesthesia.

Select narcotic analgesics, codeine, dextromethorphan, and hydrocodone, are approved for use alone or in combination to suppress chemically or mechanically stimulated coughing.

ADVERSE EFFECTS

The most common effects produced by the narcotic analgesics include mental confusion, nausea, vomiting, dry mouth, constipation, and urinary retention. In sensitive individuals, histamine release produces hypotension and allergic reactions ranging from itching, skin rashes, and wheals to anaphylaxis. Therefore, it is important to determine whether patients are allergic to any narcotic agent before one is administered. The most serious adverse effects associated with the chronic use of narcotic analgesics are the development of **tolerance** and **physical dependency.** Tolerance quickly develops to the euphoria, analgesia, sedation, and respiratory depression produced by the narcotic analgesics. With chronic use, the dose must be increased continually to achieve the desired pharmacologic response (analgesia, euphoria). Patients are considered tolerant to opiates if they are taking more than 60 mg of morphine a day (or an equivalent analgesic dose of another opioid). At sufficiently large doses, even tolerant individuals die from severe respiratory depression. Although the onset of tolerance varies with the analgesic, cross-tolerance occurs with all narcotic analgesics, including codeine. On the other hand, tolerance seldom develops to the annoying spasmogenic effects of constipation and urinary retention. Even infants exposed to narcotic drugs through the placental blood have been born physically dependent on these drugs.

Although physical dependence and tolerance are consequences of long-term narcotic use, these conditions alone do not indicate addiction. **Addiction** is a disease state that results from a complex interaction of behavior, genetics, psychology, and neurobiology in which the individual responds to the opiate euphoria, the rush or high, as an enhanced reward. This response is reinforced by the use of short-acting narcotics through which the high can be experienced more often with repeated use. Once addiction has developed, the narcotic must be continually administered to avoid the onset of withdrawal symptoms (abstinence syndrome). Narcotic addiction is not limited to individuals who abuse heroin or morphine (street abuse). Medical professionals, who have access to narcotic analgesics, may become addicted as well.

The abstinence syndrome associated with narcotic analgesics gradually develops over the 72 hours following the last exposure to a narcotic ("fix"). During the initial period of withdrawal, sweating, yawning, restlessness, insomnia, and tremors occur. As the syndrome reaches its peak, blood pressure and irritability increase, accompanied by vomiting and diarrhea. Excessive sweating, gooseflesh, chills, and skeletal muscle cramps develop toward the end of the withdrawal period. Individuals who are addicted to the narcotic analgesics usually survive the withdrawal period. Administration of a narcotic at any time during the withdrawal period will suppress the abstinence syndrome. Other CNS drugs such as barbiturates, alcohol, or amphetamines cannot suppress narcotic withdrawal. However, when acute withdrawal has occurred, sometimes clonidine is administered to reduce the autonomic symptoms, and benzodiazepines are given to reduce the irritability, anxiety, and insomnia while the patient is being managed through the crisis.

In the treatment of narcotic addiction, methadone is particularly useful because it satisfies an addict's narcotic hunger so that the individual actually becomes acclimated to methadone. Methadone does not produce severe withdrawal symptoms, and the symptoms occur gradually during the 6- to 7-week maintenance compared to 72 hours for other narcotics. Because oral methadone is half as potent as parenteral methadone, it is easier to withdraw patients from methadone gradually without incurring a severe abstinence syndrome. Levomethadyl acetate is another drug that is used only for the management of opiate dependence, ie, treatment of narcotic addiction.

ACUTE NARCOTIC POISONING

Narcotic overdose, or acute poisoning, frequently occurs from accidental ingestion (children), attempted suicide, or exposure of a fetus during pregnancy. The symptoms of poisoning include coma, respiratory depression, cyanosis, hypotension, and a fall in body temperature. Once patients receive adequate ventilatory support, the poisoning can be treated with specific narcotic antagonists.

SPECIAL FORMULATIONS

Today there are a number of novel formulations designed to improve patient compliance or achieve analgesia even when high doses are required (eg, pain accompanying cancer). Opioids can be given orally, rectally, subcutaneously, intravenously, intraspinally, transdermally, and transmucosally. Patients must be instructed on the use of nasal sprays or transdermal patches. Practice preparation and application using these systems is essential to obtain good compliance, especially in older patients. For transdermal patch application, the area should be clear of hair. Shaving is not the method of choice because it could irritate the skin and promote absorption of greater amounts of drug. Creams, lotions, and soaps, which could irritate the skin or prevent patch adhesion, should not be used. Fever or high temperatures of climate can cause the patch to release more drug, resulting in toxicity. Patients should be instructed to clearly identify those times when they may be in hotter climates than usual so that dose adjustment can be considered.

Fentanyl is available as a lozenge called an *Oralet* to induce conscious sedation prior to therapeutic procedures. The Oralet is placed in the patient's mouth and the patient is instructed to suck (now chew) the medication. This permits transmucosal absorption of the drug in order to achieve appropriate peak blood concentrations. Another transmucosal preparation of fentanyl, known as *Actiq*, is available for the treatment of breakthrough cancer pain.

CAUTIONS AND CONTRAINDICATIONS

Narcotic analgesics should be used with caution in patients with bronchial asthma, heavy pulmonary secretions, convulsive disorders, biliary obstruction, or head injuries. In these cases, narcotic analgesics may worsen the existing condition. Ambulatory and elderly patients should be warned about the drowsiness that may accompany the use of narcotic analgesics in the acute (early) exposure to these drugs. Since narcotic analgesics will cross the placental barrier and affect the fetus, chronic use of these drugs by the mother during pregnancy should be avoided. It is not uncommon for narcotic analgesics to be administered to reduce the pain associated with labor and thus facilitate delivery. Short-term exposure of the fetus at term (from use of these drugs at parturition) presents relatively little potential danger to the newborn.

Because of their adverse effects and the potential of physical dependency, narcotic analgesics should never be used when a nonnarcotic analgesic can relieve the pain. Whenever narcotic analgesics are to be administered intravenously, naloxone should be readily available.

DRUG INTERACTIONS

Very few specific drug interactions occur with the narcotic analgesics. Narcotic analgesics potentiate the depression of any CNS-depressant drug (sedative-hypnotics, alcohol, and general anesthetics). Meperidine undergoes an unusual, potentially fatal, reaction when used in the presence of MAO inhibitors. Sweating, hypotension, or hypertension may occur in patients taking meperidine with pargyline, phenelzine, or tranylcypromine concomitantly. Dextromethorphan has been reported to undergo a similar interaction with phenelzine. As a result, dextromethorphan should not be given to patients who are receiving MAO inhibitors. Rifampin and phenytoin have been associated with reduction in the plasma concentrations of methadone sufficient to induce withdrawal symptoms.

CONSIDERATIONS FOR THE RESPIRATORY CARE PRACTITIONER

Narcotic analgesics are frequently administered on a repeated schedule (every 4 to 8 hours) to relieve moderate to severe pain. For full analgesic effect, the drug must be taken before intense pain occurs. It is important, therefore, that narcotic analgesics be administered on time, as scheduled. Adherence to the prescribed schedule ensures that patients have an adequate blood level of drug to sustain an analgesic effect. If the next dose of drug is significantly delayed, the pain will recur and may be enhanced by psychological factors associated with anticipation of discomfort.

The respiratory care practitioner may encounter patients receiving nebulized morphine for the treatment of pain associated with cancer. For such treatment the pharmacist prepares the morphine dose prior to patient administration; it is not a commercially available preparation. The morphine dosage is customized to the patient's status; however, administration prior to peak pain dictates the dosing schedule for the patient.

The respiratory care practitioner should always remember the potential for orthostatic hypotension from narcotic analgesics. If the patient needs to be moved from one location to another, the patient should first be moved from a lying to a sitting position. Allow the patient's blood pressure to accommodate the change in position before having the patient stand. Once the patient is standing, again wait a minute or two to allow for the blood pressure to accommodate before having the patient walk to a different location. Whether working in inpatient, outpatient, or home-care settings, the respiratory care practitioner is in the position to remind patients to take drugs, especially opioids, as prescribed. The patient must not change the dose or dose interval unless instructed by the physician. The respiratory care practitioner may observe the signs and symptoms of a drug reaction or drug interaction that should be brought to the physician's attention.

Narcotic analgesics are CNS depressants at any dose. Thse drugs cause hypoventilation. It is therefore important to monitor vital signs, especially respiration rate, when patients, in particular the elderly, are receiving these drugs. Dose adjustment may be indicated by decreased blood pressure or respiratry rate and tidal volume; cardiovascular or respiratory depression is an indication that the patient has been overmedicated. Shortness of breath or difficulty breathing should be reported to the physician immediately. Hypersensitivity to these drugs is a contraindication for their use. Patients with depressed respiratory function such as chronic obstructive pulmonary disorder (COPD), emphysema, or severe asthma will exhibit respiratory distress from narcotic-induced respiratory depression. Any elevation in body temperature, such as fever, which is not associated with flu or cold, should be considered as a potential side effect and should be reported to the physician.

Although opioid analgesics are frequently used in a controlled environment such as a hosptial or rehabilitation center, there is considerable opportunity for outpatient (unsupervised) use of prescription as well as over-the-counter analgesics. This potentiates the opportunity for adverse reactions to develop. Alcohol and CNS depressants enhance the narcotic depressant cffects and work to depress cardiorespiratory function.

USE IN PREGNANCY

Drugs in this class have been designated Pregnancy Category C or NR, not rated. Adequate studies in humans have not been conducted to establish safety in pregnancy. However, the potential benefit to the pregnant patient may outweigh the risks.

NARCOTIC ANTAGONISTS

Narcotic antagonists are drugs that attach to the opioid receptors and displace the narcotic analgesic. Narcotic displacement rapidly reverses life-threatening respiratory depression. There are two types of narcotic antagonists—pure antagonists and partial antagonists (Table 14-5). Pure antagonists, such as naloxone and nalmefene, are competitive blocking drugs. Naloxone occupies the opioid receptors but has no agonist activity (stimulation); it inhibits the narcotic analgesic from attaching to the receptors but does not produce any pharmacologic action of its own. Partial antagonists, such as butorphanol, nalbuphine, and pentazocine, have two actions on the respiratory system. These drugs produce weak morphine-like effects in normal individuals, resulting in respiratory depression. In cases of acute narcotic poisoning, however, partial antagonists reverse the respiratory depression. Partial antagonists bind with the receptors and produce little or no stimulation of the receptors that mediate respiratory depression. Today, the drug of choice in the treatment of acute narcotic poisonings is naloxone because it does not produce any respiratory depression.

Table 14-5

Narcotic Antagonists Used to Treat Narcotic Analgesic Respiratory Depression or Addiction

Drug (Trade Name)	Type of Antagonist	Adult Dose
Treatment of Respiratory Depression		
Naloxone (Narcan)	Pure	0.4–2 mg repeated at 3-min intervals IM, SC, IV
Nalmefene (Revex)	Pure	Individualized dose by weight
Treatment of Addiction		
Naltrexone (ReVia)	Pure	Only after the patient has been opioid-free for 7–10 days; maintenance dose 50 mg every 24 h
Methadone	—	15–20 mg PO initially; 40 mg for those dependent on high narcotic doses
Levomethadyl (Orlaam)	—	Maintenance dose 60–90 mg three times a week

ANTITUSSIVE NARCOTICS AND EXPECTORANTS

Antitussives. Among the narcotic antitussive drugs, codeine, hydrocodone, hydromorphone, and noscapine are natural derivatives of opium, whereas dextromethorphan is a synthetic product. Among these narcotic drugs, dextromethorphan or very small amounts of codeine have a recognized therapeutic value. Codeine, in analgesic doses in particular, has come under close scrutiny because of its potential for misuse.

The adult antitussive dose of codeine is 10 to 20 mg every 4 to 6 hours. For dextromethorphan, a dose of 15 to 30 mg is recommended over the same time interval. For children 6 to 12 years of age, one-half the adult dose is usually recommended. Table 14-6 compares antitussive doses for the narcotic antitussive drugs. These drugs are considered effective for the treatment of a nonproductive cough that is unable to mobilize mucus. Dextromethorphan is frequently found as the principal drug in over-the-counter cough and cold preparations.

Cough suppression may be only one objective in relieving the symptoms of a

Table 14-6

Comparative Doses of Narcotic Antitussive Drugs

Antitussive Drug	Adult Oral Antitussive Dose
Codeine	10–20 mg every 4–6 h
Dextromethorphan	15–30 mg every 4–8 h
Hydrocodone	5 mg every 4–6 h
Hydromorphone	1 mg every 3–4 h

cold. Additional objectives of therapy include relieving nasal congestion, reducing pain and fever, and promoting bed rest through sedation. It is not surprising, therefore, that agents such as expectorants, antihistaminics, sympathomimetics, and alcohol are present in various combinations in over-the-counter cold and cough preparations. When codeine or hydrocodone is present, the cold preparation may be classified as Schedule III or Schedule V because other active ingredients (such as antihistaminics, sympathomimetic amines) result in a preparation with a lower potential for abuse.

Although not considered an antitussive drug, lidocaine (1% to 2%) is a local anesthetic administered in a hand-held nebulizer to suppress coughing in respiratory care patients. The local anesthetic acts topically, at the point of contact with source of the irritation, to inhibit the conduction of impulses to the central nervous system and reduce coughing.

Coughing is essential to good bronchial hygiene because it periodically permits a high-speed expiration, which mobilizes retained secretions. An effective cough can occur only if the patient has adequate inspiratory volume. Patients who experience pain during inspiration (such as posttrauma, postsurgery, or during pleural inflammation) interrupt inspiration and coughing as a result of experiencing pain. This causes mucus accumulation in the bronchial tree, and more serious respiratory problems may develop. Therefore, it is not uncommon for a narcotic analgesic to be given to dampen the patient's reaction to involuntary control of respiratory and coughing. The dose of the narcotic analgesic is selected to avoid spasm of bronchial smooth muscle.

Expectorants are neither opioids nor narcotics. Expectorants are presented here because they are often combined with antitussive drugs to alter the volume and viscosity of mucus retained in the respiratory tract. Expectorants are mucokinetic; that is, they promote the discharge of mucus from the respiratory tract, thus reducing chest congestion and potential infection by removing the environment for pathogenic microorganism growth. There are two classes of expectorants: mucolytic expectorants and stimulant expectorants.

Mucolytic expectorants, such as acetylcysteine *(Mucosil),* are presented in the chapter on Bronchodilator Drugs and the Treatment of Asthma (Chapter 19). These drugs attack sulfur (sulfhydryl) bonds within the mucopolysaccharide component of mucus. As the mucus is broken into smaller mucopolysaccharide chains, the viscosity is reduced, with the goal of making the mucus easier for the patient to mobilize from the respiratory tree.

Stimulant expectorants, as the name implies, irritate the gastric mucosa, resulting in a reflex vagal stimulation of bronchial glands to produce more secretions. Even though these expectorants cause more bronchial secretion, the quality of the secretion is altered. In a well-hydrated patient, water will be incorporated into the bronchial secretions, thus making the secretions less viscous and easier to move. This is the reason why patients are encouraged to "push fluids" such as water or fruit juices rich in water content. Expectorants may be administered by mouth and absorbed into the circulation through the gastrointestinal system (vagal reflex), or they may be aerosolized or nebulized and delivered directly to the respiratory mucosa (topical stimulation).

Stimulant expectorants commonly found in combination with OTC antitussive products include ammonium chloride, guaifenesin, and terpin hydrate. Guaifenesin, also known as glycerol guaiacolate, is believed to decrease the adhesiveness of mucus (by reducing surface tension), making it easier for the patient to mobilize. There is some doubt that traditional expectorants such as ammonium chloride, terpin hydrate, and menthols are clinically effective in altering mucus production. Nevertheless, these drugs are still found in recommended and alternative medications for the treatment of cough, cold, and mucus.

Other active substances commonly found in combination with cough suppressants and expectorant are sympathomimetic amines (ephedrine, phenylephrine, and pseudoephedrine), which are combined with antitussive drugs to produce nasal decongestion by constricting nasal blood vessels. The antihistamines that are H_1 antagonists, such as chlorpheniramine and pyrilamine, exert an anticholinergic action, which may decrease secretion of mucus, whereas alcohol may act as a CNS depressant.

It is not unusual to find that liquid preparations contain alcohol, some in excess of 15%. (Consider the possible CNS interactions that may occur when these products are used in addition to other prescription medications.) Table 14-4 lists examples of combination cold preparations that contain a narcotic antitussive as the principal active drug. Note the concentration of the antitussive product as well as the types of additional pharmacologic agents in each preparation. Although this is not an exhaustive list of available products, notice the various amounts of alcohol present in even pediatric liquid preparations. It is no wonder some of these products are recommended for bedtime use; they certainly can promote sleep.

Note to the Respiratory Care Practitioner

An effective method of thinning retained secretions in respiratory patients is administration of nebulized saline (salt water).

Aerosolized alcohol has been used to decrease mucus surface tension and decrease viscosity. It is used on occasion as a defoaming agent in the treatment of pulmonary edema.

Chapter 14 Review

UNDERSTANDING TERMINOLOGY

Answer the following questions.

1. What is a narcotic?
2. Describe an antitussive effect.
3. Define narcotic antagonist.

Match the definition or description in the left column with the appropriate term in the right column.

4. The opposite of euphoria.   a. ADH
5. Naturally occurring within the body.   b. analgesic
6. Production of only a small   c. anuria
   amount of urine.
                                          d. dysphoria
7. Vomiting.
                                          e. emesis
8. Production of no urine.
                                          f. oliguria
9. A substance that inhibits one's
   reaction to pain.   g. endogenous
10. Antidiuretic hormone.

ACQUIRING KNOWLEDGE

Answer the following questions.

11. What types of pain are relieved by narcotic analgesics?
12. What are the therapeutic uses of narcotic analgesics?
13. What is the proposed mechanism of action of narcotic analgesics?
14. What effects do the narcotic analgesics have on the CNS?
15. How might these effects be involved in other drug interactions? What drugs might potentiate CNS respiratory depression?
16. What is the spasmogenic action of the narcotic analgesics?
17. Why does urine retention occur with the use of narcotic analgesics?
18. Are all narcotic analgesics administered orally? Why or why not?
19. What adverse effects are associated with narcotic analgesics?

APPLYING KNOWLEDGE ON THE JOB

Answer the following questions.

20. One of your responsibilities is to alert the physician about patients with prescriptions that have potential precautions or drug interactions. What

would you recommend with each of the following prescriptions for the patients in question?

   a. Patient A has been prescribed codeine for severe headaches. Pharmacy records indicate that the patient also takes *Metaprel,* a bronchodilator prescribed for bronchial asthma.

   b. Patient B has been prescribed morphine for severe postoperative pain. You note in reviewing his chart that he also takes the drug *Moduretic,* a diuretic, for hypertension.

   c. Patient C has been prescribed *Demerol* for a muscle injury. She's already taking *Nardil* for depression.

21. For each of the following adult patients, how much narcotic is needed to produce the desired effect?

   a. Patient A has been prescribed codeine for dental pain.

   b. Patient B has been prescribed a cough preparation containing codeine.

   c. Patient C had been prescribed *Dilaudid* for pain associated with cancer.

   d. Patient D has bronchitis and has been prescribed *Dilaudid* for his painful cough.

Additional Reading

Bedder MD. Epidural opioid therapy for chronic nonmalignant pain: A critique of current experience. *J Pain Symptom Manage* 1996;11(6):353.

Dejo RA. Drug therapy for back pain. Which drugs help which patients. *Spine* 1996; 21(24):2840.

Goldstein FJ. Preemptive analgesia: A research review. *MEDSURG Nursing* 1995;4(4):305.

Kress JP. Sedating critically ill ventilated patients: A pharmacologic primer. *J Crit Ill* 1997;12(5):287.

Louie K. Management of intractable cough. *J Palliat Care* 1992;8(4):46.

St. Marie B. Chemical abuse and pain management. *J Intra Nurs* 1996; 19(5):247.

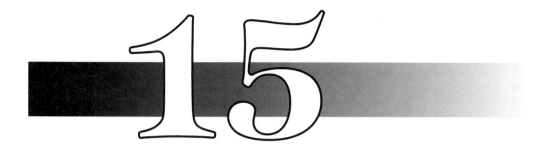

Cardiac Physiology and Pathology

Henry Hitner, PhD
Barbara Nagle, PhD

Chapter Focus

This chapter describes the basic physiological concepts of normal heart function and the diseases that commonly affect the heart. It also explains how these disease states affect cardiac function.

Chapter Terminology

angina pectoris: Chest pain caused by insufficient blood flow to the heart.

arteriosclerosis: Hardening or fibrosis of the arteries.

atherosclerosis: Accumulation of fatty deposits in the walls of arteries.

AV: Atrioventricular.

CAD: Coronary artery disease.

CHF: Congestive heart failure.

conduction system: Specialized cardiac tissue that regulates the activity of the heart.

electrocardiogram (ECG):   Recording of the electrical activity of the heart.

myocardial infarction (MI):   Heart attack.

myocardium: Heart muscle.

SA: Sinoatrial.

Chapter Objectives

After studying this chapter, you should be able to:

- Describe normal cardiac function related to contractility, blood flow, and neuronal control.
- Explain the consequences of congestive heart failure on the cardiovascular system.
- Describe the development and progression of coronary artery disease.

The heart is a muscle whose main function is to generate the force that moves the blood through the circulatory system. Occasionally, efficient heart function becomes impaired and results in a life-threatening situation. Fortunately, however, several classes of drugs are therapeutically useful in alleviating many cardiac conditions.

Cardiac Function

To understand the action of the different classes of drugs that affect the heart, it is convenient to divide it into three functional parts: cardiac muscle, conduction system, and nerve supply.

CARDIAC MUSCLE

The pumping ability of the heart depends on the arrangement of the heart muscle **(myocardium)** into a system of four chambers. Contraction of the chambers increases pressure within the ventricles and forces the blood through a system of valves and out into the general circulation. This is illustrated in Figure 15-1.

The blood supply to the myocardium is routed via the corinary arteries that branch off the aorta immediately after the aorta leaves the heart. Under normal conditions, blood flow in the coronary arteries is dependent on the force of myocardial contractions. Any interference with the normal function of the myocardium or with the normal flow of blood to the myocardium results in a decreased capacity of the heart to contract.

CONDUCTION SYSTEM

The **conduction system** of the heart is composed of a specialized type of muscle tissue that is located in specific areas of the heart. The conduction system is illustrated in Figure 15-2.

Conduction tissue has a unique characteristic, known as autorhythmicity. This characteristic enables the heart to initiate its own electrical stimulation. Normally, an electrical impulse is generated within the sinoatrial **(SA)** node. This impulse continues through the atrioventricular **(AV)** node into the common bundle of His, through the left and right bundle branches and Purkinje fibers. This movement

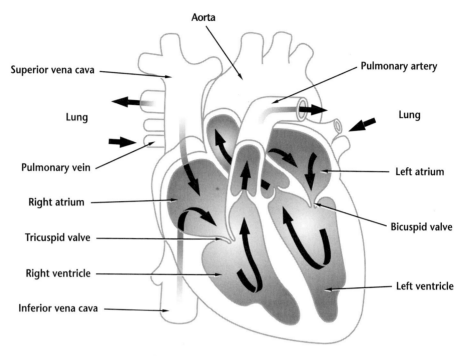

Figure 15-1
Blood flow through the cardiac chambers and valves.

results in contraction of the atria followed by contraction of the ventricles. Thus, the conduction system is responsible for coordinating the contractions of the heart chambers.

A recording of the electrical activity of the conduction system results in a characteristic waveform known as the **electrocardiogram (ECG).** The pattern of the ECG reflects depolarization (sodium ions entering the cell) and repolarization (potassium ions leaving the cell) of cardiac tissue. Depolarization of the atria produces the P wave of the ECG. The PR interval is the time required for passage of an electrical impulse from the SA node through the AV node. Depolarization of the ventricles produces the QRS wave (AV node through Purkinje fibers). Repolarization of the ventricles produces the ST segment and the T wave. A normal ECG is shown in Figure 15-2.

NERVE SUPPLY

The heart receives its nerve supply from both divisions of the autonomic nervous system. Because the heart possesses the ability to initiate its own heartbeat, the function of the autonomic nervous system is to regulate the rate and force of contraction of the heart. Sympathetic nerves release norepinephrine at the nerve endings, increasing heart rate (positive chronotropic action) and force of contraction

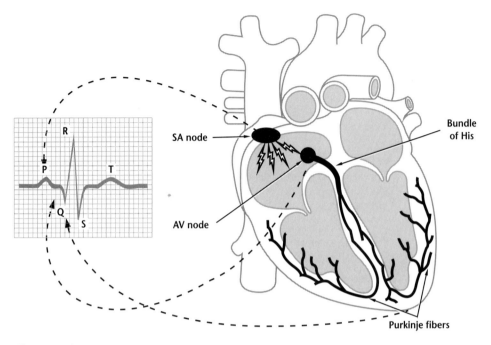

Figure 15-2
Relationship between the cardiac conduction system and electrocardiogram.

(positive inotropic action). Parasympathetic nerves release acetylcholine at the nerve endings, decreasing heart rate (negative chronotropic action) and force of contraction (negative inotropic action). Each division opposes the other, and, depending on the level of body activity, one division adjusts its activity so that homeostatic conditions are maintained.

Main Diseases of the Heart

The two most common diseases affecting the heart are congestive heart failure **(CHF)** and coronary artery disease **(CAD).**

CONGESTIVE HEART FAILURE

In congestive heart failure, the contractile ability of the heart to pump blood is decreased so that the heart pumps out less blood than it receives. Blood accumulates inside the chambers, causing enlargement (dilation) of the heart. Consequently, there is less blood circulating in the blood vessels to supply the body organs. The kidneys—particularly sensitive to a decrease in blood flow—respond by retaining more water and electrolytes, leading to fluid retention and general edema.

When the left side of the heart fails, fluid accumulates in the lungs (pulmonary edema) and interferes with gas exchange, resulting in shortness of breath. When the right side fails, fluid accumulates in the abdominal organs (ascites) and lower extremities. Failure of one side of the heart is usually followed by failure of the other side, resulting in total heart failure. Congestive heart failure is treated with cardiac glycosides, diuretics, and a variety of vasodilator drugs.

CORONARY ARTERY DISEASE

Coronary artery disease is a general term for several types of cardiac disease. An insufficient flow of blood through the coronary arteries to the heart is a common factor in all these diseases.

Arteriosclerosis   Arteriosclerosis is a disease of the aging process in which there is a hardening (fibrosis) and narrowing of the arteries. These changes result in a decreased blood flow. One type of arteriosclerosis, in which fatty deposits (plaques) accumulate within the walls of the arteries, is known as **atherosclerosis.** The coronary arteries are particularly prone to both conditions, and, as stated earlier, any abnormal decrease in coronary blood flow decreases the function of the heart.

Angina Pectoris   Angina pectoris refers to the clinical condition characterized by chest pain caused by insufficient coronary blood flow. Arteriosclerosis, atherosclerosis, and coronary artery spasms appear to be the causes of angina pectoris. Attacks of angina, usually caused by physical exertion or psychological stress, are relieved by rest and a class of drugs known as the vasodilators, or antianginal drugs.

Myocardial Infarction   Heart attack **(myocardial infarction, or MI)** is the leading cause of death in industrialized nations. When an area of the myocardium is deprived of its blood supply (ischemia), the muscle cells die (necrosis), resulting in an area of dead cells known as an infarct. Complete blockage, or thrombosis, of one of the coronary arteries is usually responsible for a myocardial infarction.

Large infarcts usually result in sudden death, whereas lesser infarcts undergo a healing process in which the dead muscle cells are replaced by connective (scar) tissue. Consequently, after an attack, the amount of contractile tissue of the heart is permanently reduced. Secondary complications commonly involve the development of congestive heart failure or disturbances of the conduction system (cardiac arrhythmias). Treatment for a myocardial infarction is aimed at allowing the heart to rest and undergo its normal healing process while treating any complications.

Chapter 15 Review

UNDERSTANDING TERMINOLOGY

Test your understanding of the material in this chapter by answering the following questions.

1. What is the difference between angina pectoris and myocardial infarction?

2. What do the following abbreviations stand for: AV, CAD, CHF, ECG, SA?

3. Differentiate between arteriosclerosis and atherosclerosis.

ACQUIRING KNOWLEDGE

Answer the following questions.

4. Describe the path of blood flow through the cardiac chambers. Which ventricle forces the blood into the general circulation (aorta)?

5. How is the blood supplied to the myocardium?

6. What makes the cardiac conduction system unique? Where is the conduction system located?

7. Describe the path of an electrical impulse that is generated at the SA node.

8. Name the characteristic parts of a normal ECG. What can an ECG tell you about cardiac functions?

9. What would a lengthened PR interval indicate? What does a widened QRS complex suggest?

10. How do the divisions of the autonomic nervous system (ANS) affect cardiac function?

11. How might congestive heart failure affect the function of the heart?

12. How can coronary heart disease contribute to the development of a myocardial infarction?

APPLYING KNOWLEDGE ON THE JOB

Select the most likely diagnosis for the following case studies.

13. A patient is brought to the emergency room in a collapsed state. She has shortness of breath and low blood pressure, and she is making a gurgling sound with each breath.

14. During a scheduled office visit, Mrs. Jones explains that after she climbs stairs, she has to sit down and rest for a while. One day last week, when there was no place to sit, she felt some pain and discomfort in her chest.

15. Your grandfather is complaining of extreme weakness and fatigue. You notice that his ankles are swollen and that he can't put his shoes on.

16. The rescue squad brings in a patient who is complaining of a sharp pain radiating down his left arm. He is extremely fatigued, short of breath, and has a very rapid heart rate. The ECG records a serious cardiac arrhythmia.

Additional Reading

Caplan M, Ranieri C. What's his ECG telling you? *RN* 1989;Feb:42.
Echocardiography: A practical primer. *Emerg Med* 1996;289(11):83.
Miracle V, Sims JM. Normal sinus rhythm. *Nursing* 1996;26(5):50.
Owen A. Tracking the rise and fall of cardiac enzymes. *Nursing* 1995;25(4):34.

Internet Activities

Contact **MedicineNet (http://www.medicinenet.com)** and find "Heart Attack" (letter AH@) and "Pericarditis" (letter AP@) under the "Disease and Treatment" main heading. Both articles provide extremely useful background information on the causes, symptoms, and treatment options for these common cardiac conditions.

Cardiac Glycosides and the Treatment of Congestive Heart Failure

Henry Hitner, PhD
Barbara Nagle, PhD

Chapter Focus

This chapter describes the pharmacology of the cardiac glycosides that are used to treat congestive heart failure (CHF). It explains how glycosides increase the force of cardiac contractions to relieve the symptoms of heart failure and discusses the roles of diuretic and vasodilator drugs in the management of CHF.

Chapter Terminology

adenosine triphosphatase (ATPase):   Enzyme that energizes the sodium/potassium pump and is inhibited by glycosides.

cardiac glycoside: Drug obtained from plants of the genus *Digitalis*.

congestive heart failure (CHF):   Condition in which the heart is unable to pump sufficient blood to the tissues of the body.

digitalization: Method of dosage with cardiac glycosides that rapidly produces effective drug levels.

ectopic beat: Extra heartbeat.

hypercalcemia: High serum calcium.

hyperkalemia: High serum potassium.

hypokalemia: Low serum potassium.

maintenance dose: Daily dosage of glycoside that maintains effective drug levels in the blood.

Chapter Objectives

After studying this chapter, you should be able to:

- Describe the symptoms of CHF.
- List two cardiac glycosides and explain their mechanisms of action.
- Differentiate between digitalization and maintenance in relationship to drug administration.
- Explain the effects of potassium and calcium on the actions of the glycosides.
- Describe five adverse effects caused by glycosides.
- Explain the role of diuretics and vasodilators in the treatment of CHF.

Congestive heart failure occurs when the heart is unable to pump sufficient blood to the tissues of the body. When blood accumulates in the heart, lungs, and veins of the lower extremities, the condition is referred to as congestion. Congestion may cause formation of blood clots in the veins (venous thrombosis), pulmonary edema that interferes with breathing, and cardiac arrhythmias, which can lead to sudden death.

When congestive heart failure occurs, the body tries to reverse the effects of heart failure by stimulating compensatory reflexes involving the sympathetic nervous system. Sympathetic reflexes release norepinephrine and epinephrine, which cause vasoconstriction and increase heart rate and force of contractions. These effects are an attempt to increase blood flow and relieve the congestion. Also, the kidneys respond by retaining sodium and water, which increases blood volume and blood pressure. Unfortunately, these compensatory responses do not usually reverse heart failure, and with time, they further weaken the heart. Individuals with congestive heart failure usually have the following symptoms: tiredness, fatigue, shortness of breath, rapid heartbeat, and peripheral edema.

Drug therapy involves the use of **cardiac glycosides,** which increase the force of myocardial contractions; diuretics, which eliminate excess sodium and water; and vasodilator drugs, which indirectly increase the amount of blood pumped by the heart (cardiac output).

Cardiac Glycosides

The cardiac glycosides are a group of compounds obtained from the plant leaves of *Digitalis purpurea* and *Digitalis lanata*. These compounds, known as glycosides, are similar in chemical and pharmacologic properties. Individual glycosides differ mainly in their rates of absorption and durations of action.

PHARMACOLOGIC EFFECTS

The unique and main pharmacologic effect of the glycosides is to increase the force of myocardial contractions in CHF without causing an increase in oxygen consumption. The efficiency of the heart is improved, restoring normal blood circulation. Kidney function increases as a result of the added blood flow and glomerular filtration rate. This increase results in elimination of the excess fluid and electrolytes associated with edema. The glycosides produce a dramatic relief of the symptoms and hemodynamic disturbances caused by congestive heart failure.

The glycosides also decrease heart rate and atrioventricular (AV) conduction. These effects are caused by stimulation of the vagus nerve. In addition, the glycosides have a direct depressant action on the AV node. They produce several characteristic changes in the ECG that can be observed. At therapeutic doses, there is depression of the ST segment, and there are changes in the T wave. In addition, there is lengthening of the PR interval, which reflects slower conduction through the AV node. At higher doses, the decreased conduction through the AV node can lead to various degrees of heart block.

Special Considerations Before glycosides are administered, a patient's pulse should be taken to ensure that the heart rate is between 60 and 100 beats per minute. If the rate is below 60 or above 100, the attending physician should be consulted before the drug is given. In addition, the heart rhythm should be normal.

MECHANISM OF ACTION

Cardiac glycosides increase the force of myocardial contractions by accelerating the entry of calcium ions inside cardiac muscle cells. First, the glycosides inhibit the enzyme **adenosine triphosphatase (ATPase),** which energizes the sodium-potassium pump. Normally, the sodium-potassium pump removes sodium from inside the cell (after depolarization) and brings potassium back into the cell (after repolarization). Inhibition of ATPase leads to accumulation of sodium ions inside heart muscle cells. Second, the increase of sodium ions inside the heart muscle is believed to stimulate an exchange mechanism whereby cells can get rid of excess sodium ions by exchanging them for calcium ions. Thus, calcium levels increase inside the heart muscle, and this increases the formation of actinomyosin, resulting in greater myocardial contraction.

After treatment with the glycosides, a congested heart contracts more forcefully within a shorter period of time. This change increases the amount of blood pumped out of the heart and improves blood circulation, which relieves the congestion of heart failure.

PHARMACOKINETICS

In acute CHF, the administration of glycosides normally follows a sequence known as digitalization and maintenance. During **digitalization,** glycosides are administered (PO or IV) at doses and intervals that rapidly produce an effective blood level. Subsequent daily **maintenance doses** are lower and adjusted to maintain a therapeutic level of glycoside in the blood.

Digoxin and digitoxin are two of the most widely used preparations. Both can be administered orally or intravenously, depending on the urgency of the situation. Food may delay absorption of the glycosides but usually does not interfere with the extent of absorption. Digoxin is not bound significantly to plasma proteins and is excreted mostly unmetabolized by the urinary tract. The half-life of digoxin is normally 1.5 to 2.0 days, but it may be prolonged in older patients.

Digitoxin is more lipid soluble than is digoxin and requires metabolism by the liver. Digitoxin metabolites are excreted by way of the urinary and GI tracts. The half-life of digitoxin is normally 5 to 7 days.

The cardiac glycosides have a low therapeutic index. When serum levels increase above the therapeutic range, adverse and toxic effects frequently occur. Glycosides also are slowly metabolized and excreted. For these reasons, serum drug levels are routinely performed to measure the amount of drug in patients and to adjust the dosage, if necessary. Table 16-1 lists the main glycoside preparations.

SERUM ELECTROLYTE LEVELS AND GLYCOSIDE ACTION

Glycosides are affected by changes in the serum electrolytes, particularly potassium and calcium. **Hypokalemia** (low serum potassium) sensitizes the heart to the toxic effects of the glycosides. Decrease in serum potassium may cause an increased incidence of arrhythmias, which can lead to ventricular fibrillation and sudden death. Administration of potassium salts is required to restore normal electrolyte levels during these crises. In contrast, **hyperkalemia** (high serum potassium) antagonizes the therapeutic effects of the glycosides. **Hypercalcemia** (high serum calcium) enhances the action of the glycosides and also can lead to arrhythmias.

Many patients with congestive heart failure are also treated with diuretics to reduce the edema associated with this condition. It is important that these patients receive adequate amounts of potassium in their diets to counterbalance the excretion of potassium caused by diuretics. Fruit juice, bananas, and vegetables are good sources of dietary potassium. In addition, there are commercial preparations of potassium supplements such as K-Lyte or Slow-K.

Table 16-1

Commonly Used Cardiac Glycosides

Drug (Trade Name)	Route	Oral Dose for Maintenance	Peak Effect (h)
Digitoxin (Purodigin)	PO, IV	0.05–0.2 mg	8–12
Digoxin (Lanoxin)	PO, IV	0.125–0.5 mg	6

ADVERSE AND TOXIC EFFECTS

The major adverse effects of the glycosides are caused by overdose. Mild symptoms include nausea, vomiting, headache, visual disturbances, and rashes. Dose reduction is usually sufficient to relieve these symptoms. The serious toxic effects involve the development of cardiac arrhythmias. Usually, there is an appearance of extra heartbeats **(ectopic beats).** Most common are premature ventricular contractions (PVCs). An increase in these contractions can lead to ventricular tachycardia, ventricular fibrillation, and cardiac arrest. Treatment involves stopping the glycoside and administering potassium and antiarrhythmic drugs to restore the normal cardiac rhythm.

In serious cardiac glycoside intoxication, an antidote is available to reduce the severity of toxicity. Digoxin Immune Fab *(Digibind)* is a preparation of antidigoxin antibodies that are administered parenterally. The antibodies bind up the glycoside drug and make it unavailable to produce its pharmacologic effects. The symptoms and severity of toxicity are usually reduced within 30 to 60 minutes. The antibody-glycoside drug complex is eliminated in the urine. The main indication for Digoxin Immune Fab is treatment of life-threatening glycoside intoxication.

CLINICAL INDICATIONS

The main use of cardiac glycosides is the treatment of congestive heart failure, to increase the force of contractions. These drugs are also used in some cases of atrial fibrillation and atrial tachycardia. The effect of the glycosides in slowing conduction through the AV node results in fewer electrical impulses reaching the ventricles. Consequently, the ventricular rate decreases toward a normal rhythm.

DRUG INTERACTIONS

Antacids, laxatives, kaolinpectin *(Kaopectate),* and cholestyramine *(Questran)* can decrease the absorption of glycosides from the GI tract. The antiarrhythmic drug quinidine increases glycoside plasma levels, and reduction in glycoside dosage is usually required when these two drugs are used together. The calcium channel blockers verapamil and diltiazem and any of the β blockers decrease heart rate and force of contraction. These drugs may depress cardiac function and precipitate CHF, thus counteracting the therapeutic effectiveness of the glycosides. Diuretics (thiazides and organic acids) and cardiac glycosides cause loss of potassium. When these drugs are used together, they may cause hypokalemia and increased glycoside toxicity.

Diuretic Therapy of CHF

The main effect produced by diuretics is the elimination of excess sodium and water by the urinary tract. Sodium and water retention is the main cause of excess blood volume and edema, which contribute to the congestion and circulatory disturbances of congestive heart failure. Diuretics, used alone or in combination with cardiac glycosides in the treatment of this condition, rapidly decrease excess blood volume and congestion, allowing the heart to function more efficiently. Thiazide diuretics, which give a mild to moderate diuretic effect, are frequently used. The organic acids, such as furosemide *(Lasix)*, are indicated when a more potent diuretic effect is required. In acute congestive heart failure, the organic acids are administered parenterally for rapid relief of edema and pulmonary congestion.

VASODILATOR THERAPY OF CHF

The main effect of vasodilator drugs is to relax or dilate blood vessels, both arteries and veins. Vasodilation lowers peripheral resistance and blood pressure. These changes decrease cardiac work and oxygen consumption. The heart is able to pump more blood (increased cardiac output) with less effort. Drugs that primarily dilate arteries or arterioles have a greater effect in lowering blood pressure. This effect is referred to as decreasing the afterload of the heart, which, simply stated, means that the heart doesn't have to work as hard in order to pump blood after the blood pressure has been lowered. Drugs that primarily dilate veins (vasodilators) mainly decrease venous return of blood back to the heart. This is referred to as decreasing the preload; this also reduces cardiac work. A few drugs dilate both arteries and veins and produce a balanced vasodilation that decreases both pre- and afterload.

Vasodilator therapy of CHF has been shown to be very beneficial, especially with the drug class known as the angiotensin-converting enzyme inhibitors. These drugs have become the preferred agents for the treatment of CHF. There is less risk of toxicity with vasodilators than with cardiac glycosides. Vasodilator drugs are used alone and in combination with diuretics and cardiac glycosides. The therapeutic actions of some of the vasodilator drugs are summarized in Table 16-2.

Table 16-2
Vasodilator Drugs Used in Congestive Heart Failure

Vasodilator	*Main Effect*	*Effect on Heart*
Angiotensin-conversing enzyme inhibitors Captopril (Capoten) Enalopril (Vasotec) Linsinopril (Prinvil, Zestril)	Decreases formation of angiotensin (potent vasoconstrictor formed in the blood) and produces dilation of arteriolar and venous vessels	Increased cardiac output
Hydralazine (Apresoline)	Dilates arteriolar more than venous vessels	Increased cardiac output
Nitroglycerin	Dilates venous more than arteriolar vessels	Decreased venous return and work of the heart
Prazosin (Minipress)	Dilates arteriolar and venous vessels	Increased cardiac output
Sodium nitroprusside (Nipride)	Dilates arteriolar and venous vessels	Increased cardiac output

Chapter 16 Review

UNDERSTANDING TERMINOLOGY

Answer the following questions.

1. Define CHF.
2. What are ectopic beats?
3. Differentiate between hyperkalemia and hypokalemia.

ACQUIRING KNOWLEDGE

Answer the following questions.

4. What is the main action of cardiac glycosides on the myocardium?
5. Explain the effect of digitalis on heart rate.
6. Explain the clinical importance of digitalization and tell how digitalization differs from maintenance.
7. What are the more serious adverse effects of digitalis? Discuss the factors that increase their development.
8. What precautions should be observed before administration of the cardiac glycosides?
9. How do the cardiac glycosides differ from each other?
10. What changes can be observed in an ECG at therapeutic doses? At toxic doses?
11. What role do diuretics play in the treatment of congestive heart failure?
12. Explain why vasodilator drugs are beneficial in the treatment of congestive heart failure.

APPLYING KNOWLEDGE ON THE JOB

Answer the following questions.

13. Mrs. McNally is a 65-year-old woman who presents at the clinic where you're working with complaints of increased shortness of breath and swelling of her feet. Her past medical history includes a diagnosis of hypertension and a moderate degree of renal failure. Pertinent lab findings show a slightly decreased potassium level of 3.2 mmol/L (normal 3.5–5 mmol/L) and an increased serum creatinine of 2.1 mg/dL (normal 0.8–1.5 mg/dL). The physician's diagnosis is acute congestive heart failure. The physician's course of therapy includes doubling Mrs. McNally's dose of hydrochlorothiazide from 25 mg to 50 mg daily and prescribing digoxin, 0.25 mg twice daily for 2 days and then 0.25 mg daily.

    a. What is the most likely electrolyte disturbance that may occur in this patient?

       b. What are the terms used to describe the administration of digoxin, twice daily for 2 days then once daily thereafter?

       c. What does the increased level of serum creatinine suggest about this patient's renal function?

14. Outline the steps to be taken in severe cardiac glycoside intoxication.

15. Explain the rationale behind the use of digoxin in the treatment of atrial fibrillation.

Additional Reading

Ahrens SG. Managing heart failure: A blueprint for success. *Nursing* 1995;25(12):26.

Blumenfeld JD, Laragh JH. Diagnosis and management of heart failure. *Hosp Med* 1997;33(3):36.

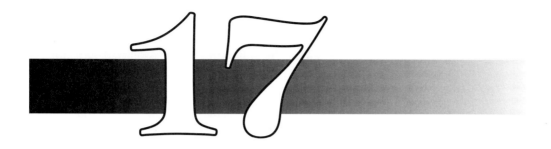

Anticoagulants and Coagulants

HENRY HITNER, PhD
BARBARA NAGLE, PhD

Chapter Focus

This chapter describes drugs that alter circulating substances in the blood, thus influencing the ability of the blood to form clots.

Chapter Terminology

alopecia: Baldness or hair loss.

coagulation: Process by which the blood changes from a liquid to a solid "plug" as a reaction to local tissue injury; normal blood clot formation.

hematuria: Appearance of blood or red blood cells in the urine.

hemorrhage: Loss of blood from blood vessels.

hemorrhagic disease of the newborn (HDN): Hemorrhaging in a newborn due to lack of vitamin K and coagulation factors.

infarction: Area of tissue that has died because of a sudden lack of blood supply.

mucopolysaccharide: Naturally occurring substance formed by the combination of protein with carbohydrates (saccharides).

thrombocyte: Cell in the blood, commonly called a platelet, which is necessary for coagulation.

thromboembolism: Clots that jam a blood vessel; formed by the action of platelets and other coagulation factors in the blood.

thrombophlebitis: Inflammation of the walls of the veins, associated with clot formation.

thrombus: Clot formed by the action of coagulation factors and circulating blood cells.

Chapter Objectives

After studying this chapter, you should be able to:

- Describe the mechanism by which a blood clot forms and is dissolved.
- Explain the two ways the commonly used anticoagulants inhibit clot formation.
- Explain why heparin must be administered by injection.
- Describe the primary response to anticoagulant overdose.
- Explain when clot dissolution is clinically useful.
- Explain how the respiratory care practitioner encounters the effects of anticoagulant treatment therapy.
- Describe when products are used to promote clotting.

Clot formation is essential to survival. Usually, a blood clot acts as a seal that prevents the further loss of blood, oxygen, and nutrients from a wounded area. In addition, factors present in the clot promote wound healing by signaling other cells (phagocytes) to carry off waste products and dead cells that accumulate at the site of injury. This protective mechanism (hemostasis) is always functioning to maintain homeostasis. Occasionally, the mechanism of clot formation becomes too active, or the blood vessels become too narrow (atherosclerosis) to allow the clots to pass through easily. As a result, clots may become jammed in blood vessels, forming a **thromboembolism,** which prevents the normal flow of blood to other tissues. The heart, the lungs, and the brain are especially susceptible to damage caused by a loss or reduction in blood flow subsequent to thrombosis. Anticoagulants are used to prevent venous clotting in patients who have thromboembolic disorders because these drugs interfere with the ability of the blood to form stable clots.

Coagulation

To understand how the anticoagulant drugs work, the process of normal blood clot formation **(coagulation)** must be understood. Many substances in the blood, such as platelets and clotting factors (see Table 17-1), are responsible for initiating coagulation.

Table 17-1

Anticoagulant Drugs That Affect Coagulation Factor Activity or Formation

Clotting Factor	Common Name	Vitamin K Dependent	Anticoagulant Action
I	Fibrinogen	No	—
II	Prothrombin	Yes	Oral anticoagulants
III	Thromboplastin, tissue factor	No	Heparin
IV	Calcium ions	No	Edetic acid, oxalic acid
V	Proaccelerin, labile factor	No	—
VI	[No name]	—	—
VII	Proconvertin	Yes	Oral anticoagulants
VIII	Antihemophilic factor (AHF)	No	—
IX	Plasma thromboplastin component (PTC), Christmas factor	Yes	Oral anticoagulants
X	Stuart factor, Stuart-Prower factor	Yes	Oral anticoagulants
XI	Plasma thromboplastin antecedent, PTA	No	—
XII	Hegeman factor	No	—
XIII	Fibrin-stabilizing factor, FSF	No	—

When an injury occurs, platelets (**thrombocytes**) immediately migrate to the damaged area. Because platelets stick to each other (aggregation) and to the vessel walls (adhesion), they form a plug around the injured tissue. Subsequently, clotting factors reach the platelet plug and interact with each other to form a stable blood clot. Figure 17-1 illustrates the sequence of clotting factor interaction. A stable blood clot is produced in three stages:

1. A substance known as thromboplastin is produced.
2. Thromboplastin converts prothrombin to thrombin.
3. Thrombin converts fibrinogen to fibrin. (Fibrin is the primary element of a blood clot.)

Thromboplastin is produced by two different mechanisms—the intrinsic and extrinsic systems. The intrinsic system requires many clotting factors and platelets to stimulate production of thromboplastin. In contrast, the extrinsic system requires factor VII and tissue extract, a substance that is released from injured cells. Regardless of the pathway involved, once thromboplastin is produced, clotting proceeds automatically, but the factors necessary for clot formation require calcium ions in order to function efficiently.

Stage 4 is the body's ability to dissolve clots once their function has ended. In stage 4, fibrinolysin acts on the fibrin elements to produce a more soluble product. These four stages are part of the coagulation and clot resolution processes.

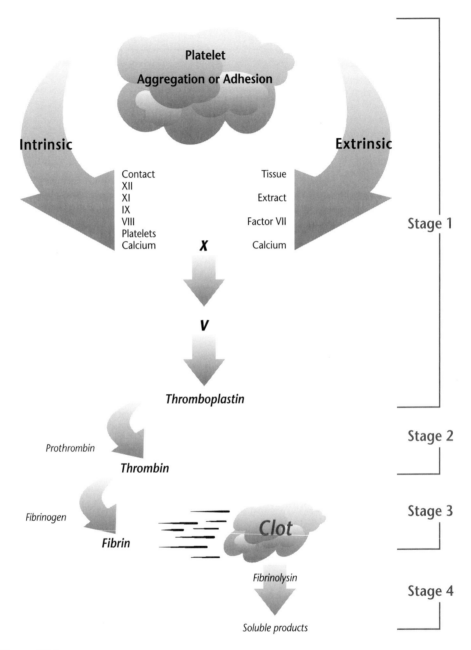

Figure 17-1
The stages of coagulation and clot resolution.

Anticoagulants

Two classes of anticoagulants are most frequently used today—the coumarin derivatives and heparin. Anticoagulant drugs may interfere with normal clotting at several sites; however, there are only two mechanisms through which the clinically useful anticoagulants produce their pharmacologic response. Anticoagulants such as heparin inhibit the function of the preformed clotting factors. The coumarin derivatives prevent the synthesis of normal clotting factors. The mechanism of anticoagulant action determines the onset and the duration of drug action.

Heparin and coumarin derivatives are most frequently employed to prevent venous thrombosis, especially pulmonary embolism. Therefore, these agents are used in the therapy of myocardial infarction, **thrombophlebitis** (inflammation of the walls of the veins), and stroke. The oral anticoagulants are the drugs of choice because they are relatively inexpensive, can be taken easily by patients, and are not associated with painful administration. However, heparin is always the preferred drug when an anticoagulant must be given to a pregnant woman. Heparin does not cross the placenta and cannot affect the developing fetus. Other uses of anticoagulants include clot suppression before blood transfusion and during open-heart surgery.

HEPARIN

Because it complexes with certain circulating clotting factors and inhibits their function, heparin is considered a peripherally acting anticoagulant. Heparin inhibits thrombin activity so that fibrin cannot be formed. In addition, heparin inhibits thromboplastin activity so that more thrombin cannot be generated. Finally, heparin interferes with platelet aggregation. As long as heparin is in contact with these substances, coagulation is depressed, and clot formation is inhibited.

Route of Administration   Heparin cannot be given orally because it is destroyed by gastric acid. Therefore, heparin is usually administered intravenously or subcutaneously. Intramuscular injection should be avoided because painful hematomas may occur. The onset of action with heparin is rapid, usually within 5 minutes, and the duration of action is 2 to 4 hours. Heparin may be administered with a heparin lock.

Heparin is a **mucopolysaccharide** obtained from the lungs and intestinal tissue of cattle or pigs. Drugs derived from animal sources must undergo a standard biological assay to determine their purity, quality, and potency. Drugs such as heparin are administered in units of activity rather than in milligrams. One hundred USP units correspond to approximately 1 mg of commercially prepared heparin.

Low-Molecular-Weight Heparins   Today there are also a few low-molecular-weight heparins available. Working from the porcine heparin, fragments of the endogenous mucopolysaccharide are removed that contain full anticoagulant activity. In this regard, these heparins are smaller, that is, are a lower molecular weight than the full parent molecule. Ardeparin, enoxaparin, and dalteparin exert their primary effect on inhibition of factor X, thrombin, and antithrombin III. Although fragments of the same parent, these drugs are not interchangeable. There is variability in the activity, and there is no conversion to assure bioequivalent dosing.

Lipolysis   In addition to the anticoagulant action, heparin and ardeparin have the ability to clear fatty molecules from the plasma. Heparin stimulates an enzyme (lipoprotein lipase) that hydrolyzes the triglycerides in the blood. This enzyme reaction reduces large fat molecules in the plasma. This effect has no influence on heparin's anticoagulant action, and its physiological importance is not fully understood. Eventually, heparin is metabolized by the liver or excreted unchanged into the urine. Patients with renal impairment or kidney disease tend to accumulate heparin because they cannot efficiently clear it from the blood.

Glycosaminoglycan   Although it is not a heparin derivative, *Danaproid* is a low-molecular-weight glycosaminoglycan that is extracted from porcine mucosa. It is a parenterally administered anticoagulant that selectively inhibits factors III, II, and Xa.

Adverse Effects   The major toxicity associated with the use of heparin is **hemorrhage.** At high levels, heparin causes bleeding to occur in mucous membranes (**petechiae**) and open wounds, such as scratches, cuts, and abrasions. If hemorrhage occurs in the GI membranes, patients' blood pressure and hematocrit may fall even though there are no external signs of bleeding. The dose and frequency of administration should be reduced when hemorrhage is evident. Use in elderly patients requires special attention because enoxaparin elimination may be delayed. Anemia has been reported with ardeparin and enoxaparin.

Protamine sulfate is the specific antidote in heparin toxicity. Each milligram of protamine sulfate will neutralize 90 to 120 USP units of heparin, 1 mg of enoxaparin, or 100 IU of ardeparin or dalteparin. Protamine binds to the heparin molecules and inhibits the anticoagulant action. Administration of heparin or protamine should always be accompanied by coagulation tests to determine the degree of clot suppression that is present (see "Monitoring Coagulation"). Other side effects seen with any chronic heparin use include hypersensitivity, fever, **alopecia** (hair loss), osteoporosis, and thrombocytopenia (decrease in the number of blood platelets). Although these effects have been reported, they are considered to be relatively uncommon.

COUMARIN DERIVATIVES

The coumarin derivatives include dicumarol and warfarin sodium (see Table 17-2). Dicumarol (bishydroxycoumarin) was originally discovered as a product of spoiled sweet clover. Cattle that grazed on the contaminated clover developed hemorrhagic disease. In addition, people who drank the milk from these cows de-

Table 17-2

Comparison of Some Commonly Employed Anticoagulant Drugs

Drug (Trade Name)	Daily Maintenance Dose	Coagulation Test Used to Monitor the Therapeutic Response
Ardeparin (Normiflo)	50 anti-Xa units/kg every 12 h up to 14 days	Routine blood and platelet counts
Anisindione (Miradon)	25–250 mg PO	Prothrombin time (protime, PT) or INR
Dalteparin (Fragmin)	2500 IU/day, 1–2 h before surgery, up to 10 days postsurgery	Routine blood and platelet counts
Danaparoid (Orgaran)	750 mg BID 1–4 h presurgery, up to 14 days postsurgery	Routine blood and platelet counts
Dicumarol	25–200 mg PO	Prothrombin time (protime, PT) or INR
Enoxaparin (Lovenox)	30 mg BID pre–knee surgery, up to 12 days postsurgery	Routine blood and platelet counts
Enoxaparin	40 mg QD for abdominal surgery	Routine blood and platelet counts
Heparin sodium injection	10,000–12,000 units initially followed by 15,000–20,000 units every 12 h SC; 5000–10,000 units every 4–6 h IV	Whole blood clotting time; activated partial thromboplastin time (APTT)
Heparin sodium lock flush solution (Heparin Lock Flush, Hep-Lock)	Not intended for therapeutic use; used for maintenance of indwelling IV catheters	—
Warfarin sodium (Coumadin)	2–10 mg PO	Prothrombin time (protime, PT) or INR

veloped hemorrhages because they ingested the active anticoagulant substance. The coumarins are significantly different from heparin because they can be administered orally. For this reason, these drugs are usually referred to as the oral anticoagulants. The oral anticoagulant of choice is warfarin sodium.

The onset of anticoagulant activity with the coumarins is slow, 12 to 72 hours. Several days may be required to produce a significant amount of nonreactive clotting factors. Similarly, the duration of action is long (2 to 10 days), even after drug administration has been discontinued. The oral anticoagulants are highly bound to plasma proteins and are eventually metabolized by the liver. Both of these factors are responsible for the many drug interactions that occur with these drugs.

Adverse Effects   Hemorrhage is always the major toxicity associated with the use of an anticoagulant. **Hematuria** (blood or red blood cells in the urine), bleeding of the gums, and petechiae are common side effects that reflect local hemorrhaging. In the presence of hemorrhage, the action of the coumarins cannot be rapidly reversed by merely discontinuing the drug. The antidote for overdose includes 2.5 to 25 mg of vitamin K_1 (phytonadione) given parenterally (usually IM, SC). Because the mechanism of action involves synthetic pathways in the liver, administration of phytonadione cannot be expected to produce immediate results. The counteraction of phytonadione is evident by monitoring prothrombin time within 2 hours after the antidote is given. In severe hemorrhage, fresh whole blood or plasma may also be administered to provide a full complement of normal clotting factors.

Other side effects accompanying the use of oral anticoagulants include nausea, diarrhea, urticaria, and alopecia. To reduce GI distress, large doses of oral anticoagulants may be administered in divided doses.

Contraindications   Anticoagulants of any type are contraindicated in patients with subacute bacterial endocarditis, ulcerative lesions (GI), visceral carcinoma, threatened abortion, severe hypertension, and recent surgery on the brain or spinal cord. Any patient with active bleeding tendencies should not receive anticoagulants. The oral anticoagulants should not be used in patients known to be vitamin K deficient.

The most important contraindication for the oral anticoagulants concerns the use of these drugs during pregnancy. The oral anticoagulants cross the placenta and may produce hemorrhaging in the fetus because the fetus is dependent on the mother for its source of vitamin K and coagulation factors. Administration of oral anticoagulants during pregnancy will result in a phenomenon known as **hemorrhagic disease of the newborn (HDN).** Vitamin K_1 (phytonadione) is administered to the mother (prophylaxis) or to the newborn (treatment) when HDN is anticipated.

VITAMIN K DERIVATIVES

Natural vitamin K promotes synthesis of prothrombin (factor II), proconvertin (factor VII), plasma thromboplastin component (factor IX), and Stuart factor (X). Synthetic derivatives of vitamin K are available. Vitamin K_1 (phytonadione) and vitamin K_3 (menadione) are fat soluble, whereas vitamin K_4 (menadiol) is water soluble. Selection of the appropriate vitamin for treatment of oral anticoagulant overdose or HDN is based on the degree of activity and onset of action. Phytonadione may be the drug of choice because it has the same degree of activity as the naturally occurring vitamin and may have a better margin of safety.

CHELATORS

Several drugs inhibit coagulation by interfering with essential ions in the blood. Chelating drugs, such as edetic acid (EDTA, ethylenediaminetetraacetic acid) and oxalic acid, bind calcium ions so that the coagulation scheme is interrupted. These agents are not routinely employed as systemic anticoagulants. However, oxalic acid in particular is present in commercially prepared test tubes to prevent the coagulation of blood taken for routine hematologic tests.

ASPIRIN AND DIPYRIDAMOLE

These two drugs prevent the formation of a clot (antithrombotic) primarily by interfering with the intrinsic or extrinsic system of coagulation. Aspirin (1 g per day) and dipyridamole (*Persantine,* 75 to 100 mg QID) produce an anticoagulant effect by strongly inhibiting platelet aggregation. This effect may be a potential danger in patients who are prone to GI bleeding or ingest large doses of aspirin. These agents are presently being tried as systemic anticoagulants in selected surgical procedures, such as heart surgery, and in prevention of postoperative clotting complications of cardiac valve replacement. These drugs are being tried alone or in combination to prevent myocardial reinfarction and death. Daily aspirin (325 mg) has been shown to produce clinically significant reductions in reinfarction and death following myocardial infarction in men. However, the clinical benefit has not been demonstrated in women after myocardial infarction. It also prevents transient ischemic attacks (TIAs) in stroke patients but has no action on the formed clot.

CLINICAL INDICATIONS

Among the heparins available today, the full mucopolysaccharide referred to as heparin is approved for the broadest spectrum of use. Heparin is approved for the prophylaxis and treatment of venous thrombosis and emboli associated with peripheral arteries and atrial fibrillation. It is also indicated for prevention of postoperative deep vein thrombosis (DVT) and pulmonary embolism in patients undergoing major abdominal surgery or who are at risk of developing thromboembolic disease. It is used to prevent clotting during cardiovascular surgery, transfusions, dialysis, and extracorporeal circulation and in the diagnosis and treatment of disseminated intravascular coagulation.

Glycosaminoglycan and low-molecular-weight heparins are approved for use in prevention of DVT in selective procedures as follows: ardeparin (knee replacement), danaparoid (hip replacement), dalteparin (abdominal surgery), and enoxaparin (knee and hip replacement and abdominal surgery). For these parenteral anticoagulants the dose must be customized to the patient within recommended guidelines for time of administration (Table 17-2).

Oral anticoagulants are approved for use in the prophylaxis and treatment of venous thrombosis, pulmonary embolism, and atrial fibrillation with embolization.

DRUG INTERACTIONS

Heparin undergoes fewer drug interactions than do the oral anticoagulants. Any drugs that are known to affect platelet aggregation will probably cause increased bleeding when taken concomitantly with heparin. Such drugs include nonsteroidal antiinflammatory drugs (aspirin, ibuprofen, indomethacin, phenylbutazone), dextran, and high doses of penicillin. Digitalis and tetracyclines have been reported to counteract the anticoagulant action of heparin. The mechanism of this action is not known.

The oral anticoagulants have the greatest potential for clinically significant interactions with other medications. These drugs are associated with three major sites where interaction may occur. Oral anticoagulants may be displaced from plasma protein binding sites, which may increase their plasma concentrations and toxicity. In addition, any drug that interferes with liver metabolism may increase or decrease the response of the oral anticoagulants. Finally, because they are taken by mouth, absorption of oral anticoagulants may be inhibited by other oral medications that bind to the anticoagulants. Several drugs, some available over the counter, such as acetaminophen, have been associated with increased bleeding from the oral anticoagulants, but the mechanism or site of action has not yet been determined. Table 17-3 describes numerous drug interactions that occur with anticoagulant drugs. Careful monitoring and appropriate dosage adjustments will ensure the safety of combination drug therapy in patients who receive anticoagulants.

Table 17-3
Drug Interactions with Anticoagulant Drugs

Interacts with	Response	Interacts with	Response
Heparins			
Aspirin		Digitalis	Decreased anticoagulant action
Cephalosporins		Nicotine	
Dextran		Antihistamines	
Dipyridamole		Tetracyclines	
Ibuprofen	Increased bleeding		
Indomethacin		Oral anticoagulants platelet inhibitors (NSAIDs)	False protime values, enhances anticoagulation
NSAIDs			
Penicillin (high doses)			
Oral Anticoagulants			
Chloral hydrate		Amiodarone	
Clofibrate	Increased bleeding via protein binding displacement	Chloramphenical	
Diflunisal		Cimetidine	
Ethacrynic acid		Co-trimoxazole	
Naldixic acid		Ifosfamide	
Penicillins		Lovastatin	Increased bleeding because of decreased liver metabolism of the anticoagulants
Salicylates		Methylphenidate	
Alteplase		Omeprazole	
Antibiotics	Increased bleeding time because of decreased availability of vitamin K	Phenylbutazone	
Kanamycin		Propofenone	
Neomycin			
Sulfonamides		Quinidine	
Tetracyclines		Quinine	
Vitamin E		Quinine	
		Sulfamethoxazole trimethoprim	

Table 17-3 (continued)
Drug Interactions with Anticoagulant Drugs

Interacts with	Response	Interacts with	Response
Oral Anticoagulants (continued)			
Aspirin Cephalosporins Dipyridamole Heparin Quinidine Quinine Steroids Sulfinpyrazone	Increased bleeding because of decreased platelet aggregation, suppression of prothrombin formation, interference with other clotting mechanisms	Alcohol Barbiturates Carbamazepine Ethchlorvynol Glutethimide Griseofulvin Nafcillin Rifampin	Decreased anticoagulant effect via increased liver metabolism of the anticoagulant
Acetaminophen Androgens β-blockers Chlorpropamine Clofibrate Corticosteroids Cyclophosphamide Danazol Dextrothyroxine Disulfiram Erythromycin Fluconazole Glucagon Hydantoins Influenza vaccine Isoniazid Ketoconazole Miconazole Quinolones Propoxyphene Propranolol Ranitidine Streptokinase Tamoxifen Thyroid hormone Sulindac	Increased bleeding by unknown mechanism	Aluminum hydroxide Cholestyramine Colestipol Sulcralfate	Decreased anticoagulant effect via decreased oral absorption of the anticoagulant
		Oral contraceptives Estrogens Vitamin K	Decreased anticoagulant effect via stimulation of clotting factor synthesis
		Adrenal corticosteroids Ethacrynic acid Indomethacin Phenylbutazone Potassium products Salicylates	Ulcerogenic effects
		Ascorbic acid Cholestyramine Estrogens Ethanol Ethchlorvynol Griseofulvin Nafcillin Oral contraceptives Spironolactone Thiazide diuretics Vitamin K Sucralfate	Decreased anticoagulant effect of warfarin or anisindione by a variety of mechanisms

SPECIAL CONSIDERATIONS

Patients receiving anticoagulant therapy should be instructed to be attentive to the appearance of bruises, bleeding gums, hematuria, or unusually heavy menstrual flow because these are signs of an increased bleeding tendency. In addition, patients should be cautioned to avoid the concomitant use of alcohol or drugs that alter platelet function, such as over-the-counter products containing aspirin or sali-cylates.

Ideally, anticoagulant therapy should be administered at the same time daily. Whenever medications are added to or deleted from the regimen of patients receiving an anticoagulant, the patients' coagulation status is subject to change. Patients should therefore be carefully observed for signs of increased bleeding or hemorrhage. Fever or rash that develops during anticoagulant therapy should be regarded as an indication of potential complication. Patients must be advised to adhere strictly to the prescribed dose schedule for oral anticoagulants. Oral medication should not be discontinued unless on the specific advice of the treating physician. Heparin is often administered by intermittent intravenous infusion. When blood is drawn, especially for the purpose of evaluating patients' coagulation status, samples should always be taken from the arm opposite the IV line to avoid false activated partial thromboplastin time (APTT) values.

Monitoring Coagulation

The dosage of any anticoagulant is individualized to the patient. The therapeutic dosage is established and maintained by evaluation of the patient's clotting time. Once a patient is stabilized, coagulation may be monitored every 4 to 6 weeks. To avoid the danger of hemorrhage from too much anticoagulant, the coagulability of the blood should be measured before more drug is administered. Among the tests used to monitor coagulation status are whole blood clotting time, partial thromboplastin time (PTT), prothrombin time, and the international normalized ratio (INR). The INR is being used because commercial thromboplastin responses to anticoagulants vary greatly between batches. The INR calibrates the commercial rabbit thromboplastins against an international human reference standard.

The effect of heparin is most frequently assessed with the whole blood clotting time and the APTT. These tests are usually performed 1 hour before the next scheduled dose of heparin. Generally, the PTT is maintained at twice the normal value when heparin is employed. Because of their selective inhibition of coagulation factors that are associated with the APTT monitoring reagents, the low-molecular-weight (LMW) drugs cannot be monitored accurately. The therapeutic effect of the LMW drugs is assessed by routine total blood and platelet counts and urinalysis throughout therapy.

The oral anticoagulants must be monitored with the one-stage prothrombin time or protime (PT) or the INR. Because of the long onset of action of these drugs, the initial dose cannot be changed for 3 to 5 days. It takes this long to achieve the peak anticoagulant response. During this time, periodic protime evaluation indicates the degree of clot suppression. The PT may be maintained at 1.2 to 1.5 times the control, which may be a 2 to 4 INR value. Heparin is known to interfere with accurate protime determinations when it is administered in conjunction with oral anticoagulants.

Thrombolytic Enzymes

Thrombolytic enzymes are used to dissolve preformed blood clots. These enzymes stimulate the synthesis of fibrinolysin, which breaks the clot into soluble products *(see Figure 17-1)*. This class of drugs includes urokinase *(Abbokinase)*, streptokinase *(Strepase)*, anistreplase *(Eminase)*, alteplase *(Activase)*, and reteplase *(Retevase)*. Alteplase, also referred to as tPA, or tissue plasminogen activator, and reteplase are thrombolytic enzymes produced through the biotechnology of recombinant DNA. Alteplase binds to fibrin within the clot, stimulates conversion of plasminogen to plasmin, and initiates clot dissolution (fibrinolysis). Reteplase is derived from the alteplase glycoprotein.

Thrombolytic enzymes are used to lyse pulmonary emboli and coronary artery thromboses during acute myocardial infarction. To receive maximum benefit, the enzymes must be administered as soon as possible following indications that a clot or infarct has occurred. For the treatment of acute myocardial **infarction,** the timing of drug administration for successful clot resolution is usually within 1 to 6 hours from the onset of symptoms. For pulmonary embolism, the time for initiation of therapy may be up to a few days.

ADVERSE EFFECTS

The major adverse effect associated with the use of thrombolytic enzymes is hemorrhage. Concomitant use of heparin, oral anticoagulants, or drugs known to alter platelet function (aspirin and nonsteroidal antiinflammatory drugs) is not recommended because of the increased risk of bleeding. Because these drugs are enzymes, mild allergic reactions have occurred in patients during use. Allergic reactions include skin rash, itching, nausea, headache, fever, bronchospasm, or musculoskeletal pain. Although severe allergic reactions to enzyme therapy may require discontinuation of therapy, milder reactions are usually controlled with antihistamine or corticosteroid therapy. Contraindications to the use of thrombolytic drugs include conditions such as active internal bleeding, cerebral vascular accident (CVA) within the past 2 months, intracranial or intraspinal surgery, or intracranial tumors. Alteplase and reteplase have been associated with cardiogenic shock, arrhythmias, and recurrent ischemia among the reported adverse effects; however, these are frequent sequelae of myocardial infarction and may or may not be attributable to the drug.

CLINICAL INDICATIONS

Thrombolytic enzymes are approved for use in the management of acute myocardial infarction, acute ischemic stroke, and pulmonary embolism. Streptokinase is also approved for lysis of deep vein thrombi. Streptokinase and urokinase have been used for clearance of occluded arteriovenous cannulas or IV catheters obstructed by clotted blood or fibrin. Currently, urokinase is not commercially available.

Coagulants/Hemostatics

There are occasions when an agent is required to decrease the incidence or severity of hemorrhage. The use of vitamin K_1 and protamine sulfate as specific antidotes for anticoagulant overdose has been discussed. A limited number of substances may be useful in arresting bleeding arising from other causes. In particular, aminocaproic acid *(Amicar)* inhibits fibrinolysin activation in situations where excessive clot dissolution is occurring. Orally or intravenously, aminocaproic acid promotes clotting and appears to concentrate in the newly formed **thrombus** (clot) so no dissolution can occur. The major danger with the use of aminocaproic acid is the production of a generalized thrombosis. Otherwise, the side effects include headache, diarrhea, cramps, and rash.

Thrombin *(Thrombogen, Thrombostat)*, obtained from cattle, is a direct activator of fibrin formation. This plasma protein initiates clot formation when applied topically to actively oozing injuries. Thrombin is never administered intravenously because of the potential danger of generalized thrombosis or antigenic reactions.

HEMOSTATIC SPONGES

Three popular preparations of gelatin or cellulose sponges are employed to soak up excess blood and fluids and control bleeding in procedures in which suturing is ineffective or impractical. Such procedures include oral, dental, ophthalmic, and prostatic surgery. Gelatin sponge *(Gelfoam)*, gelatin film *(Gelfilm)*, and oxidized cellulose *(Oxycel, Surgicel, Hemo-Pak)* expand in contact with large amounts of blood. These gauze or sponge preparations also permit clotting to occur along their surfaces when used as wound dressings and surgical packings. These agents are applied topically to control hemorrhage in situations such as amputation, resection of the internal organs, and certain neurologic surgery. Most of these packings ultimately are absorbed by the body with little or no deleterious effect. Oxidized cellulose, in particular, cannot be used as a permanent implant because it interferes with bone regeneration. It may also induce cyst formation and reduce epithelialization (healing) of surface wounds.

Special Considerations for the Respiratory Care Practitioner

Drugs that affect coagulation do not directly affect treatment or maintenance of respiratory care being delivered by the respiratory care practitioner. Respiratory patients receiving chronic anticoagulant therapy have a predisposition to bleed (delayed clot formation) at the injection site when blood samples are drawn. For the respiratory care practitioner, this may be encountered during periodic blood collection for monitoring oxygen and carbon dioxide tension. Otherwise, these drugs serve to protect the integrity of respiratory function by minimizing the potential for developing clots within the cardiorespiratory system.

Because many of the anticoagulants are used in a controlled hospital setting, close patient observation minimizes the risk associated with the onset of adverse reactions. In the hospital environment it is assumed that drug interactions that potentiate bleeding, such as platelet inhibitors (aspirin, NSAIDs), are minimized by frequent chart review by the medical-pharmacy team. Patients certainly may continue to take oral anticoagulants on an outpatient basis for chronic prophylaxis of emboli. Therefore, it becomes necessary to provide clear instruction not only to the patient but to relatives and friends who may participate in home care of the patient. Adverse reactions with this class of drugs are potentially life threatening and need to be communicated to the doctor immediately. Before undergoing dental work or other surgery, the patient should confer with the physician monitoring anticoagulant therapy.

Chapter 17 Review

UNDERSTANDING TERMINOLOGY

Match the description in the left column with the appropriate term in the right column.

1. Several blood clots together that form a plug.
2. Hair loss or baldness.
3. Inflammation of the walls of the veins because of blood clots.
4. The appearance of red blood cells or blood in the urine.
5. A blood clot.

a. alopecia
b. hematuria
c. thromboembolism
d. thrombophlebitis
e. thrombus

ACQUIRING KNOWLEDGE

Test your understanding of the material in this chapter by answering the following questions.

6. What are the major stages of coagulation?

7. Explain the action of antithrombotic drugs.

8. How does heparin differ from the oral anticoagulants?

9. What factors permit heparin to have a rapid onset of action?

10. How do the oral anticoagulants exert an antithrombotic effect? What coagulation factors are affected? Why do the oral anticoagulants have a long onset of action?

11. Name two specific contraindications to the use of warfarin sodium.

12. What effects does aspirin have on anticoagulant therapy?

13. Explain the major toxicity associated with anticoagulant therapy.

14. Why isn't vitamin K_1 useful in heparin overdose?

15. How can the effects of the oral anticoagulants or heparin be monitored before the next scheduled dose is given?

16. When is heparin preferred over the coumarins?

17. What are three contraindications to the use of anticoagulants?

Additional Reading

Avery C. Improvement in heparin prophylaxis. *Nursing Times* 1995;91(20):11.

Harrison M. Central venous catheters, a review of the literature. *Nurs Stand* 1997;11(17):43.

Herman WW. Current perspectives on dental patients receiving coumarin anticoagulant therapy. *JADA* 1997;128(3):317.

Kay R. Low molecular weight heparin for the treatment of acute ischemic stroke. *N Engl J Med* 1995;333(24):1588.

Normal EM. Low dose heparin in pediatric IVs. *Am J Nurs* 1997;97:161.

Stevenson AL. International normalized ratio in anticoagulant therapy: Understanding the issues. *Am J Crit Care* 1997;6(2):88.

Internet Activities

Pharmacology quizzes, case studies, discussions, and journal clubs are available on the internet on the topics of anticoagulants, heparin, treatment of stroke, and use of these drugs during pregnancy. Two providers of this information include the search engine AltaVista and the Web site of PharmInfonet.

1. At **www.altavista.com** enter "anticoagulants" into the search box. You will be provided with more than 5000 relevant titles. Scroll down the titles until you

reach "Anticoagulants, antithrombotics and Thrombolytics, Question #." Click on the titles that are numbered questions 4, 6, 7, and 9. These quizzes are supported by the pharmacology department at the University of Iowa. Each question about heparin and oral anticoagulants will provide multiple-choice answers. After reviewing this chapter, select the most appropriate answer. The computer will indicate whether the choice was correct. Incorrect answers will provide a prompt "See correct answers" to explain why each answer was true or false.

2. At **www.altavista.com** enter "anticoagulants" into the search box. Scroll down until you reach the title "Virtual Phlebotomy-anticoagulants." This Web page will present the complications of drawing blood when the patient is receiving anticoagulants. It also describes correct phlebotomy technique when bleeding occurs.

3. Continue to scroll through these titles until you reach "Anticoagulants (systemic)." Click on this Web site to enter "The Virtual Medical Center" supported by mediconsult.com.

4. Enter **www.PharmInfo.com** to reach the Web site maintained by the Pharmaceutical Information net (PharmInfonet). At the home page, go to the left panel and select "Disease Centers, thrombolytics." When the next screen is presented, read through the actions of this drug class. Continue down the page until you reach "Case Report: heparin-induced thrombocytopenia." Click on this title to access a case presentation and discussion on this patient.

Antiallergic and Antihistaminic Drugs

HENRY HITNER, PhD
BARBARA NAGLE, PhD

Chapter Focus

This chapter describes the drugs that reduce the symptoms produced by seasonal allergies. Many of these drugs are readily available as over-the-counter products that selectively influence the histamine response by interacting with histamine receptors (but not histamine receptors located in the gastrointestinal tract).

Chapter Terminology

antiallergic: Drug that prevents mast cells from releasing histamine and other vasoactive substances.

antigen: Substance, usually protein or carbohydrate, that is capable of stimulating an immune response.

antihistamine: Drug that blocks the action of histamine at the target organ.

asthma: Inflammation of the bronchioles associated with constriction of smooth muscle, wheezing, and edema.

controller: Drug that prevents the onset of symptoms (or disease) as a result of exposure before the reactive process can take place.

drug fever: A fever induced by use of certain drugs.

eczematoid dermatitis: Condition in which lesions on the skin ooze and develop scaly crusts.

erythema: Redness of the skin, often a result of capillary dilation.

histamine: Substance that interacts with tissues to produce most of the symptoms of allergy.

histamine cephalgia: Headache caused by dilation of cerebral blood vessels due to histamine release.

rhinitis: Inflammation of the lining of the nose associated with one or more of the following symptoms: nasal congestion, rhinorrhea, sneezing, or itching.

rhinitis medicamentosa: Rebound congestion caused by extended use of decongestants.

sensitize: To induce or develop a reaction to naturally occurring substances (allergens) as a result of repeated exposure.

xerostomia: Dryness of the oral cavity resulting from inhibition of the natural moistening action of salivary gland secretions or increased secretion of salivary mucus rather than serous material.

Chapter Objectives

After studying this chapter, you should be able to:

- Explain the reactions produced by histamine released in response to allergic reactions.
- Describe the difference in action between an antihistamine and a drug that is effective in the prophylactic management of asthma.
- Describe two specific therapeutic uses of antihistamines that result from an action on the CNS yet are not associated with allergic responses.
- Describe three side effects of antihistamines that are extensions of their therapeutic activity.
- Describe three examples of first- and second-generation antihistamines and the characteristic difference between the two groups.
- Describe allergic rhinitis and its treatment.
- Describe rhinitis medicamentosa and how to prevent and treat this condition.

Sneezing, coughing, itching, headache, and nasal congestion often indicate that people are experiencing an allergic reaction. Severe allergic reactions can result in respiratory and cardiovascular failure (anaphylaxis). The symptoms of an allergic reaction indicate that individuals have become **sensitized** to certain antigens in the environment. **Antigens** are substances such as pollen, mold, dust, and insect venom that stimulate the production of antibodies in the blood and tissues. In certain (sensitized) people, repeated exposure to these antigens results in allergic reactions because of antigen-antibody interactions. People who suffer from **asthma,** an inflammation of the bronchioles associated with construction of smooth muscle, wheezing and edema, are highly sensitive to antigenic stimulation. Allergic reactions that occur in asthmatic people severely restrict their ability to breathe.

Once an antigen has initiated an allergic reaction, certain cells in the body (mast cells) release active substances into the blood. The most important substance released is **histamine,** which interacts with other cells to produce most of the symptoms of allergy. Drugs that block only the tissue action of histamine are known as **antihistamines.** Such drugs alleviate the annoying discomfort that accompanies most allergic reactions.

In contrast, drugs that prevent mast cells from releasing histamine ae considered **antiallergic** agents. Antiallergic drugs also block the action of other active substances (serotonin and bradykinin). Antiallergic drugs are valuable in the prophylactic therapy of asthma because they help prevent future allergic reactions.

Action of Histamine

Histamine is found throughout the body in the mast cells and basophilic white blood cells. The largest concentrations of mast cells are in the lungs, the GI tract, and the skin. When an antigen comes into contact with the skin or lungs or enters the bloodstream of sensitized individuals, the mast cells and basophils immediately release histamine into the blood. Histamine then interacts with the membrane receptors in certain tissues to produce the symptoms of allergy.

Two types of receptors are associated with histamine: H_1 and H_2 receptors. Histamine interacts with the H_1 receptors, located on blood vessels, bronchiolar smooth muscle, and intestinal smooth muscle, to mediate allergic reactions. The intensity of the allergic symptoms is proportional to the amount of histamine released.

The H_2 receptors are located within the stomach, heart, blood vessels, and uterine tissue. The most important response mediated by H_2 receptors is increased secretion of gastric acid. This response is not usually associated with allergies. However, the action of H_2 receptors is clinically important in the management of GI distress due to acid production.

VASCULAR EFFECTS

Histamine usually produces a transient drop in blood pressure because it dilates small blood vessels and capillaries. With large histamine concentrations, this drop can result in hypotension and circulatory collapse. Dilation of cerebral blood vessels stimulates pain receptors in the skull. This action explains the throbbing headache known as **histamine cephalgia** and may explain the headaches commonly associated with some red wines. Capillary dilation in the skin results in a localized redness called **erythema.**

In addition, histamine causes fluids and proteins to leak out of the capillaries. When capillary leakage occurs in the nasal mucous membranes, nasal congestion occurs. When capillary leakage occurs in the skin, edema, wheals, or hives are produced. Itching and pain occur because histamine irritates sensory nerve endings.

Table 18-1
Physiological Responses Following Histamine Stimulation

System or Tissue	Histamine Effect	Receptor	Physiological Response
Blood pressure	Decreased	H_1, H_2	Hypotension
Heart rate	Increased	H_2	Rapid heartbeat
Bronchioles	Constriction	H_1	Breathing difficulty
Intestine	Contraction	H_1	Constipation/diarrhea
Skin capillaries	Redness, edema, itching	H_1	Response of Lewis
Gastric acid secretion	Increased	H_2	Nausea, heartburn

The erythema and edema produced by histamine in the skin are known as the response of Lewis.

EXTRAVASCULAR SMOOTH MUSCLE EFFECTS

Histamine produces contraction of the smooth muscle of the intestine and bronchioles by stimulating H_1 receptors. Contraction of intestinal smooth muscle results in disturbances of intestinal activity. Contraction of the bronchiolar smooth muscle results in bronchoconstriction, which makes breathing difficult.

Human beings are more sensitive to the bronchiolar constriction produced by histamine than to the disturbances of intestinal activity. In particular, people who have pulmonary diseases (asthma, chronic bronchitis, and emphysema) may be unusually sensitive to the respiratory actions of histamine. It is also thought that there is a higher incidence of people who have gastrointestinal reflex who also have asthma.

CARDIAC EFFECTS

Histamine produces several effects on the heart that are directly related to the amount of histamine present. Histamine usually produces rapid heartbeat. However, at high levels of histamine (histamine shock), cardiac conduction is impaired. Such impairment may lead to the development of arrhythmias and cardiovascular collapse. The major effects of histamine are summarized in Table 18-1.

Antiallergic Agents

Allergic reactions can be blocked in two ways. As shown in Figure 18-1, the mast cells can be prevented from releasing their contents, or the H_1 receptors can be blocked from interacting with histamine. Cromolyn sodium *(Intal, Nasalcrom)* selectively prevents the release of histamine from the mast cells. Cromolyn sodium is not a bronchodilator, a smooth muscle relaxant, or a histamine-receptor antagonist. Because this drug has no effect on histamine receptors, cromolyn sodium must be administered before histamine release has begun.

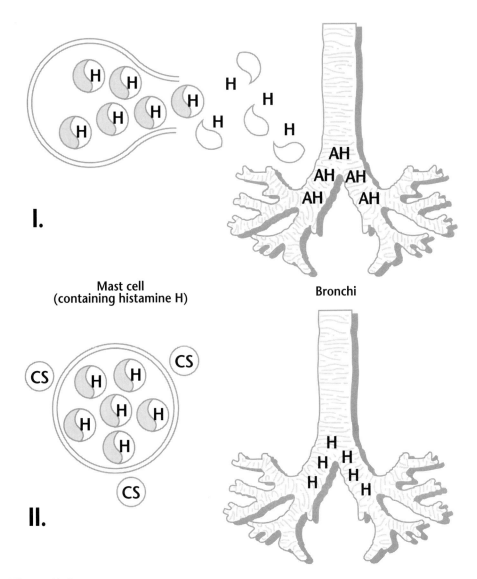

Figure 18-1
Site of action of antihistaminic antiallergic drugs. **I.** Antihistaminic drugs (AH) specifically block histamine (H_1) receptors. **II.** Antiallergic drugs such as cromolyn sodium (CS) prevent the release of histamine (H) from the mast cells.

Drugs like cromolyn sodium that prevent the onset of symptoms or disease as a result of exposure before the reactive process can take place are called **controllers.** Cromolyn sodium is inhaled and reaches the pulmonary mast cells before any antigens can induce an allergic reaction.

ROUTES OF ADMINISTRATION

Cromolyn is available as a dry powder inhaler *(Spinhaler)*, as a solution for inhalation *(Intal)* or nasal spray *(Nasalcrom)*, and as an oral concentrate *(Gastrocrom)*. Indications for use and dosages are presented in Table 18-2. Nasalcrom is available over-the-counter, but the other formulations require a prescription. The spinhaler and nasamatic devices have instructions for proper use. These instructions must be reinforced in order to assure proper use. The oral capsule formulation, which contains a measured dose, is opened, and the powder is dissolved in a glass of hot water. The full glass of liquid must be consumed to receive the proper dose. Fruit juice, milk, or food will inhibit dissolution and absorption of the drug and, therefore, should not be consumed until one-half hour after dosing.

CLINICAL INDICATIONS

Cromolyn is currently used as a prophylactic adjunct, or controller, in the management of chronic bronchial asthma and allergic rhinitis to prevent bronchospasms. Pulmonary function tests must demonstrate that the patient has a bronchodilator-reversible component to the airway obstruction for cromolyn to be of any benefit. Patients must be compliant with dosing at regular repeated intervals; otherwise, the drug cannot achieve a satisfactory response. Regular use of cromolyn for 3 to 4 weeks is required to have the maximum "controlling effect." Oral cromolyn improves diarrhea, flushing, headaches, urticaria, abdominal pain, and nausea in some patients with mastocytosis. In this condition, mast cells accumulate in organs and tissues in excessive amounts. Patients may experience symptoms associated with excessive histamine release, from pruritis to peptic ulcer and chronic diarrhea.

ADVERSE EFFECTS AND CONTRAINDICATIONS

Adverse effects are minimal and include wheezing, nasal itching, nasal burning, nausea, drowsiness, and headache. Occasionally, bronchospasms occur because the micronized powder irritates the lung membranes. Cromolyn is contraindicated in patients who develop hypersensitivity to the drug.

Table 18-2

Indications for Use of Cromolyn Sodium

Formulation	Prophylaxis Indication	Dose
Nebulization solution, inhalation capsules, and Aerosol	Severe bronchial asthma, exercise-induced bronchospasm	20 mg inhaled 4 times daily at regular intervals; one 20-mg capsule or 20 mg of nebulizer solution 1 h before exercise
Nasal solution	Allergic rhinitis	One spray in each nostril 3–6 times a day at regular intervals
Oral	Mastocytosis	Two capsules 4 times a day 30 min before meals and at bedtime

Antihistaminic Agents

Antihistaminic drugs are used to relieve acute reactions in which histamine has already been released. All of the antihistamines available specifically block histamine from interfacing with its H_1 receptors. Therefore, the H_1-mediated allergic responses of histamine are prevented. Antihistaminic drugs are usually administered orally (see Table 18-3) because they are absorbed well from the intestinal tract.

Table 18-3

Frequently Used Antihistaminic Drugs*

Drugs†	*Trade Name*	*Sedative Dose*	*Adult Oral*	*Child Oral*	*Adult Parenteral*
Astemizole***§	Hismanal	—	10 mg/day	10 mg/day‡	—
Azatadine	Optimine	—	1–2 mg BID	1–2 mg BID	—
Brompheniramine	Dimetapp¶	—	Do not exceed 40 mg/day	0.5 mg/kg every 4–6 h	5–20 mg IM, SC
Cetirizine***	Zyrtec	—	5 or 10 mg once a day		
Chlorpheniramine	Aller-Chlor, Chlor-Trimeton¶	—	2–4 mg every 4–6 h	1–2 mg every 4–6 h‡	5–20 mg IV, IM, SC
Clemastine	Tavist¶	—	1.34–2.68 mg BID	0.67–1.34 mg BID‡	—
Cyproheptadine	Periactin	—	4–20 mg/day	2–4 mg BID, TID	—
Dexchlorpheniramine	Polaramine	—	2 mg every 4–6 h	0.5–1 mg every 4–6 h‡	—
Dimenhydrinate	Dramamine	—	50–100 mg every 4–6 h; do not exceed 400 mg/day	25–50 mg every 6–8 h up to 150 mg/day	50 mg IV, IM
Diphenhydramine	Benadryl¶	50 mg at bedtime	25–50 mg every 4–8 h	12.5–25 mg TID, QID	10–50 mg IV, IM up to a maximum of 400 mg/day
Fexofenadine***	Allegra	—	60 mg BID		
Hydroxyzine	Atarax, Vistaril	50–100 mg before anesthesia	25 mg TID, QID	50–100 mg daily in divided doses‡	
Loratadine***	Claritin	—	10 mg daily	10 mg daily	—

Continued

Table 18-3 (continued)

Frequently Used Antihistaminic Drugs*

Drugs†	Trade Name	Recommended Doses			
		Sedative Dose	Adult Oral	Child Oral	Adult Parenteral
Meclizine	Antivert, Bonine	—	25–100 mg/day	—	—
Methdilazine	Tacaryl	—	8 mg BID, QID	4 mg BID, QID	—
Phenindamine	Nolahist	—	25 mg every 4–6 h; do not exceed 150 mg/day	12.5 mg every 4–6 h; do not exceed 75 mg in 24 h	—
Promethazine	Phenergan	25–50 mg at bedtime	12.5 mg QID or 25 mg at bedtime	6.25–12.5 mg TID or 25 mg at bedtime	25 mg IV, IM
Pyriamine (4 mg) pheniramine (4 mg) phenotoloxamine (4 mg)	Poly-Histine Elixir	—	10 mL every 4 h PO	2.5–5 mL every 4 h PO	—
Terfenadine§,***		—	60 mg BID	60 mg BID‡	—
Trimeprazine	Temaril	—	2.5 mg QID	2.5 mg TID	—
Tripelennamine	PBZ, PBZ-SR	—	25–50 mg every 4–6 h up to 600 mg/day	5 mg/kg/day up to 300 mg/day	—
Triprolidine (2.5 mg), pseudoephedrine (60 mg)	Actagen, Actifed¶	—	1 dose every 4–8 h PO up to 4 doses/day	—	—

† All drugs are used for acute allergy (urticaria, rhinitis, hay fever, contact dermatitis, and pruritus) except for dimenhydrinate, which is used to prevent motion sickness, and meclizine, which is used for motion sickness and vertigo. Diphenhydramine is also used as an antiemetic.

* Not an inclusive list of trade names.

‡ Dose for these drugs is set for children as young as 2–6 years and 6–12 years of age. Experience younger than 2 years has not been established.

¶ Available OTC plus prescription; all other products prescription only.

§ No longer manufactured.

*** Second-generation antihistamines.

A few antihistaminics are available for parenteral administration. These drugs are rapidly metabolized by the liver, necessitating repeated drug administration (usually two to four times a day) to maintain a therapeutic response. First-generation antihistamines include chloropheniramine (Chlortrimeton), clemastine (Tavist), diphenhydramine (Benadryl), and promethazine (Phenergan). These agents are characterized by a nonselective interaction with peripheral and central histamine receptors. For this reason, these early antihistamines produce the same spectrum of therapeutic responses, varying only in their degree of activity. These drugs can be used interchangeably and frequently cause sedation along with relief of allergy symptoms. In addition to inhibiting the actions of histamine, these drugs possess local anesthetic and anticholinergic activity. Through a local anesthetic action, antihistamines can depress sensory nerve activity and thus relieve itching and pain. Diphenhydramine (Benadryl) is still considered an antihistamine of choice.

Dimenhydrinate (Dramamine) exerts a unique action in the brain to relieve vertigo and motion sickness and the nausea that accompanies them. Cyproheptadine (Periactin) and azatadine (Optimine) have the ability to inhibit the actions of histamine and serotonin. For this reason, these two drugs may offer a wider range of relief in highly sensitized individuals.

The second generation of antihistamines, which includes astemizole (Hismanal), cetirizine (Zyrtec), fexofenadine (Allegra), loratadine (Claritin), and terfenadine (Seldane), appeared to be more selective for peripheral H_1 receptors. These agents are not as sedating or drying and demonstrate equal or better antiallergic activity as compared to the older drugs. An added advantage is that patients who may become refractory to a particular first-generation antihistamine may find relief with the second-generation drugs.

CLINICAL INDICATIONS

Antihistamines are frequently used in acute allergic reactions including urticaria, hay fever, insect bites, rhinitis, and dermatitis. Because of their inherent sedation, antihistamines may be used to induce sleep in over-the-counter sleeping aids (eg, Nytol) or to relieve motion sickness (eg, Dramamine). Certain antihistamines—chlorpromazine, perfenazine (Trilafon), prochlorperazine (Compazine), promethazine (Phenergan), and triflupromazine (Vesprin)—are extremely effective in reducing nausea and vomiting. These drugs are used as adjunct pre- and postoperative medications to minimize anesthetic irritability and facilitate patient recovery.

Antihistamines are frequently found in cold remedies and cough syrups because of their ability to dry nasal secretions. The anticholinergic component of H_1 antagonists provides relief from symptoms associated with the common cold as well as allergic reactions such as runny nose. In addition, sedation caused by an antihistamine in a multiingredient cold product aids recovery by promoting bed rest. Examples of over-the-counter cold and allergy products that contain antihistaminics are given in Table 18-4.

ADVERSE REACTIONS

Antihistaminics generally produce similar side effects but differ in the predominance or intensity of one side effect over another. The most common side effects produced by the antihistaminics are drowsiness and sedation. Another frequently occurring side effect is dry mouth **(xerostomia).** At any dose, most of these drugs exert an anticholinergic effect that dries the mucous linings of the mouth and nasal passages. This side effect is therapeutically useful in treating the common cold. Other adverse effects include hypotension, rapid heartbeat, anorexia, epigastric distress, and urinary retention.

Table 18-4

Over-the-Counter Cold and Allergy Preparations That Contain Antihistaminics*

Product Name	Antihistamine	Form	Other Active Ingredients
Drixoral Syrup	2 mg brompheniramine	Syrup	Pseudoephedrine 30 mg
Allerest Maximum Strength 12-hour caplets	12 mg chlorpheniramine	Caplet	Pseudoephedrine 75 mg
Caladryl	1% diphenhydramine	Cream	Calamine, camphor, parabens 8%
Tylenol Multisymptom Hot Medication	4 mg chlorpheniramine	Powder	Acetaminophen 650 mg, dextromethorphan 30 mg, pseudoephedrine 60 mg
Dimetane Decongestant	4 mg brompheniramine	Capsule	Phenylephrine 10 mg
Dristan Cold Multisymptom Formulation	2 mg chlorpheniramine	Tablet	Acetaminophen 325 mg, phenylephrine 5 mg
Nyquil Nighttime Cold/Flu Medicine Liquid	1.25 mg doxylamine/mL	Liquid	Alcohol 25%, acetaminophen 157 mg, dextromethorphan 5mg, pseudoephedrine 10 mg
Sting-eze	diphenhydramine		Benzocaine, camphor, eucalyptol, phenol
Triaminic Nite Light	1.0 mg chlorpheniramine/ 5 mL	Syrup	Pseudoephedrine 15 mg, dextromethorphan 7.5 mg
Ziradryl	1% diphenhydramine	Lotion	Alcohol, camphor, parabens, zinc oxide 2%

* Not an inclusive list of available products.

Within the class of antihistamines, diphenhydramine (Benadryl), promethazine (Phenergan), and hydroxyzine (Vistaril) reportedly cause sedation most often, whereas chlorpheniramine (Chlortrimeton) produces less sedation. In unusual circumstances, patients may become nervous and unable to sleep (insomnia) while taking chlorpheniramine. In patients over 60 years of age, paradoxical stimulation rather than sedation can occur and may warrant dose reduction to eliminate this adverse experience.

Several second-generation products were placed on the market in an attempt to reduce, or eliminate, drowsiness. Astemizole (Hismanal) and terfenadine (Seldane) were the first of these agents. These drugs were metabolized in the microsomal (P_{450}) system and interacted with other medications, leading to elevated plasma concentrations of the antihistamine. These increased levels led to cardiac arrhythmias, such as prolonged QT intervals. Cardiac arrhythmia, arrest, and some deaths occurred in patients taking these drugs. These agents were withdrawn from the market.

Cetirizine (Zyrtec) has some sedation qualities but less than many of the older antihistamines. It is administered once daily and has not been associated with any cardiac problems. Loratadine (Claritin) and fexofenadine (allegra) are second-generation antihistamines. They produce less sedation than any of the other antihistamines. They have not been associated with any cardiac problems.

CAUTIONS AND CONTRAINDICATIONS

Because of their anticholinergic activity, antihistaminic drugs should be used with caution in patients with cardiovascular disease or hypertension or patients predisposed to developing an increase in intraocular pressure or urinary retention. Antihistaminics should not be used by patients with a known hypersensitivity to antihistaminics or patients with narrow-angle glaucoma, stenosing peptic ulcer, or prostatic hypertrophy. Antihistaminics should not be used in newborn or premature infants because these patients are more susceptible to the adverse effects. Similarly, antihistaminics should not be used by nursing mothers because these drugs are excreted into breast milk and thus passed into the newborn. These drugs should not be given to dehydrated children because dystonia (abnormal tissue tone) may occur. Phenothiazine antihistaminics such as promethazine *(Phenergan)* are contraindicated for use in patients with CNS depression or a history of phenothiazine-induced jaundice.

Antihistaminics are found as active agents in many ointments, sprays, and cream preparations to be used on the skin. The prolonged indiscriminate use of topical antihistaminic preparations can lead to the development of hypersensitivity in some people. This hypersensitivity may range from rashes to **eczematoid dermatitis,** in which lesions on the skin surface ooze and develop scaly crusts. Antihistaminics may also produce **drug fever,** which will subside only when the drug is stopped. The mechanism of this drug-induced fever is not known. Antihistaminics are not harmless drugs, even though they may be found in many over-the-counter products (Table 18-4).

Antihistamines should not be used when testing patients for allergic reactions. This applies to skin testing when attempting to determine allergic responses. Antihistamines will mask the response.

The potential for adverse effects increases when any individual takes three to five medications *or more* daily, and older patients are likely to be taking multiple medications. Patients taking multiple medications, including the elderly, are more likely to experience dizziness, excessive sedation, paradoxical stimulation, or confusion with these drugs. Medications that affect the cardiovascular or central nervous system may predispose patients to developing mental confusion. In addition, the availability of antihistamines in over-the-counter preparations contributes additional seasonal exposure, as in winter colds and spring and fall allergies. Even with appropriate magnification in eyeglasses, it is often difficult for patients to read the fine print on packaging that identifies the contents of over-the-counter products.

Antihistamines are not recommended for use during pregnancy. Animal studies have demonstrated abnormalities in the offspring with certain antihistamines. Convulsions in newborns after human exposure to antihistamines in the third trimester have been reported. Safe use during pregnancy has not been established.

DRUG INTERACTIONS

In general, antihistaminics interact with many drugs. Some antibiotics, muscle relaxants (curare), and narcotic analgesics (morphine) cause the release of histamine from mast cells. If patients are taking such a drug, it is not unusual for an antihistaminic to be given to counteract the effects of histamine. Drugs that depress the activity of the CNS (sedatives, tranquilizers, and alcohol) increase the incidence of drowsiness when taken with antihistaminics. This synergistic effect is most likely to occur with over-the-counter products (Table 18-4) that contain an antihistaminic in addition to alcohol as an active ingredient.

Macrolide antibiotics—erythromycin, clarithromycin, and troleandomycin—and antifungals—ketoconazole, itraconazole, and miconazolem—elevate the plasma levels of loratadine. The mechanism of interaction is inhibition of hepatic metabolism. Although these drugs significantly increase the plasma concentration of loratadine, this antihistamine does not appear to produce clinically significant adverse effects at higher blood levels, as did terfenadine and astemizole. Table 18-5 describes potential drug interactions that can occur with antihistaminics.

Table 18-5
Drug Interactions with Antihistaminic Drugs

Drug	Response
Antibiotics:† azithromycin, clarithromycin, erythromycin, troleandomycin	Increase plasma concentrations of astemizole, loratadine, and terfenadine through inhibition of hepatic metabolism
Anticholinergics: atropine	Increase nervousness, insomnia, and constipation
Anticoagulants: coumarins	Delay absorption of anticoagulant
Antidepressants: imipramine	Increase anticholinergic effect, urinary retention, and intraocular pressure
Antifungals:† fluconazole, itraconazole, ketoconazole, miconazole	Increase plasma concentrations of astemizole, loratadine, and terfenadine through inhibition of hepatic metabolism
Cimetidine	Increases the plasma concentration of loratadine
CNS depressants: alcohol, barbiturates, hypnotics, narcotic analgesics, phenothiazines, tranquilizers	Increase drowsiness, sedation, and lethargy
Corticosteroids: oral drugs	Increase risk of glaucoma in susceptible patients
HIV protease inhibitors:† indinavir, nelfinavir, ritonavir, saquanavir	Increase terfenadine plasma concentrations through inhibition of hepatic metabolism
MAO* inhibitors: amphetamines, tranylcypromine	Intensify the drying effects of antihistaminics and may cause hypotension with phenothiazines
Serotonin release inhibitors, Sparfloxacin, Zileuton	Increase terfenadine plasma concentrations through inhibition of hepatic metabolism†

* *Abbreviation:* MAO, monoamine oxidase.
† Predisposes the patient to QT interval prolongation and/or potentially life-threatening cardiotoxicity with astemizole and terfenadine.

GUIDELINES FOR USE

Antihistamines provide symptomatic relief for a variety of acute and chronic conditions when used at the recommended dose and at regular approved intervals. Because these products are widely available over-the-counter, patients frequently assume the drugs have less potential for producing adverse effects. In all cases where the antihistamine is available over the counter and by prescription, the formulation of the OTC product contains the active agent, only in a lower amount than at the prescription level. Therefore, with children, the elderly, and hectic working adults, it becomes extremely easy for patients to take multiple doses, which result in levels comparable to the prescription antihistamines. Whenever possible, respiratory care professionals (RCPs) should review the following facts with patients who are using antihistamines or cromolyn.

PATIENT INSTRUCTION

Special formulations should be reviewed with patients to assure that they use the product in such a manner that the designated amount of drug is delivered appropriately.

Sustained-release (SR) preparations should not be chewed or crushed. These capsules should not be opened to divide the dose. The pellets are coated to release the drug at a variety of time intervals, which cannot be determined by the patient. SR preparations should be swallowed intact with water.

Oral capsules of cromolyn are designed to be opened so the powder can be dissolved in hot water. Patients should be reminded not to take fruit juice, milk, or food with the drug because they will interfere with drug absorption.

Instructions for use of the spinhaler and nasal inhalation are included in the product package. Patients should receive instructions by a health care professional, such as an RCP, demonstrating the insertion of the capsule in order to facilitate compliance with dosing.

DOSING SCHEDULE

The time of dosing should be provided in writing if necessary to assure adequate drug absorption. Oral cromolyn should be taken 30 minutes before meals to avoid any delay in drug absorption.

DOSING WITH MEALS

Oral antihistamines may cause gastric upset in some patients. Patients may take antihistamines with meals to minimize the irritation.

ADVERSE EFFECTS

Patients should be instructed to avoid prolonged exposure to sunlight because antihistamines may produce photosensitivity. Even with nonsedating antihistamines, patients should be reminded to avoid alcohol and CNS depressants, which could potentiate adverse effects. This includes OTC preparations for relief of coughs, colds, flu, and allergy. Any product designated "elixir" contains alcohol in amounts that can interact with antihistamine effects.

NOTIFY THE PHYSICIAN

The physician must be notified immediately if the patient develops involuntary muscle spasms, wheezing, or edema. These may be signs of extrapyramidal reactions or hypersensitivity, respectively.

Patients should be instructed to notify the physician immediately if their medical history changes or they develop signs and symptoms of glaucoma, peptic ulcer, or urinary retention.

USE IN PREGNANCY

Antihistamines are designated as Pregnancy Category B or C. They are not recommended for use in pregnancy because the safety for use in human beings has not been established. The physician should be notified if the patient becomes pregnant during therapy.

Corticosteroids

ALLERGIC RHINITIS

In addition to antihistamines and antiallergic drugs such as cromolyn, corticosteroids may also be needed for the treatment of allergic **rhinitis.** Allergic rhinitis is the most common chronic allergic respiratory disease. It affects about 20% of the United States population. Allergic rhinitis is one of three different types of rhinitis. Rhinitis can be divided into allergic rhinitis with seasonal or perennial types, infectious rhinitis, and noninfectious, nonallergic rhinitis.

Intranasal corticosteroids work against the inflammation-causing factors of allergic rhinitis. Corticosteroids inhibit inflammatory cell and mediator activity as noted in Chapter 20 on Adrenal Steroids. They reduce vascular permeability and edema of the nasal mucosa.

Intranasal corticosteroids have a number of advantages. They relieve all nasal symptoms of allergic rhinitis, have an excellent safety profile, and are dosed once or twice daily. The effects are localized, which limits exposure and limits the risk of systemic effects. Commonly used intranasal corticosteroids are found in Table 18-6.

ADMINISTRATION

A common problem associated with the use of intranasal steroid is trauma to the nasal passages during drug administration. To avoid this problem it is best to instruct the patient to administer medication to the right nostril using the right

Table 18-6
Nasal Corticosteroid Sprays

Generic Name	Trade Name	Dose per Inhalation	Base Initial Adult Dosage	Pediatric Indication
Beclomethasone	Beconase AQ	42 μg	1–2 sprays per nostril twice daily	Children >6 years
	Vancenase AQ 84 μg Double Strength	84 μg	1–2 sprays per nostril daily	Children >6 years
Budesonide	Rhinocort	32 μg	2 sprays per nostril twice daily or 4 sprays per nostril daily	Children >6 years
Flunisolide	Nasarel	25 μg	2 sprays per nostril twice daily	Children >6 years
Fluticasone propionate	Flonase	50 μg	2 sprays per nostril daily or 1 spray per nostril twice daily	Children >4 years
Mometasone furoate monohydrate	Nasonex	50 μg	2 sprays per nostril daily	Children >12 years
Triamcinolone acetonide	Nasacort	55 μg	2 sprays per nostril daily	Children >6 years

hand and to the left nostril using the left hand. Crossing over from left to right tends to twist the inhaler and lead to nasal trauma.

Nasal Decongestants

This group of medications was reviewed in Chapter 6, Drugs Affecting the Sympathetic Nervous System. As α-adrenergic drugs, they can constrict blood vessels in the mucous membranes of the nasal sinuses, producing a decongestant effect. For allergic rhinitis, intranasal decongestants, such as phenylephrine (Neo-Synephrine) or oxymetazoline (Afrin) can be used.

RHINITIS MEDICAMENTOSA

Although intranasal decongestant may have some benefit, the use should be limited to 3 to 5 days. Longer use can result in rebound congestion, known as **rhinitis medicamentosa.** In this condition, congestion becomes so severe that it is difficult to breathe through the nose. Inhalations become more and more frequent as the person attempts to keep the nasal passages open.

The use of nasal decongestants can be in response to allergic rhinitis or to the use of other medications as shown in Table 18-7. These medications may cause nasal congestion as an adverse effect, and the topical decongestants can be used in response to that adverse effect. Because these topical nasal decongestants are available over the counter, self-treatment is available without input from any health care professional. The mechanism by which rhinitis medicamentosa occurs is not known. The physical change involved is the production of edema leading to nasal swelling and nasal obstruction.

The best way to manage rhinitis medicamentosa is to prevent it from occurring. Encouraging your patients to limit the use of nasal decongestants to 3 to 5 days will help avoid the problem. The first step is to explain to the patient the cause of the congestion. The patient must understand why the condition has developed and what he or she must do to successfully discontinue the use of the nasal decongestant.

The second way is to discontinue the topical decongestant. This can be done immediately but may result in the patient having considerable discomfort for the first 4 to 7 days. The use of saline nasal spray may be very helpful during this period. Occasionally, inhaled nasal steroids may be used during the initial period to decrease the inflammation associated with rhinitis medicamentosa.

Another method is to slowly decrease the use of the topical decongestant. Begin by reducing the use of decongestant in one nostril by using saline for every other dose. Once the first nostril is on saline only, then begin using saline on the other nostril.

Table 18-7
Medications That May Cause Nasal Congestion

Vasodilators (vasodilation leads to tissue edema and nasal congestion)
  Methyldopa
  Clonidine
  Reserpine
  Hydralazine
  Propranolol
Psychotherapeutic agents (α-adrenergic blockers leading to vasodilation)
  Amitriptyline
  Thioridazine
Oral contraceptives and estrogens
Cocaine
Cromolyn sodium

Chapter 18 Review

UNDERSTANDING TERMINOLOGY

Test your understanding of the material in this chapter by answering the following questions.

1. What is the difference between an antiallergic and an antihistaminic drug?
2. Differentiate between erythema and dermatitis.
3. Define prophylaxis.
4. Define xerostomia.

ACQUIRING KNOWLEDGE

Answer the following questions.

5. Where is histamine located in the body? What stimulates histamine release?
6. What are the effects of histamine on various tissues?
7. How does cromolyn sodium produce its antiallergic response? When is cromolyn sodium used?
8. How do the antihistaminics prevent the action of histamine? What receptors are involved in allergic reactions?
9. What other pharmacologic actions do antihistaminics produce?
10. Why are antihistaminics found in over-the-counter products? What are two examples?
11. What adverse effects are associated with antihistaminic use?
12. What drugs commonly interact with antihistaminics?

APPLYING KNOWLEDGE ON THE JOB

Answer the following questions.

13. Mrs. Lewis calls the clinic where you are working. She says when she was in the clinic 2 days ago, the doctor diagnosed her illness as allergic rhinitis and gave her prescriptions for *Nasalcrom* and *Chlor-Trimeton*. She claims she has used *Nasalcrom* for the past 48 hours without any relief of her nasal symptoms. "My nose is running like a faucet with this pollen count so high. I didn't fill the *Chlor-Trimeton* prescription because I have to work and can't tolerate the drowsiness." What should you tell her?
14. Six months later, during cold season, Mrs. Lewis calls the office for a refill on her *Nasalcrom*. She says she has a terrible cold with a runny nose, and the *Nasalcrom* worked so well when she used it during hay fever season, she wants to use it now. What should you do?
15. Your patient is experiencing rhinitis medicamentosa. How would you explain this condition to your patient, and what would you recommend?

Additional Reading

Cross S. Rhinitis management. *Pract Nurse* 1997;13(5):262.
Mathewson HS. Drug capsule: Antihistamines and asthma. *Respir Care* 1996;41(3):212.

Internet Activities

"Healthline" is a Web site maintained by the American Academy of Family Physicians (AAFP) in order to provide patients and medical associates access to current information on a variety of diseases. The AAFP has developed information for the public about a broad range of medical problems that family physicians are trained to treat. Through this site you can find Patient Information Handouts on more than 200 health topics, *Good Health Newsletter* with tips for preventative medicine, and publications, including brief reviews, that provide reliable information to the public. Go onto this Web site by typing **www.healthline.com.** Go to the bottom of the Web page and select "Patient Information." The next Web page will provide a user-friendly menu with four categories: The Body, Treatments, Common Conditions/Diseases/Disorders, and Healthy Living. Select "Allergies" to access a brief review on the treatment of allergic conjunctivitis with antihistamines.

You can also enter this site by typing **www.healthline.com/articles.** You will be provided a number of current articles from "Nonsedating Antihistamines" to "Allergic Rhinitis, symptoms, cost of treatment, and primary reason for school absence in children"; just click and read. Most articles are limited to two pages. Through this Web site, you can also read current topics covered in the *Journal of Family Practice.*

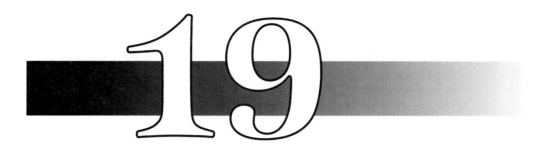

Bronchodilator Drugs and the Treatment of Asthma

HENRY HITNER, PhD
BARBARA NAGLE, PhD

Chapter Focus

This chapter describes the common diseases that affect the respiratory system and the pharmacology of drugs used to treat these conditions. It also explains the role of the autonomic nervous system in asthma and how different bronchodilators interact with this system. In addition, it describes how corticosteroids, mucolytics, and the new antileukotriene drugs are used to affect respiratory function.

Chapter Terminology

asthma: Respiratory disease characterized by bronchoconstriction, shortness of breath, and wheezing.

bronchodilator: Drug that relaxes bronchial smooth muscle and dilates the respiratory passages.

chemical mediator: Substance formed by mast cells, certain blood cells, and other body cells that is released during inflammatory and allergic reactions.

chronic bronchitis: Respiratory condition caused by chronic irritation that increases secretion of mucus and causes degeneration of the respiratory lining.

controllers: Medications that are used to prevent acute asthmatic attacks. These are primarily used as prophylactic measures.

COPD: Chronic obstructive pulmonary disease, usually caused by emphysema and chronic bronchitis.

emphysema: Disease process causing destruction of the walls of the alveolar sacs.

leukotrienes: Formerly known as slow-reacting substances of anaphylaxis (SRA-A), these are 1000 times more potent than histamine as a bronchoconstrictor. It is a derivative of arachidonic acid.

mucolytic: Drug that liquefies bronchial secretions.

prostaglandins: Series of chemical mediators that are released by most body cells and are often involved in disease processes. It is a derivative of arachidonic acid.

relievers: Medications that quickly relieve the patient's symptoms. These are used during an acute asthmatic attack.

Chapter Objectives

After studying this chapter, you should be able to:

- Describe chronic obstructive pulmonary disease (COPD) and asthma.
- List four respiratory components affected by asthma.
- List three chemical mediators involved in asthma.
- Describe the mechanism of action and main pharmacological effects of the three types of bronchodilators.
- Explain the role of corticosteroids, cromolyn, antileukotrienes, and mucolytics in respiratory therapy.

The respiratory system plays a vital role in the exchange of the respiratory gases, oxygen (O_2) and carbon dioxide (CO_2). Functionally, the respiratory system consists of a series of anatomic tubes (trachea, bronchi, bronchioles, and alveolar ducts) that conduct air to and from the air sacs (alveoli) of the lungs. Each alveolus is surrounded by a network of capillaries. Both the alveoli and the capillaries consist of a single cell layer that allows rapid diffusion of O_2 into the blood and equally rapid diffusion of CO_2 out of the blood.

The respiratory passageways are composed of smooth muscle and cartilage (C-rings). The smooth muscle controls the size of the lumen of the respiratory passages. The autonomic nervous system regulates the contraction of the smooth muscle. Stimulation of the sympathetic nervous system, mainly through the release of epinephrine from the adrenal gland and the subsequent stimulation of β_2 receptors, produces smooth muscle relaxation (bronchodilation). Parasympathetic stimulation (ACh) produces contraction (bronchoconstriction). **Bronchodilators** are drugs that relax bronchial smooth muscle and dilate respiratory passages.

Respiratory Diseases

Any disease process or condition that interferes with respiratory exchange causes serious alterations in the levels of the gases in the blood O_2 and CO_2. The most common causes of respiratory difficulties are chronic obstructive pulmonary disease and asthma.

CHRONIC OBSTRUCTIVE PULMONARY DISEASE (COPD)

COPD is a relatively common respiratory condition that is caused by emphysema and chronic bronchitis. Both conditions cause irreversible changes to the respiratory system. **Chronic bronchitis** is caused by chronic irritation of the respiratory tract. Cigarette smoke and other environmental pollutants increase and thicken respiratory secretions of mucus. These secretions interfere with gas exchange, resulting in eventual fibrotic changes in the respiratory lining. Chronic cough, increased susceptibility to infection, and restriction of physical activity are characteristics of this condition. Drug therapy can provide some relief, but it cannot reverse the fibrosis and other physical changes in the respiratory lining.

EMPHYSEMA

Emphysema is a disease process involving destruction of the alveolar walls. Consequently, there is an enlargement of the air spaces within the lungs. Individuals with emphysema have difficulty expelling air from the lungs. Respiratory gas exchange is reduced, and shortness of breath occurs. Irreversible lung damage takes place, forcing the individuals to restrict daily activities. Treatment involves respiratory exercises designed to increase the efficiency of respiration, oxygen therapy, and medications. Bronchodilators and mucolytic agents are used to dilate the bronchi and to promote expectoration of bronchial secretions.

ASTHMA

Asthma is a chronic inflammatory lung disorder characterized by shortness of breath and wheezing. These effects are caused by inflammation and bronchoconstriction of the respiratory airways. Many factors can cause asthma in susceptible individuals. These factors include respiratory irritants (dust and noxious chemicals), exercise (particularly in cold weather), respiratory tract infections, aspirin and related drugs, and, most commonly, development of an allergy to foreign proteins (pollen, animal dander, etc.).

In allergic asthma, individuals develop antibodies to the foreign protein (antigen). After exposure to the antigen, an antigen-antibody reaction occurs in the respiratory tract, precipitating an asthmatic attack. The immediate result is shortness of breath, wheezing, and the terrifying feeling of suffocation. Relief of asthmatic attacks involves use of drugs that relax respiratory smooth muscle (bronchodilators) and drugs that produce antiinflammatory effects on the respiratory passageways.

Exercise-induced asthma (EIA) is defined as a transient increase in airway resistance following 6 to 8 minutes of vigorous exercise. The type, intensity, and duration of the exercise as well as the environment influence the onset and severity of EIA. Sports that require continuous exertion and cold, dry air, in particular, can trigger EIA. Proper conditioning, adequate warm-up, and preexercise treatment with β_2-adrenergic agonists or other antiinflammatory medications can reduce the incidence of EIA.

Aspirin-induced asthma (AIA) is a mucosal inflammatory disease combined with precipitation of asthma and rhinitis following ingestion of aspirin and most nonsteroidal antiinflammatory drugs (NSAIDs). The attack usually occurs within a few hours of aspirin or NSAID ingestion and is accompanied by profuse rhinorrhea, conjunctival and periorbital edema, and vasomotor flushing of the head and neck in addition to the asthmatic attack. Aspirin and NSAIDs inhibit the synthesis of certain prostaglandins that are important for maintaining bronchial tone while increasing the synthesis of other arachidonic acid derivatives, particularly leukotrienes, that promote bronchoconstriction. Most individuals with AIA have asthma, and treatment of AIA is similar to the treatment of asthma in general. Individuals with AIA should avoid ingestion of aspirin, NSAIDs, and other drugs that inhibit the synthesis of prostaglandins.

Asthma has several components in addition to the characteristic inflammation, bronchoconstriction, and wheezing. There is usually mucosal edema and increased production of bronchial mucus. Ciliary activity of the respiratory tract is usually depressed.

The decrease in ciliary activity interferes with the clearing of mucus and other debris from the lower respiratory airways. Most importantly, asthma is a chronic inflammatory condition of the respiratory airways. It should be treated primarily with antiinflammatory agents to prevent acute attacks.

CHEMICAL MEDIATORS

During an inflammatory reaction, **chemical mediators** are formed and released from injured tissue, mast cells, and leukocytes located within the respiratory tract. These mediators are responsible for most of the symptoms and complications of asthma. The chemical mediators involved include histamine, eosinophilic chemotactic factor of anaphylaxis (ECF-A), and various arachidonic acid derivatives, especially derivatives known as the **leukotrienes.** Several leukotrienes combine to form what was formerly known as the slow-reacting substance of anaphylaxis (SRS-A), which is an important mediator of inflammation. Recent advances in molecular biology have identified additional mediators that are referred to as cytokines. Tumor necrosis factor and several other cytokine mediators, known as interleukins, are currently undergoing intense investigation. The large number of chemical mediators involved in asthma presents a complicated situation both for the understanding of the disease and for its treatment.

Histamine   Whenever there is injury or insult to body tissue, histamine is rapidly released from mast cells. The pharmacology of histamine was presented in Chapter 18. In the respiratory tract, histamine causes bronchoconstriction, increased vascular permeability that contributes to mucosal edema, and infiltration of leukocytes, particularly eosinophils. Antihistamines are usually not used in asthma but may be helpful if there is an allergic component.

Eosinophilic Chemotactic Factor of Anaphylaxis   Eosinophilic chemotactic factor (ECF-A) is also released by mast cells and functions to attract eosinophils to the site of cell injury or irritation. Eosinophils are part of the general inflammatory and allergic reaction that often occurs in the lining of the respiratory tract in asthma. The inflammatory and allergic reactions worsen and prolong the asthmatic process. When this occurs, antiinflammatory corticosteroid drugs are used to suppress the inflammatory process.

Prostaglandins   The arachidonic cascade results in the production of many chemical mediators. The **prostaglandins** are some of those chemical mediators produced by almost all body cells. When cells are irritated or injured, various prostaglandins are rapidly formed and released by the cell membranes. The prostaglandins produce numerous biological effects, including effects on smooth muscle, secretion of mucus, and the inflammatory process.

Leukotrienes   The leukotrienes (LT) are another product of the arachidonic cascade. During anaphylaxis (a severe allergic reaction) and asthma, the mast cells produce and release several different leukotrienes. The most important of these are referred to as LTB, LTC, LTD, and LTE. Leukotrienes are extremely potent inflammatory agents and bronchoconstrictors that have a long duration of action, much greater than that of histamine. In addition, leukotrienes promote mucosal edema, secretion of mucus, and leukocyte infiltration. Leukotrienes are considered to be important mediators involved in asthma. There has been an intense search by drug companies to discover drugs that block the production of the leukotrienes. Several new drugs that interfere with the action of leukotrienes, the antileukotrienes, have recently been approved for use in asthma (see below).

Role of the Autonomic Nervous System

Bronchiolar smooth muscle tone and secretion of mucus are normally influenced by the sympathetic and parasympathetic divisions of the autonomic nervous system. Sympathetic stimulation by epinephrine (β_2 receptor) produces bronchodilation. Parasympathetic activation, via the vagus nerve and release of acetylcholine, produces bronchoconstriction and increased secretion of mucus. Noxious irritants of the respiratory tract stimulate vagal reflexes that result in parasympathetic activation. It has been suggested that in asthmatics there is a predominance or hyperactivity of the parasympathetic division. This factor may be important and may contribute to the increased sensitivity and hyperreactivity of the asthmatic airway.

The general approach to the treatment of asthma is to give drugs that increase sympathetic activity or decrease parasympathetic activity (anticholinergic drugs). Research has shown that in certain cells, sympathetic activation stimulates the formation of an intracellular nucleotide called cyclic adenosine monophosphate, or cyclic AMP. Parasympathetic activation stimulates the formation of another nucleotide, cyclic guanosine monophosphate, or cyclic GMP.

Cyclic AMP appears to be responsible for mediating the effects of sympathetic stimulation to produce bronchodilation. Also, during asthma, the formation and release of mediators (histamine, leukotrienes, and ECF-A) from mast cells is inhibited by increased levels of cyclic AMP. Cyclic GMP appears to be responsible for mediating the effects of parasympathetic stimulation to produce bronchoconstriction, secretion of mucus, and increased release of mediators from mast cells.

In summary, the current approach to the treatment of asthma takes into account that in patients with asthma, there may be increased parasympathetic activity, which increases intracellular levels of cyclic GMP. The high levels of cyclic GMP result in release of mast cell mediators that cause bronchoconstriction, increased secretion of mucus, mucosal edema, and leukocyte infiltration. Treatment of asthma is aimed at increasing intracellular levels of cyclic AMP with sympathomimetics and other drugs. As levels of cyclic AMP increase in bronchial smooth muscle and mast cells, there is relaxation of smooth muscle (bronchodilation) and inhibition of release of the mast cell mediators that cause inflammation. These effects give relief from the asthmatic attack and help prevent further complications. The main drugs used to treat asthma are the corticosteroids and the antileukotrienes that reduce and control inflammation and other drugs, such as the bronchodilators, used primarily to relieve acute attacks.

Bronchodilator Drugs

A number of different drug classes are used in the treatment of asthma. Bronchodilators include β-adrenergic drugs (sympathomimetics), theophylline, and anticholinergic drugs. Some of these drugs are also referred to as "reliever" drugs. Steroids, antileukotrienes, and other antiinflammatory drugs are referred to as "controller" drugs. **Reliever** drugs relieve bronchospasm while **controller** drugs prevent asthmatic attacks.

β-ADRENERGIC DRUGS

Sympathetic stimulation of bronchial smooth muscle causes bronchodilation. This effect is mediated by the β_2-adrenergic receptors. Consequently, drugs that stimulate the β_2 receptors produce bronchodilation.

Epinephrine (which is normally released from the adrenal gland) and isoproterenol are two potent β-receptor stimulators. These drugs stimulate both β_1 (heart) and β_2 (smooth muscle) receptors. As a consequence, increased heart rate and other sympathetic effects occur in addition to bronchodilation. Overuse of these drugs may cause tachycardia and cardiac arrhythmias.

Adrenergic drugs that selectively stimulate the β_2 receptors at therapeutic doses are available. These drugs are preferred over the older drugs, which stimulate both β_1 and β_2 receptors. However, at higher than therapeutic doses or in susceptible individuals, the selective β_2 drugs may also cause some β_1-receptor and cardiac stimulation.

There are several other advantages of the newer selective β_2 drugs over older drugs such as epinephrine. The newer drugs can be administered orally and by metered-dose inhaler (MDI), whereas the older drugs are administered only by subcutaneous injection or MDI. Also, the duration of action of the newer drugs is much longer (several hours), and therefore, they provide longer protection with fewer drug administrations. However, epinephrine is still used in the treatment of acute asthmatic attacks, for which it is usually administered by subcutaneous injection. The β-adrenergic drugs used in the treatment of asthma are presented in Table 19-1.

Patients who experience infrequent asthmatic attacks usually carry an MDI and inhale the drug when they experience difficulty in breathing. Patients who experience more frequent asthmatic attacks usually use the inhalers or take one of the oral preparations on a regular basis. Currently, the inhalation route is the preferred method of administration. Albuterol is most commonly used as a reliever via MDI. Its onset of action is 5 to 10 minutes. Salmeterol is a long-acting β_2 agonist administered by MDI. This drug has a slow onset of action but is more potent that most other β_2 drugs. It is particularly useful for nocturnal asthma, exercise-induced asthma, and as adjunctive therapy in patients with poor asthma control who also take steroids.

In severe acute asthma, it make be necessary to provide the patient with a continuous nebulization of a β_2 agonist. Albuterol can be administered at a dose of 15 mg/h to adults in an acute situation.

The most common adverse effects of the adrenergic drugs are CNS stimulation, including respiratory stimulation, restlessness, apprehension, tremors, and anxiety. Cardiac stimulation resulting in tachycardia and arrhythmias may also occur. The selective β_2 drugs produce fewer CNS and cardiovascular effects than epinephrine and isoproterenol.

Table 19-1

Sympathomimetic (β-Adrenergic) Bronchodilator Drugs

Drug (Trade Name)	Adult Dose	Peak Effect/Duration of Action (Minutes)
Adrenergic Drugs		
Epinephrine Injection, USP	0.2–0.5 mg (1:1000) SC PRN	5–60
Epinephrine Mist	2–3 oral inhalations every 3–4 h	5–60
Isoproterenol *(Medihaler-Iso, Mistometer)*	2–3 oral inhalations every 3–4 h	10–60
Subjective β-2 Drugs		
Albuterol *(Proventil, Ventolin)*	2–4 mg PO TID, QID	120–480
	2 oral inhalations every 4–6 h	30–300
Bitolterol *(Tornalate)*	2–3 oral inhalations every 6 h	360–480
Isoetharine *(Bronkometer)*	2–3 oral inhalations every 3 h	15–120
Metaproterenol *(Alupent)*	10–20 mg PO TID, QID 2–3 oral	90–480
	inhalations every 6 h	30–360
Pirbuterol *(Maxair)*	2 oral inhalations every 6 h	360–480
Terbutaline *(Brethine, Bricanyl)*	2.5–5 mg PO TID	120–480
	0.25–0.5 mg SC	15–240
	2 oral inhalations every 4–6 h	30–300
Salmeterol *(Severent)*	2 oral inhalations every 12 h	60–720

THEOPHYLLINE

Xanthine compounds—including caffeine, theophylline, and theobromine—are found naturally in tea, cocoa, and coffee. Theophylline is the only xanthine used in the treatment of asthma and COPD. Theophylline inhibits an intracellular enzyme, phosphodiesterase, that normally inactivates cyclic AMP. By inhibiting phosphodiesterase, levels of cyclic AMP increase in bronchiolar smooth muscle and in mast cells. As discussed, cyclic AMP produces bronchodilation and inhibits the release of mediators from mast cells. Consequently, both β-adrenergic drugs and theophylline increase cyclic AMP levels, which are important in the control and treatment of asthma. As a bronchodilator, theophylline is less potent than the β_2 drugs and can cause serious CNS and cardiac adverse effects when the plasma concentrations exceed the narrow therapeutic range.

Theophylline can be administered orally, rectally, or intravenously. There is significant patient variability in regard to absorption and metabolism. Therefore, the dose must be adjusted carefully. Plasma concentrations of theophylline are periodically determined to ensure that theophylline levels are in the therapeutic range (10 to 20 µg/mL). Concentrations below the therapeutic range are ineffective, and concentrations above this range cause toxicity.

Dosing of theophylline can be very difficult. In fact, some clinicians believe it should be restricted to pulmonologists and allergists because of all of the drug interactions and resulting dosing adjustments. Theophylline is an example of a drug whose metabolism changes as we grow. In children the dosing is as high as 24 mg/kg/day. Over time, it is reduced to 10 mg/kg/day in adults because of the decrease in metabolism.

Theophylline interacts with many antibiotics and anticonvulsants that require substantial changes in dosing. Whenever medications are added or discontinued from a patient's regimen it is important to make sure that the primary prescriber is made aware.

Numerous preparations of theophylline, including extended-release tablets, are available. Aminophylline is a water-soluble preparation of theophylline that is used for intravenous administration, usually during acute asthmatic attacks. Theophylline can be administered in combination with sympathomimetics in situations where one drug is unable to control the asthmatic condition alone.

The most frequent side effects from oral administration of theophylline are nausea and vomiting. Because theophylline produces vasodilation, some patients experience flushing, headache, and hypotension. Caution is necessary in patients with existing cardiovascular disease because theophylline may cause excessive cardiac stimulation. Theophylline also stimulates the CNS and may cause restlessness, insomnia, tremors, and convulsions, especially when plasma levels are above the therapeutic range.

ANTICHOLINERGIC DRUGS

Anticholinergic drugs (atropine-like) are not widely used in the treatment of asthma. Although they do produce some bronchodilation, they tend to dry mucous membranes. However, in patients in whom other bronchodilators cannot be used or are not effective, administration of anticholinergic drugs by aerosol may produce bronchodilation and offer some relief. By blocking the actions of acetylcholine (which increases intracellular levels of cyclic GMP), the anticholinergic drugs decrease intracellular levels of cyclic GMP.

Ipratropium Bromide (Atrovent) Ipratropium is a derivative of atropine and is the only anticholinergic drug used for asthma and COPD. Compared to the β$_2$ drugs, ipratropium is less potent. Ipratropium is administered by oral inhalation. It has a slow onset but prolonged duration of action (6 hours). It is poorly absorbed into the systemic circulation and therefore causes few adverse effects. Excessive drying of the mouth and upper respiratory passages may cause discomfort and is the most common side effect. Use can also lead to tachycardia.

Ipratropium is available in several different dosage forms. It is available as a nebulizing solution, and this is the common form used in an emergency room or for patients who are too young to use an MDI. It is available as an MDI and also as a nasal inhaler for use in rhinitis. It is important to note that the MDI contains peanut oil as one of the ingredients, and so this should not be used by patients allergic to peanuts.

Corticosteroids

The general pharmacology of the glucocorticoids is detailed in Chapter 20, Adrenal Steroids. One of the main uses of these drugs is for treatment of inflammatory and allergic conditions such as asthma. The major effect of steroids in the treatment of asthma is to inhibit the inflammatory response that occurs in the respiratory airways. Steroids are used systemically in acute asthmatic conditions and by inhalation in the chronic control of asthma. Steroids are frequently used with bronchodilators, which usually allows a reduction of the dosage of the bronchodilator drug.

During acute asthmatic attacks, steroids are administered either parenterally or orally to achieve effective drug levels rapidly. Prednisone (Deltasone), orally, is widely used in these situations. Steroids have the potential to produce a large number of adverse effects, some of which can be serious. For this reason, steroids should be used with caution and at the lowest effective dosages.

Steroids are most commonly administered by oral inhalation for the chronic control of asthma. The advantage of inhalation is that lower dosages of steroid are delivered directly into the respiratory tract. Use of this route greatly reduces systemic absorption and the adverse effects associated with steroid use. Corticosteroids available for inhalation are listed in Table 19-2. Recently, a new dosage form has become available. Budesonide is now available as an inhalation suspension for nebulization. This will allow for use of inhaled steroids in younger patients who cannot coordinate MDIs.

Table 19-2
Corticosteroids Administered by Aerosol Inhalation

Drug (Trade Name)	Usual Dose
Beclomethasone (Beclovent, Vanceril)	2 inhalations QID
Budesonide (Pulmicort) Turbohaler	1–2 oral inhalations BID
Budesonide (Pulmacort Respules) inhalation suspension	0.5 mg daily or 0.25 mg BID
Flunisolide (Aerobid)	2 inhalations BID
Fluticasone (Flovent)	1–2 oral inhalations BID
Triamcinolone (Azmacort)	2 inhalations QID

Adverse Effects Adverse effects associated with steroid use include fluid retention, muscle wasting, metabolic disturbances, and increased susceptibility to infection. There has been concern about the effects of inhaled steroids on growth. This does not appear to be a problem with the newer steroids such as budesonide and fluticasone. These effects are not usually observed with inhalation therapy. However, steroids increase the incidence of oral infections (usually fungal infections), and they can cause cough, hoarseness, and other vocal chord disturbances. The incidence of these adverse effects can be reduced by rinsing the mouth with water after inhalation to minimize the amount of steroid that remains in the oral cavity.

Nonsteroidal Antiinflammatory Drugs

CROMOLYN SODIUM

Allergic conditions involve the interaction of an antigen (foreign protein) and an antibody (produced by the body). This interaction causes mast cells to release histamine and other chemical mediators, which then trigger an asthmatic attack. Cromolyn sodium is a drug that interferes with the antigen-antibody reaction to release mast cell mediators. The drug is taken prophylactically (before allergic exposure) on a regular basis. Cromolyn is also useful in certain types of nonallergic asthma.

Administration of cromolyn is by inhalation, three to four times per day. It is available as a nasal spray (Nasalcrom) for allergic rhinitis, as an oral inhaler (Cromolyn Sodium Inhalation, USP), or as a nebulizing solution. Cromolyn is not a bronchodilator, and it has no use in the treatment of acute asthma. The therapeutic effect to prevent asthmatic attacks requires several weeks to fully develop.

The most frequent adverse effects are nasal stinging, nasal irritation, headache, and bad taste. In addition, allergic reactions have occurred involving rash, hives, cough, and angioedema.

Nedocromil (Tilade) is a drug similar to cromolyn in mechanism and pharmacologic effect. It is administered by oral inhalation, usually two inhalations four times per day.

ANTILEUKOTRIENE DRUGS

A major focus of asthma research has been to discover drugs that interfere with the formation of the prostaglandin derivatives known as leukotrienes, more specifically referred to as the cysteinyl leukotrienes (LTC, LTD, LTE). These substances are formed from the lipoxygenation of arachidonic acid by the enzyme 5-lipoxygenase. These compounds, formed and released by mast cells, eosinophils, and airway epithelial cells, cause bronchoconstriction, mucus production, inflammation, and airway hyperactivity. Recently, several new drugs were approved that interfere with leukotriene (LT) activity either by blocking the leukotriene receptor or by inhibiting the enzyme (5-lipoxygenase) that is required for the synthesis of leukotrienes.

Zafirlukast (Accolate) is a competitive receptor antagonist at the LTD and LTE receptor. The drug is administered orally 20 mg BID and is well absorbed. Food significantly reduces drug absorption. The most common adverse reactions are headache, nausea, diarrhea, dizziness, and liver function abnormalities (increased serum transaminase levels).

Montelukast (Singulair) is a specific LTD receptor (referred to as cys-LT-1 receptor) antagonist. The drug is administered orally, usually 10 mg once a day for adults, 5 mg once a day (chewable tablet) for children 6 to 14 years of age, and 4 mg daily for ages 2 to 5 years. The drug is rapidly absorbed and not affected by the presence of food. Montelukast has not been reported to affect liver function. Headache, GI disturbances, and dizziness are the reported adverse effects.

Zileuton (Zyflo) blocks the formation of leukotrienes by inhibiting an enzyme, 5-lipoxygenase, that is required in their synthesis. The drug is administered 600 mg orally four times a day and is unaffected by food. The drug can elevate liver function tests. All of the drugs in this class have been associated with reports of development of a granulomatous, necrotizing vasculitis (Churg-Strauss syndrome).

The exact therapeutic role for the antileukotriene drugs has yet to be established. These drugs may be used as alternatives to the corticosteroids and nonsteroidal agents or used in combination with these same drugs. Use of the antileukotrienes does facilitate a reduction in the need and dosage for β_2 and corticosteroid drugs and also minimizes the adverse effects of these drugs. These are of particular use in aspirin-induced asthma. The antileukotriene drugs are summarized in Table 19-3.

Table 19-3
Antileukotriene Drugs

Drug (Trade Name)	Usual Daily Dose	Mechanism of Action
Zafirlukast (Accolate)	20 mg oral BID	LT receptor blocker
Montelukast (Singulair)	Adults: 10 mg oral	LT receptor blocker
Zileuton (Zyflo)	600 mg QID	5-Lipoxygenase inhibitor

LT = leukotriene

Mucolytics

Mucolytics are chemical agents that liquefy bronchial mucus. In various conditions, such as asthma, bronchitis, and respiratory infections, the production of mucus increases. In these situations the mucus thickens and also contains glycoproteins, cellular debris, and inflammatory exudate. During respiratory infections, the mucus becomes purulent. These changes in the mucus make it difficult for the respiratory tract to remove it by way of ciliary action. The upward movement of mucus by the cilia is often referred to as the mucociliary escalator system. When increased production and thickening of mucus contribute to airway obstruction and interfere with normal respiration, mucolytics are administered by aerosol to thin or liquefy secretions. Then, the mucus and other respiratory secretions can be removed by coughing or a suction apparatus. Acetylcysteine is a widely used mucolytic. It is also important that patients be adequately hydrated because water itself can help liquefy and mobilize secretions.

Acetylcysteine (Mucosil) contains a chemical group (sulfhydryl) that breaks apart the glycoproteins in bronchial secretions. This action decreases the viscosity (resistance to flow) of bronchial secretions and promotes easier mobilization and removal. Acetylcysteine is irritating to the respiratory tract and can cause bronchospasm. For this reason, a bronchodilator is added to the inhalation mixture. Administration is usually by nebulization, three or four times a day as a 10% or 20% solution, followed by postural drainage and tracheal suction when necessary.

There are two other mucolytic agents that work in two different ways. Sodium bicarbonate, as a 2% solution, alters the pH of secretions. By increasing the pH, it weakens the bonds of mucus and reduces its viscosity. It is given by aerosol or direct tracheal irrigation. The usual dose is 2 to 5 mL. At this dose, there is no effect on the pH of the blood.

Another mucolytic agent is α-dornase (Pulmazyme). This is commonly used to reduce the viscosity of mucus in patients who have cystic fibrosis. The medication works by proteolysis, which breaks down DNA material that contributes to mucosal viscosity in these patients.

Alpha dornase does not break the bonds of DNA within cells, only extracellular DNA. Extracellular DNA is a breakdown product of many of the white cells that accumulate during the inflammatory process. This extracellular DNA is a major component of the purulent and viscous secretions in the lungs of patients with cystic fibrosis. This material is a breeding ground for bacteria that can lead to chronic and life-threatening infections.

As part of other therapies for patients with cystic fibrosis, alpha dornase 2.5 mg is nebulized orally and given daily for adults and children > 5 years old. Some patients may require therapy twice daily. This is one of the few respiatory products that requires refrigeration.

Expectorants

Dryness of the respiratory tract causes irritation and stimulates cough reflexes. The result is a dry, hacking, unproductive cough.

Expectorants are agents that stimulate the production of respiratory secretions, which then decrease the irritation and cough caused by excessive dryness of the airways. Consequently, the main use of expectorants is to increase the output of respiratory tract secretions, which indirectly suppresses cough. The expectorants include salts (ammonium chloride and potassium citrate), ipecac syrup, and guaifenesin. Expectorants are added to many cough syrups and cold medications. After oral administration, the expectorants produce their effect by first irritating the lining of the stomach. This gastric irritation stimulates gastric reflexes that increase both gastric and respiratory tract secretions. Because of the gastric irritation, expectorants may cause nausea and vomiting. There is some controversy as to the real effectiveness of expectorants.

Other Therapies Used in the Treatment of Severe Asthma

Magnesium sulfate given intravenously may be used to relax smooth muscle in the respiratory tract and may help to stabilize mast cells and prevent histamine release. However, its mechanism of action is not known.

Furosemide is a diuretic but can be used to decrease bronchoconstriction in the treatment of asthma. There are several proposed mechanisms of action. Furosemide may relax the smooth muscles of the bronchial tree. Another proposed mechanism is that it may inhibit the release of mediators such as leukotrienes and histamine. Furosemide is given by inhalation at a dose of 1 mg/kg, up to 40 mg for an adult. No significant adverse effects have been noted with the use of furosemide.

Isoflurane is an anesthetic gas that acts as a bronchodilator. It blocks the bronchoconstrictor effect of both acetylcholine and histamine. It is reserved for patients who have not responded to other forms of bronchodilator treatment. It can be used only for short periods because it has cardiac and neurologic side effects. Isoflurane is reviewed in Chapter 13.

Investigational Therapies

Immunoglobulin E (IgE) is produced when a body responds to an antigen. The IgE attaches to the mast cell and causes the release of its mediators. Investigational studies have used a monoclonal antibody that binds with the IgE before it can connect with the mast cell to prevent the release of mediators of inflammation.

Currently, this is available only as an intravenous product but is a unique way to try to prevent inflammation. Further studies will be needed to determine its true efficacy and commercial viability.

Anticytokine therapy is also an investigational treatment. Cytokines are mediators of inflammation that are released by the mast cells. Glucocorticoids are effective antiinflammatory agents but are not very specific and can have significant side effects. Interleukin-4 (IL-4) and interleukin-5 (IL-5) are two cytokines that cause chronic inflammation in asthma. By producing monoclonal antibodies that are anti-IL-4 and anti-IL-5, it may be possible to provide a method of prophylaxis, preventing lung injury.

NAEPP Guidelines

In 1991, under the auspices of the National Asthma Education and Prevention Program (NAEPP), the first Expert Panel on the Management of Asthma published *Expert Panel Report: Guidelines for the Diagnosis and Management of Asthma.* This landmark report redefined commonly held beliefs about asthma care, setting the stage for nationwide improvements in the clinical management of asthma.

The report was updated in 1997 and contains sections related to the following areas of care:

1. Pathogenesis and definitions
2. Measures of assessment and monitoring
3. Control of factors contributing to asthma severity
4. Pharmacologic therapy
5. Education for a partnership in asthma care

Information on obtaining these guidelines is listed below in the reference section.

Chapter 19 Review

UNDERSTANDING TERMINOLOGY

Match the definition or description in the left column with the appropriate term in the right column.

1. 1000 times more potent than histamine as a bronchoconstrictor

2. A disease in which patients have difficulty expelling air from the lungs; causes destruction of the walls of the alveolar sacs.

3. Characterized by shortness of breath and wheezing.

4. A drug that relaxes bronchial smooth muscle and dilates the lower respiratory passages.

5. Chronic obstructive pulmonary disease.

6. A respiratory condition caused by chronic irritation that increases secretion of mucus and causes degeneration of the respiratory lining.

7. A drug that liquefies bronchial secretions.

a. asthma
b. bronchodilator
c. chronic bronchitis
d. COPD
e. emphysema
f. mucolytic
g. Leukotrienes

ACQUIRING KNOWLEDGE

Test your understanding of the material in this chapter by answering the following questions.

8. What are some of the factors that can precipitate an asthma attack?

9. List four physiological changes that can occur in the respiratory tract during an asthma attack.

10. What chemical mediators are released from mast cells? What effects do they produce?

11. Discuss the relationship of cyclic AMP and cyclic GMP to the autonomic nervous system.

12. What effects do increasing the level of cyclic AMP or decreasing the level of cyclic GMP have on the respiratory tract during asthma?

13. Compare the pharmacologic effects of epinephrine and albuterol. What is the main indication for each?

14. Explain the mechanism of action of theophylline.
15. Discuss the indications for the use of corticosteroids. What advantage is there to using beclomethasone by inhalation?
16. Explain the mechanism of action of cromolyn. How is it administered?
17. How does acetylcysteine liquefy mucus?
18. Describe the mechanism of action of montelukast and zileuton.

APPLYING KNOWLEDGE ON THE JOB

Answer the following questions.

19. Mrs. Willard has been prescribed Ventolin plus Atrovent Inhalation Aerosol while in the hospital to treat her chronic obstructive pulmonary disease (COPD). When you walk into her room to do your afternoon assessment, you notice she is wheezing more than on admission 3 days ago. Both inhalers are due within the next half hour. Which inhaler would you administer first to provide her with the quickest relief?

20. Mr. Wiblin calls his physician's office complaining of a dry throat, raspy voice, and a couple of white, patchy areas in his throat. He requests a prescription for an antibiotic. You pull his chart and see that he was given new prescriptions for Azmacort and theophylline 1 week ago for newly diagnosed asthma. What additional questions would you ask him? Is an antibiotic appropriate for this patient? If not, why?

21. Following a bee sting, a young boy developed hives and had difficulty breathing. What drug is indicated for immediate treatment of this condition? How should it be administered?

22. Mrs. Peabody is an elderly woman who has taken theophylline for years for her asthma. Recently, she has complained of trouble sleeping, and she says her hands are shaking and her heart is pounding. What do you think is happening to her? What would be a logical course of action to take?

Additional Reading

Aronica M, Sheller JR. Inhaled steroids in asthma. *Comp Ther* 1998;24(8):378.

Fernandez E. Update on the pharmacologic approach to asthma. Part 1. Xanthine and adrenergic bronchodilators. *Respir Ther* 1984;14(4):42.

Holloway J, et al. Churg-Strauss syndrome associated with zafirlukast. *JAOA* 1998;98(5):275.

Horwitz RJ, et al. The role of leukotriene modifiers in the treatment of asthma. *Am J Respir Crit Care Med* 1998;157:1363.

Janson-Bjerklie S. Status asthmaticus. *Am J Nurs* 1990;90(9):52.

Miller LG. Update on exercise-induced asthma. *Hosp Med* 1991;27(2):29.

Rumbak MJ. Modern management of acute asthma. *Hosp Med* 1991;27(5):41.

Schaefer OP. Managing asthma in the allergic patient. *Comp Ther* 1999;25(11/12):507.

Zafirlukast for asthma. *Med Lett* 1996;38(990):111.

Montelukast for persistent asthma. *Med Lett* 1998;40(1031):71.

Levalbuterol for asthma. *Med Lett* 1999;41(1054):51.

NAEPP Guidelines 1997. National Heart, Lung and Blood Institute Information Center, P.O. Box 30105, Bethesda, MD 20824-0105.

Internet Activities

Visit the **MedicineNet** Web site (http//www.medicinenet.com) and click on the "Diseases and Treatment" heading. Highlight the letter "A" and find both the "Asthma" and "Allergic Rhinitis" subheadings. Both provide additional background and drug information concerning these two common respiratory conditions.

NAEPP publications are available at www.nhlbi.nih.gov/nhlbi/nhlbi.htm.

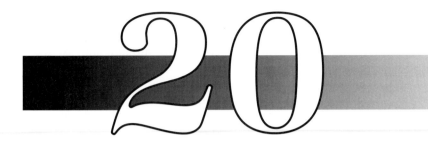

Adrenal Steroids

Henry Hitner, PhD
Barbara Nagle, PhD

Chapter Focus

This chapter describes substances that contribute to the body's natural response to injury, particularly tissue damage. It explains how these substances produce a significant physiological effect on the kidneys to capture excreted sodium ions and on muscles to conserve glucose, which acts as fuel. Adrenal steroids are normally found in the body, but with repeated exogenous use, they are associated with a state of dependency.

Chapter Terminology

catabolism: Process in which complex compounds are broken down into simpler molecules; usually associated with energy release.

glucocorticoid: Steroid produced within the adrenal cortex (or a synthetic drug) that directly influences carbohydrate metabolism and inhibits the inflammatory process.

lysosome: Part of a cell that contains enzymes capable of digesting or destroying tissue/proteins.

mineralocorticoid: Steroid produced within the adrenal cortex that directly influences sodium and potassium metabolism.

phagocytes: Cells that migrate to wounded areas to consume harmful substances introduced by the injury.

replacement therapy: Administration of a naturally occurring substance that the body is not able to produce in adequate amounts to maintain normal function.

repository preparation: Preparation of a drug, usually for intramuscular or subcutaneous injection, that is intended to leach out from the site of injection slowly so that the duration of drug action is prolonged.

steroid: Member of a large family of chemical substances (hormones, drugs) containing a structure similar to that of cortisone (tetracyclic cyclopentaphenanthrene).

tropic: Having an affinity for the designated organ, as in adrenotropic.

Chapter Objectives

After studying this chapter, you should be able to:

- Identify the two main classes of steroids.
- Describe the action of steroids on the inflammatory process.
- Describe the primary action of steroids on the renal tubules.
- Describe three adverse effects associated with chronic (routine) use of steroids.

The adrenal glands are located on the upper surface of each kidney. The glands consist of an inner part, known as the adrenal medulla, and an outer part, known as the adrenal cortex. The medulla, which is part of the sympathetic nervous system, secretes catecholamines during sympathetic activation. The cortex is composed of three separate tissue layers. Each layer releases one or more hormones that have important physiological functions, as shown in Table 20-1.

The hormones of the adrenal cortex are divided into two main classes: the glucocorticoids and the mineralocorticoids. The hormones of the adrenal cortex are generally referred to as corticosteroids or just **steroids**. A deficiency in steroid pro-

Table 20-1

Layers of the Adrenal Cortex and the Main Hormones Secreted from Each Layer

Layer	Hormones	Main Function
Glomerulosa (outer)	Aldosterone (referred to as a mineralocorticoid)	Regulates blood levels of sodium and potassium
Fasciculata (middle)	Cortisol, cortisone (referred to as glucocorticoids)	Regulate the metabolism of carbohydrates and proteins; also have potent antiinflammatory effects
Reticularis (inner)	Minute amounts of male and female sex hormones	Normal physiological function of the sex hormones from this layer not clearly understood

duction results in Addison disease. Excess steroid production results in Cushing disease. There are two primary indications for steroid administration: one is **replacement therapy** in the treatment of hormone deficiency conditions such as Addison disease; the other is treatment of inflammation.

Glucocorticoids

From the standpoint of pharmacology, the most important steroids are the **glucocorticoids.** They are used frequently in the treatment of inflammatory or allergic conditions.

REGULATING CORTISOL SECRETION

The production and secretion of cortisol is controlled by corticotropin (ACTH, adrenocorticotropic hormone), secreted by the anterior pituitary gland. The **tropic** hormones (such as corticotropin) are regulated by the releasing factors of the hypothalamus. Corticotropin stimulates the secretion of cortisol from the adrenal cortex. It is important to know which factors stimulate the hypothalamus to secrete the releasing factor for corticotropin. The main factors that influence the hypothalamus are the sleep-wake cycle (diurnal rhythm, circadian rhythm), negative feedback, and stress.

Sleep-Wake Cycle   The levels of corticotropin, and therefore of cortisol, are adjusted to each individual's sleep-wake cycle. Higher amounts of corticotropin and cortisol are secreted for availability during the waking hours, whereas lower amounts are present during sleep. The maximum secretion occurs before 8 AM, and the lowest levels occur after 4 PM. During the wake period, cortisol regulates body metabolism to meet the requirements of this active period.

Negative Feedback   Releasing factor and corticotropin stimulate the release of cortisol into the bloodstream. When the level of cortisol rises above normal, further release of corticotropin and the releasing factor is inhibited. This negative feedback maintains the day-to-day levels of cortisol at relatively constant amounts.

Stress   Stress refers to a situation in which the body is subjected to increased physical or mental demands: exercise, cold weather, infections, surgery, and anxiety are all forms of stress. Stress produces an increase in corticotropin secretion, which stimulates cortisol secretion. The increased cortisol in the blood provides the body with a greater ability to cope with the demands of stress. Stress usually raises the body's demand for muscle activity, repairing tissue, fighting infection, or just stimulating metabolic systems in preparation for activity. In order to satisfy these activities, the glucocorticoids make fuel available to the tissues.

EFFECTS OF GLUCOCORTICOIDS (CORTISOL)

The glucocorticoids regulate the metabolism of carbohydrates and proteins, particularly during stress. During periods of stress involving bodily injury (trauma or surgery), there is an increased demand for glucose. Tissues undergoing repair and wound healing use glucose almost exclusively. In addition, the brain normally uses only glucose. The main physiological effects of the glucocorticoids—producing and conserving body stores of carbohydrates (glucose)—are accomplished by two main metabolic processes: gluconeogenesis and protein **catabolism.** Both of these processes are stimulated by the glucocorticoids.

Gluconeogenesis   Gluconeogenesis is the process of making glucose. It occurs in the liver, where amino acids and glycerol are converted into glucose. Glucose synthesized in the liver is either stored (as glycogen) or immediately available in the circulating blood. The overall result is an increase in the production of glucose for use by injured tissue or by the brain.

Protein Catabolism   Catabolism is the breakdown of proteins into amino acids. This occurs mainly in skeletal muscle. The amino acids that are released can then be used by the liver to make glucose (gluconeogenesis). At the same time, glucocorticoids modulate glucose uptake by the muscle and fat cells so that more glucose remains in circulation. Glucose is also moved from collagen and connective tissue. Note: this action on muscle cells and collagen leads to tissue wasting (weakening) with high-dose, long-term use of exogenous glucocorticoids.

EFFECTS ON BLOOD CELLS

Glucocorticoids cause a decrease in the circulating levels of eosinophils, basophils, and lymphocytes. At the same time, the neutrophils, red blood cells, and platelets are increased. This contributes to the day-to-day tissue repair by reducing cells that stimulate local inflammatory responses and increasing the cells necessary for microadhesion and tissue oxygenation.

Fluid Retention   The glucocorticoids also have some mineralocorticoid activity, that is, the ability to cause the retention of sodium by the kidneys. Wherever sodium goes, water follows; therefore, water also is retained by the body. At high concentrations, sodium and water retention may lead to the development of edema and/or hypertension.

PHARMACOLOGIC EFFECTS

The most important uses of the glucocorticoids are for replacement therapy in adrenocortical insufficiency (Addison disease) and in the treatment of inflammatory conditions. The steroids that are available include the naturally occurring steroids and various synthetic preparations. All of these available steroids are either administered to achieve wide tissue distribution (systemic) or a more limited target tissue distribution (nonsystemic).

Replacement Therapy   The adrenal steroids are essential to life. In Addison disease, there is a deficiency of both glucocorticoids and mineralocorticoids. The main symptoms in Addison disease are dehydration, hypotension, and muscle weakness. Following ACTH administration, plasma cortisol and 17-hydroxycorti-costeroids (17-OHCS) are measured. When the plasma levels of these steroids do not rise or cannot be detected, primary adrenal failure, Addison disease, is present.

Cosyntropin is a synthetic peptide that corresponds to an active segment of ACTH. Although it provides the same therapeutic activity as ACTH with less allergenic potential, its formulation limits its use to diagnostic evaluation. Patients with Addison disease must receive hormone replacement as chronic systemic therapy. The naturally occurring glucocorticoids (cortisone, hydrocortisone) are used most frequently (see Table 20-2). Dosages administered are similar to the levels that normally exist in the body (20 to 30 mg per day). For patients who continue to lose sodium as a result of the lack of aldosterone, a mineralocorticoid (fludrocortisone acetate, Florinef) also must be administered along with the glucocorticoid.

Inflammation and Antiinflammatory Therapy   Inflammation is usually considered the first step in the natural process of wound healing. However, sometimes the normal inflammatory response is too intense (acute inflammatory reaction) or is prolonged (chronic inflammatory reaction) so that the inflammation itself becomes a disease process. For example, in rheumatoid arthritis, the inflammatory

Table 20-2

Comparison of Naturally Occurring and Synthetic Glucocorticoids

Drug (Product Name)	Equivalent Antiinflammatory Dose (mg)	Sodium Retention	Duration of Action (Hours)
Short-acting steroids			
Cortisone* (Cortone)	25	High	12–24
Hydrocortisone* (Cortef, Hydrocortone)	20	High	12–24
Intermediate-acting steroids			
Methylprednisolone* (Depo-Medrol, Medrol, Solu-Medrol)	4	None	24–36
Prednisolone† (Delta-Cortef, Hydeltra-TBA, Predcor 25, Predcor 50)	5	Mild	24–36
Prednisone† (Deltasone, Medicortone, Orasone, Panasol)	5	Mild	24–36
Triamcinolone† (Aristocort, Aristospan, Kenacort, Kenalog-40)	4	None	36–48
Long-acting steroids			
Betamethasone† (Celestone, Cel-U-Ject, Selestoject)	0.60	None	48–72
Dexamethasone† (Decadron, Hexadrol, Decadron-LA)	0.75	None	48–72

* Naturally occurring.
† Synthetic.

response can lead to permanent joint damage. In chronic respiratory disease, accumulated mediators of inflammation cause the bronchial tissue to become scarred and atelectic, unable to fully expand. Therefore, suppression of the inflammatory response becomes the most important therapeutic endpoint.

INFLAMMATION The inflammatory process is a normal response to injury. When tissues are damaged, proinflammatory substances (histamine, bradykinin, prostaglandins, leukotrienes, and serotonin) are released (see Figure 20-1). The prostaglandins and leukotrienes are mediators of inflammation that dilate small blood vessels (vasodilation) and increase permeability of capillary walls, causing proteins and fluid to leak out of the injured cells. As blood flow to the damaged area increases, **phagocytes** (leukocytes, mast cells) migrate to the area to consume harmful substances introduced by the injury. In the process, more leukotrienes are released, and some recruit more phagocytes to the injured area so the localized inflammatory response is amplified. Depending on the site of the inflammation (joints, head, skeletal muscle), pain receptors are stimulated by the released bradykinins, and prostaglandins G2 and H2 stimulate peripheral pain receptors directly. These prostaglandins constrict blood vessels and are further metabolized to the active substances PGE2 and PGF2a. Prostaglandin PGE2 is involved in the production of erythema (abnormal redness), edema, and pain that accompany the inflammatory process. (PGF2a is associated with uterine contraction—cramping—and vasodilation.)

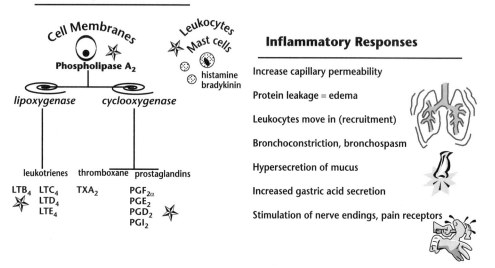

Figure 20-1
Mediators of inflammation and the site of glucocorticoid actions.

All of these effects represent the cardinal signs of inflammation: redness, swelling (edema), warmth, and pain.

ANTIINFLAMMATORY THERAPY Glucocorticoids are the most potent antiinflammatory agents available. The glucocorticoids interfere with all stages of the inflammatory response, preventing edema resulting from capillary leakage and stabilizing cell membranes (including lysosomes). Stabilization of the membranes prevents cell lysis and further cell damage. It also contributes to reducing the release of histamine from mast cells and other vasoactive substances. Glucocorticoids limit the production of proinflammatory substances. By inhibiting phospholipase A2 synthesis through lipocortins, glucocorticoids indirectly inhibit the production of prostaglandins and leukotrienes. These actions reduce vascular permeability, swelling, and edema.

Depending on the dose and duration of exposure, glucocorticoids suppress the immune system. Immunosuppression is merely an extension of the antiinflammatory response in which lymphocytes (T, B cells) and macrophages are significantly inhibited from performing their immune functions.

The naturally occurring substances cortisone and cortisol and the synthetic substances produce all of the glucocorticoid activities presented here. Slight alterations in the structure of the naturally occurring glucocorticoids result in synthetic steroids with greater antiinflammatory potency. The synthetic steroids have a longer duration of action than do the naturally occurring steroids. In addition, they produce fewer undesirable mineralocorticoid effects. Features of the glucocorticoids are compared in Table 20-2.

CLINICAL INDICATIONS

ACTH is primarily used for diagnostic evaluation of adrenocortical function. In established disorders, ACTH is used in the constellation of drug therapy for exacerbations of multiple sclerosis and hypercalcemia associated with cancer. Glucocorticoids are the drugs of choice in conditions where the endogenous hormone is not appropriately produced, as in primary and secondary adrenal cortical insufficiency.

Glucocorticoids also are approved for use in a wide range of inflammatory disorders where a degenerative process is out of control. These include rheumatic disorders, arthritis, collagen disease, specific ulcerative colitis, multiple sclerosis, severe allergic reaction, respiratory disease, and management of leukemias and lymphomas. Glucocorticoids are frequently used to treat allergies because inflammation is part of an allergic reaction. In the management of multiple sclerosis, leukemias, and lymphomas, the steroid is acting as an immunosuppressant. In the management of chronic disease, glucocorticoids are part of a selective strategy to interrupt the cycle of inflammation before irreversible damage occurs.

In addition to these FDA-approved uses of corticosteroids, there are other uses that are medically appropriate although not specifically approved by the FDA (off-label use). Such inflammatory conditions include acute mountain sickness, bacterial meningitis, COPD, Graves ophthalmopathy, respiratory distress syndrome, septic shock, and spinal cord injury.

ADMINISTRATION AND DOSAGE

Glucocorticoids may be administered orally, intramuscularly, intravenously, topically, intranasally, or by inhalation. Intravenous administration is reserved for emergencies, when prompt systemic effects are needed. Intramuscular injections are used when frequent readministration is undesirable. The preparations for IM injection include **repository preparations,** in which the glucocorticoid is slowly released from the muscle, providing a longer duration of action. In general, extended-release steroids are prepared in the acetate form rather than as the sodium succinate or sodium phosphate. Examples of injectable preparations that have a slow onset and long duration of action are presented in Table 20-3.

There is a wide range in the therapeutic dosages of the glucocorticoids. Doses must be adjusted to meet the needs of individual patients. Dosages and indications for administration of glucocorticoids are presented in Table 20-4. Short-term treatment with glucocorticoids absorbs scar tissue (keloids) when injected directly into the scarred skin. For exacerbations of chronically inflamed joints and soft tissue, the drugs may be injected into the specific area. For swollen joints, the edematous fluid is removed before the steroid is injected. Too frequent intraarticular administration can damage joint tissues, so patients are advised to decrease all stress on the inflamed joint to minimize the need for reinjection.

Topical use of the glucocorticoids is indicated in the treatment of inflammation and pruritic dermatosis. Topical steroids are available over the counter or by prescription. Over-the-counter preparations are specifically labeled for the temporary relief of minor skin irritations, itching, and rashes from eczema, dermatitis, insect bites, poison ivy, detergents, and cosmetics as well as itching in the genital and anal regions. Examples of over-the-counter topical steroids are presented in Table 20-5. These products usually contain a lesser amount of hydrocortisone than may be obtained by prescription; nevertheless, the active component is still a

Table 20-3

Examples of Extended-Release Injectable Steroids*

Glucocorticoid	Product Names
Dexamethasone acetate	Dalone LA, Decadron-LA, Decaject LA
Hydrocortisone acetate	Generic hydrocortisone preparations
Methylprednisolone acetate	depMedalone 40, Depo-Medrol, Depoject, D-Med 80
Prednisolone acetate	Articulose 50, Predalone 50
Prednisolone tebutate	Hydeltra-TBA, Predalone-TBA

* These drugs are not for intravenous use; they are administered intramuscularly, intraarticularly, and intralesionally.

Table 20-4

Doses and Indications of Adrenal Steroids*

Adrenal Steroid	Indication	Dose
Corticotropins		
ACTH (Acthar, Corticotropin)	Confirmation of adrenal responsiveness	80 units single injection or 10–25 units diluted IV over 8 h
	Multiple sclerosis	80–120 units/day IM for 2–3 weeks
Repository corticotropin	IM, SC	40–80 units every 24–72 h (IM, SC)
Corticotropin zinc (Cortrophin-Zinc)	IM only	40–80 units every 24–72 h
Copsyntrophin (Cortrosyn)	IM or IV	0.25–0.75 mg
Mineralocorticoids		
Fludrocortisone acetate (Florinef Acetate)	Addison disease	0.1–0.2 mg/day three times a week
Glucocorticoids		
Betamethasone (Celestone, Cel-U-Ject, Selestoject)	Antiinflammatory	0.6–7.2 mg daily PO; up to 9 mg IV
Cortisone (Cortisone Acetate, Cortone)	Antiinflammatory	25–300 mg/day PO
Dexamethasone (Decadron, Dexone, Dexameth)	Allergic disorders	0.75–9 mg daily PO
	Cushing syndrome	1 mg at 11 pm or 0.5 mg every 6 h for 48 h
Dexamethasone with lidocaine (Decadron with Xylocaine)	Soft tissue injection, bursitis	0.5–0.75 mL
Hydrocortisone (Cortisol, Cortef)	Antiinflammatory	20–240 mg/day PO
Hydrocortisone sodium phosphate (Hydrocortone phosphate)	Antiinflammatory	15–240 mg/day IV, IM, or SC
Hydrocortisone sodium succinate (A-Hydrocort, Solu-Cortef)	Antiinflammatory	100–500 mg every 2, 4, or 6 h IM, IV
Hydrocortisone acetate (Hydrocortone Acetate)	Intralesion, intraarticular; *not* IV	12.5–50 mg
Methylprednisolone (Medrol)	Antiinflammatory	4–48 mg/day PO or alternate-day therapy
Methylprednisolone sodium (A-Methapred, Solu-Medrol)	Antiinflammatory	10–40 mg IV over several minutes
Methylprednisolone acetate (Depo-Medrol, Duralone-40, Depoject)	Adrenalgenital syndrome	40 mg IM every 2 weeks
	Rheumatoid arthritis, dermatologic lesions	40–120 mg IM weekly
	Asthma, allergic rhinitis	80–120 mg IM
	Intraarticular	4–80 mg
Prednisone (Meticortin, Orasone, Panasol-S, Deltasone)*	Antiinflammatory, asthma	50–60 mg/day PO

Continued

Table 20-4 *(continued)*

Doses and Indications of Adrenal Steroids

Adrenal Steroid	Indication	Dose
Glucocorticoids *(continued)*		
Prednisolone (Delta-Cortef, Prelone)	Multiple sclerosis	200 mg daily PO for 7 days, then 80 mg every other day for 1 month
Prednisolone acetate (Key-Pred, Predcor, Articulose, Predaject-50)	Intralesional, intraarticular, soft tissue	4–100 mg
Triamcinolone (Aristocort, Atolone, Kenocort)	Adrenal insufficiency	4–12 mg daily PO
	Bronchial asthma	8–16 mg daily PO
	Respiratory disease	16–48 mg daily
	Tuberculous meningitis	32–48 mg
	Acute leukemia and lymphoma	16–40 mg daily PO
	Systemic lupus erythematosus	20–32 mg daily PO
	Edema	16–20 mg PO until diuresis occurs

* Not an inclusive list of products.

steroid. Adverse effects similar to those described for other steroids may accompany misuse of these drugs.

For the treatment of asthma and the management of respiratory allergies, several glucocorticoids are available as intranasal sprays or aerosol inhalants. This route of administration delivers the steroid directly to the inflamed respiratory target tissue. Although the site of action is local, all of these steroids are absorbed into the blood. High doses of some inhaled steroids may be high enough to produce systemic effects. Inhalation and intranasal administration may be the route of choice in chronic respiratory conditions in order to reduce steroid dependence,

Table 20-5

Examples of Over-the-Counter Topical Steroid Preparations

Product Name	Amount and Preparation of Hydrocortisone
Dermolate Anal-Itch	0.5% ointment, cream
CaldeCORT Rectal Itch	0.5% acetate equivalent ointment, pump spray
Cortaid	0.5% acetate equivalent ointment, lotion, pump spray
Bactine Hydrocortisone	0.5% cream
Lanacort 5	0.5% acetate equivalent cream, ointment
Gynecort, Cortef Feminine Itch	0.5% acetate equivalent cream

wean patients off other (systemic) steroids, or provide additional support to the patient's respiratory therapy regimen (such as β-adrenergic bronchodilators).

METABOLISM AND EXCRETION

No matter what route of administration is employed, glucocorticoids that enter the circulation are metabolized by the liver and then excreted in the urine. The most common urinary metabolites are the 17-hydroxycorticosteroids (17-OHCS). These can be measured from 24-hour urine collections, and they provide an estimate of glucocorticoid secretion from the adrenal cortex. In patients with adrenocortical insufficiency, these metabolites are usually very low.

ADVERSE EFFECTS

The more serious adverse effects of the glucocorticoids usually occur in patents receiving high doses or long-term treatment. The adverse reactions are an exaggeration of the normal steroidal effects and are similar to the symptoms of Cushing disease. The adverse effects are summarized in Table 20-6.

Single steroid doses should be taken before 9 am to allow drug distribution to mimic diurnal levels without suppressing available adrenocortical activity. Because large doses of steroids may cause gastrointestinal upset, patients may take these medications with meals or antacids to minimize irritation.

Diabetic patients may notice changes in blood glucose levels during home monitoring. Diabetics may have elevated blood glucose concentrations requiring dose adjustment in insulin or oral antidiabetic drugs. It is important for these patients to give full disclosure of steroid use to other physicians, such as the diabetologist or endocrinologist, in order to keep their medication history current.

Table 20-6

Adverse Effects of Long-Term Steroid Therapy

Metabolic Effect	Symptoms
Glucocorticoid	
Increased gluconeogenesis	Obesity, diabetes mellitus
Increased protein catabolism	Muscle weakness and wasting, thinning of skin (ecchymoses, striae), osteoporosis (loss of protein matrix), decreased growth (in children), decreased wound healing, increased infections (in leukopenia), peptic ulceration
Mineralocorticoid	
Sodium and water retention	Edema, increased blood volume, hypertension
Loss of potassium	Muscle weakness and cramps
Miscellaneous effects	
Androgenic effects	Hirsutism, virilism, irregular menstruation
Eye complications	Glaucoma, cataract formation
Psychological changes	Euphoria, steroid addiction, depression

Ocular exposure to steroids may cause steroid-induced glaucoma and cataracts with long-term use.

Steroids and ACTH may reduce the patient's resistance to fight local infection by suppressing the body's inflammatory process. The use of aerosols and sprays occasionally deposits amounts of steroids in the mouth and pharynx that predispose the patients to develop oral fungal infections known as thrush. *Candida albicans* is the most common microorganism that grows unchecked because the steroid is suppressing other normal oral flora and immune mechanisms in the mouth. Despite its tenacious local infection, measures can be taken to minimize this side effect. In addition, rinsing the mouth after dosing and washing the spacer and mouthpiece after use can reduce the potential for an oral fungal infection.

STEROID ADDICTION AND WITHDRAWAL

An important adverse reaction associated with long-term use is steroid addiction, which may result in mood changes (euphoria), insomnia, personality changes, and psychological dependency. This is steroid psychosis. The incidence is usually associated with larger steroid doses. Abrupt withdrawal of the steroids may lead to severe mental depression. For this reason, discontinuation of long-term or high-dose steroids must be done under medical supervision, gradually, in small decrements to avoid precipitating withdrawal symptoms and depression. The steroid dose is decreased 5 mg every 7 to 14 days until the desired dose is reached. A tapering dosage regimen is not necessary if the patient is on oral steroids for less than 1 week. Some other signs and symptoms of steriod withdrawal include malaise, headache, fatigue, lethargy, weakness, anorexia, nausea, orthostatic hypotension, dizziness, fainting, hypoglycemia, weight loss, and worsening asthma.

Alternate-Day Therapy   Steroid administration also is accomplished by alternate-day therapy (ADT). ADT is intended to reduce or eliminate the adverse effects of prolonged steroid treatment. In ADT, a short-acting steroid is administered every other day in the morning. The effects of a single dose of a intermediate-acting steroid will last into the next day. However, during the second day (no steroid administered), the patient's adrenal gland begins to function (is released from negative feedback). On the following day (third day), the steroid is again administered, and the patient's adrenal gland is once again suppressed. This therapy prevents adrenal atrophy and permanent destruction of the adrenal gland. There is also a lower incidence of other adverse effects.

Mineralocorticoids

The **mineralocorticoids** are hormones secreted by the outer layer of the adrenal gland. The main effect of the mineralocorticoid hormones is to regulate the fluid balance of the body. When there is a deficiency of mineralocorticoids, a condition known as hypoaldosteronism results. This condition usually is caused by adrenalectomy or by adrenal tumors. Replacement therapy is necessary because the mineralocorticoids are essential for life.

PHYSIOLOGICAL EFFECTS

The most important mineralocorticoid is aldosterone. Its site of action is at the distal tubules of the nephrons. The main function of the nephrons is the formation of urine, during which process many essential nutrients and ions are reabsorbed through the tubules back into the blood. Aldosterone increases the reabsorption of sodium ions. In exchange, potassium ions are transported into the urine. This process is usually referred to as sodium-potassium exchange. Water is also reabsorbed with sodium. Consequently, normal sodium and water levels (isotonic) are maintained in the blood and other body tissues.

ADMINISTRATION AND DOSAGE

Fludrocortisone (Florinef) is a potent mineralocorticoid that has a greater glucocorticoid potency than does cortisone. Although fludrocortisone has dual activity, it is usually administered in conjunction with a glucocorticoid (cortisone, hydrocortisone) to achieve total replacement therapy in primary and secondary adrenocortical insufficiency. Fludrocortisone is administered orally in doses of 0.1 to 0.2 mg per day, three times per week.

ADVERSE EFFECTS

Excessive use of the mineralocorticoids results in sodium and water retention and the loss of potassium. The major symptoms are edema, hypertension, and muscle weakness from the loss of potassium. In certain patients, the edema could lead to congestive heart failure. A physician should be notified if dizziness, continuing headaches, or swelling in the lower extremities occurs. Dose adjustment usually mitigates adverse effects. Other adverse effects include increased sweating, bruising, and allergic skin rash.

Special Considerations

Steroids are administered for their antiinflammatory activity in patients with normal adrenal function. With continued use (as well as misuse of these drugs), patients may experience changes in appearance and behavior indicative of metabolic alterations. Because steroids universally affect metabolism, patients must be observed carefully for changes in body weight, electrolyte balance, and cardiac function. The sodium retention associated with these drugs may lead to elevated blood pressure, even hypertension, and edema. Patients should be weighed daily to monitor changes in overall body weight.

Patients should be questioned about feeling fatigued or experiencing cramps and weakness in the extremities because these may be symptoms of hypokalemia.

Patients with Addison disease are often sensitive to drug effects and, therefore, often have an exaggerated response to drug therapy. Patients, especially those on high-dose therapy, should be monitored for changes in sleep patterns and mood, particularly depression or psychotic episodes.

Oral steroids should be used cautiously in patients who have GI ulceration, renal disease, congestive heart failure, ocular herpes simplex, diabetes mellitus, emotional instability, or psychotic tendencies. In all of these conditions, steroids may exacerbate the underlying disease as a direct extension of the pharmacologic actions, such as interference with protective mucoprotein production (ulcers), retention of sodium and water (congestive heart failure), and immunosuppression (herpes infection). Although steroids are ulcerogenic, it is not unusual that certain patients with gastrointestinal ulcer or colitis may be placed on a steroid regimen. In such cases, the risk of continuing degeneration outweighs the risk of short-term exposure to the steroid in order to obtain an immediate antiinflammatory response.

CONTRAINDICATIONS AND PRECAUTIONS

Steroids are contraindicated for use in patients who have systemic fungal infections and local viral (herpes) infections. Live virus vaccinations should not be given during steroid therapy. Patients receiving high-dose steroids may not have the ability to develop antibody immunity, putting them at risk for developing infection and neurologic complications. This does not apply to patients receiving physiological steroid doses as replacement therapy.

Drug Interactions

Steroids have been reported to interact with a variety of drug classes (Table 20-7). Because the glucocorticoids affect carbohydrate metabolism, it is not surprising that diabetics may have an increased insulin or oral hypoglycemic requirement during periods of steroid treatment. Steroids administered concomitantly with potassium-depleting diuretics, amphotericin B, albuterol, or digitalis may potentiate the development of hypokalemia. Patients receiving coumarin anticoagulants may have a decreased coumarin response in the presence of steroids. Prothrombin time must be monitored to ensure that patients are adequately covered.

Phenytoin, phenobarbital, and rifampin enhance the metabolism of corticosteroids, leading to reduced blood steroid levels and a decreased pharmacologic response. In patients receiving these drugs chronically, the dose of corticosteroid may require adjustment.

On the other hand, oral contraceptives inhibit steroid metabolism. Concomitant use of these drugs may lead to elevated blood steroid concentrations and may potentiate steroid toxicity.

This class of drugs has a tremendous potential for overuse and overexposure as a result of the availability of over-the-counter preparations. In addition, steroids may be prescribed concurrently by more than one treating physician. It is not un-

Table 20-7

Examples of Drug Interactions Associated with Glucocorticoids

Glucocorticoids Interact With	Response
Amphotericin B, digitalis, diuretics	Potentiate hypokalemia (possible digitalis toxicity)
Antibiotics, macrolide	Decrease methylprednisolone clearance from plasma
Coumarin anticoagulants	Inhibit response to the anticoagulants
Growth hormone (Somatrem)	Decrease growth-promoting effect of Somatrem
Insulin, oral hypoglycemics	Increase requirement for insulin or oral hypoglycemics
Isoniazid	Increase requirements for isoniazid
Oral contraceptives, estrogens, ketoconazole	Increase steroid response
Phenobarbital, phenytoin, rifampin	Increase steroid requirement because of increased steroid clearance

usual for older patients to visit orthopedists, allergists, diabetologists, pulmonologists, and rheumatologists in addition to their family physician. Therefore, it becomes important to review steroid actions that could be misinterpreted as exacerbations of other underlying conditions. It is also important to review the patient's medications before starting steroid therapy to determine if the patient is already on a steroid prescribed for a different indication.

Because of age-related reduced muscle mass, the elderly are more sensitized to the effects of steroids and should be carefully observed for changes in behavior, coordination, and strength. The muscle weakness and mental confusion produced by steroids will decrease the patient's compliance with respiratory treatment techniques and treatment schedule.

For patients receiving high doses of steroids, there is a decrease in their ability to fight local infections (immunosuppressive response). In patients with preexisting respiratory disease, this may manifest as a persistent cold, increased bronchial secretions, or recurrent fungal infections.

Patients using inhaled steroids should be instructed to rinse their mouth with water without swallowing after each dose. If the patient can "taste" the medication after dosing, it is apparent the steroid was deposited on the oral mucosa or swallowed. Proper technique, including the use of spacer devices, is critical to the effective use of aerosols and sprays and minimizes the development of oral thrush.

Patients receiving high-dose or long-term therapy should not discontinue steroids without supervision of the prescribing physician to avoid precipitating symptoms of withdrawal.

USE IN PREGNANCY

Drugs in this class have been designated Pregnancy Category C. Safety for use in pregnancy has not been established through adequate use or clinical trials in pregnant women. Steroids cross the placenta. Chronic maternal steroid use in the first trimester is known to produce cleft palate in newborns (about 1% incidence). The benefit to the mother must outweigh risk to the fetus and newborn. When clearly required, maternal steroid administration should be at the lowest effective dose for the shortest duration, and the infant should be subsequently monitored for adrenal activity. When mothers receive ACTH, the newborn should be monitored for hyperadrenalism.

Note to the Respiratory Care Practitioner

The respiratory care practitioner is in a position to observe changes in the respiratory patient that may require medical attention. The physician must be notified immediately if significant fluid retention manifested as swelling of lower extremities or unusual weight gain, muscle weakness, abdominal pain, seizures, or headache occurs. These symptoms may indicate the necessity for dose alteration or discontinuation if hypersensitivity develops. Topical steroids will more likely produce skin or ocular itching and irritation rather than the spectrum of other effects.

Chapter 20 Review

UNDERSTANDING TERMINOLOGY

Test your understanding of the material in this chapter by answering the following questions.

1. Define the term steroid.
2. Differentiate between mineralocorticoids and glucocorticoids.
3. Explain replacement therapy.

ACQUIRING KNOWLEDGE

Answer the following questions.

4. What are the two main parts of the adrenal gland?
5. Which layer of the adrenal cortex secretes the mineralocorticoids? Which layer secretes the glucocorticoids?
6. What disease results from a deficiency of the corticosteroids?
7. What three factors regulate the release of cortisol?
8. What is the importance of higher glucocorticoid secretion during injury and wound healing?
9. List the two main therapeutic uses of the glucocorticoids.
10. What are the main differences between the naturally occurring steroids and the synthetic steroids?
11. List the major adverse effect of steroid therapy. What is meant by ADT?
12. What is the function of the mineralocorticoids?
13. What are the adverse effects of excessive administration of the mineralocorticoids?

APPLYING KNOWLEDGE ON THE JOB

Answer the following questions.

14. Assume you are a pharmacy assistant in a nursing home, screening patients for contraindications and drug interactions. What is the potential drug problem—and its solution—for each of the following cases?

   a. Patient A has hypertension. He has been prescribed hydrocortisone injections for severe bursitis.

   b. Patient B is diabetic. She has been prescribed prednisolone for osteoarthritis.

15. What is the potential drug problem for each of the following patients? How would you resolve the problem?

   a. A 25-year-old woman has been prescribed betamethasone for severe psoriasis. The patient is currently taking oral contraceptives.

   b. A 16-year-old boy has been prescribed prednisone for bronchial asthma. He is an epileptic currently taking phenobarbital for seizure control.

Additional Reading

Anderson B. An overview of drug therapy in chronic adult asthma. *Adv Clin Care* 1991;6:44.
O'Neil BJ. Steroids: Drug of a new age? *Emergency* 1991;23:60.
Ruholl LH. Your body clocks: A student guide to circadian rhythms. *Imprint* 1991;38:123.

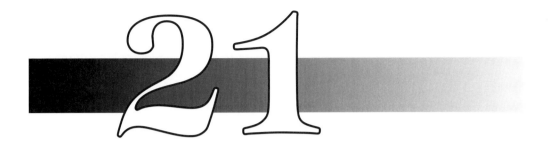

Antibacterial Agents

Henry Hitner, PhD
Barbara Nagle, PhD

Chapter Focus

This chapter describes the pharmacology of drugs used to treat bacterial infections. It explains the basic classification and identification procedures pertaining to bacteria. It also discusses the major classes of antibiotic drugs, mechanisms of antibacterial action, clinical indications, and main pharmacologic and adverse effects produced by these drugs.

Chapter Terminology

antibacterial spectrum: Bacteria that are susceptible to the antibacterial actions of a particular drug.

antibiotic: Antibacterial drug obtained from another microorganism.

antibiotic susceptibility: Identification of the antibiotics, by bacterial culture and sensitivity testing, that will be effective against specific bacteria.

antimicrobial: Antibacterial drugs obtained by chemical synthesis and not from other microorganisms.

bacteria: Single-celled microorganisms, some of which cause disease.

bacterial resistance: Ability of some bacteria to resist the actions of antibiotics.

bactericidal: Antibiotic that kills bacteria.

bacteriostatic: Antibiotic that inhibits the growth of, but does not kill, bacteria.

β-lactamases: Bacterial enzymes that inactivate penicillin and cephalosporin antibiotics.

broad-spectrum: Drug that is effective against a wide variety of both gram-positive and gram-negative pathogenic bacteria.

cephalosporinases: Bacterial enzymes that inactivate cephalosporin antibiotics.

chemoprophylaxis: Use of antibiotics to prevent infection, usually before a surgical procedure or in patients at risk for infection.

chemotherapy: Use of drugs to kill or inhibit the growth of infectious organisms or cancer cells.

gram negative: Bacteria that retain only the red stain in a Gram stain.

gram positive: Bacteria that retain only the blue stain in a Gram stain.

Gram stain: Method of staining and identifying bacteria using crystal violet (blue) and safranin (red) stains.

pathogenic: Type of bacteria that cause disease.

penicillinase: Bacterial enzymes that inactivate penicillin antibiotics.

Chapter Objectives

After studying this chapter, you should be able to:

- Explain the use of the Gram stain in bacterial identification.
- Explain the mechanism of antibacterial action for each of the major drug classes: penicillins, cephalosporins, aminoglycosides, tetracyclines, sulfonamides, macrolides, fluoroquinolones, and the drugs used to treat tuberculosis.
- List one drug from each major drug class and two characteristic adverse effects from each drug class.

Microbiology is the study of microscopic organisms of either animal (bacteria and protozoa) or plant (fungi and molds) origin. **Bacteria** are single-cell organisms that are found virtually everywhere. Bacteria that cause disease are called **pathogenic,** and those that do not are nonpathogenic.

There are no bacteria in the internal environment of the body. However, there are many different types of bacteria, including pathogens, in the external areas, such as the mouth, GI tract, nose, upper respiratory passages, and skin. Therefore, the potential for bacterial invasion always exists. However, even when bacteria enter the body, the normal body defense mechanisms (skin, leukocytes, immune system) function to protect and prevent the development of infection. When the skin or other body tissues break down, bacteria penetrate into the internal body tissues and set up areas of infection. Bacteria produce toxins that cause inflammation, tissue damage, fever, and other symptoms associated with infection.

Morphology of Bacteria

There are thousands of different types of bacteria. Bacteria are generally classified by shape and arrangement. The basic bacterial shapes are spherical (cocci), rod-like (bacilli), and curved rods (spirilla). Some of the bacterial arrangements are in pairs (diplo), chains (strepto), or clusters (staphylo). Table 21-1 illustrates some of the more common bacterial arrangements.

It is necessary to stain bacteria in order to visualize and identify them. One of the most important bacteriologic stains is the **Gram stain,** which contains two dyes: crystal violet (blue) and safranin (red). Bacteria that retain only the blue stain are classified as **gram positive,** whereas bacteria that retain only the red stain are **gram negative.** It is important to distinguish gram-positive from gram-negative organisms. The response to antibiotic therapy varies with the type of bacteria involved. Gram stains aid the accurate diagnosis and proper treatment of bacterial infections.

The normal procedure for bacterial identification involves taking some material from the infected area (throat swab, sputum, or urine) and growing the bacteria in a culture medium. After 24 to 48 hours the bacteria are stained. Identification is based on morphology and biochemical characteristics. Newer biochemical diagnostic techniques are available for the immediate identification of some organisms.

In addition to identification, it is frequently important to determine which chemotherapeutic drugs will be most effective against the specific bacteria that are causing the infection. Identification of the antibiotics that are effective against specific bacteria is referred to as **antibiotic susceptibility.** Two of the simplest methods to determine antibiotic susceptibility are the disk test and serial dilution. In each

Table 21-1

Bacterial Morphology and Some Common Bacterial Arrangements

Bacterial Form	*Bacterial Arrangement*	*Classification*
Cocci		
Pairs		Diplococci
Chains		Streptococci
Clusters		Staphylococci
Bacilli		
Straight		Bacilli
Short curved		Vibrio
Spirillum		
Twisted		Spirilla
Twisted		Borrelia
Twisted		Treponema

case, the bacteria are cultured in media that contain varous antibacterial drugs. The drug with the greatest sensitivity will produce the greatest inhibition of bacterial growth. This screening method indicates which drug should produce the best clinical results in eradicating the infection. Bacterial identification and determination of antibiotic susceptibility are commonly referred to as culture and sensitivity testing.

Chemotherapy

Chemotherapy refers to the use of drugs to kill or to inhibit the growth of infectious organisms or cancerous cells. Chemotherapy is indicated when normal body defense mechanisms are inadequate to control infection.

Antibacterial agents are divided into two main types: bactericidal and bacteriostatic. **Bactericidal** drugs are lethal; that is, they actually kill the bacteria. **Bacteriostatic** drugs inhibit the reproduction (growth) of bacteria. With bacteriostatic drugs, elimination of the pathogenic bacteria depends on phagocytosis by host leukocytes and macrophages and other actions of the immune system.

SOURCES OF ANTIBACTERIAL DRUGS

Antibacterial drugs are obtained from two major sources: soil microorganisms and chemical synthesis. Bacteria and other microorganisms naturally produce substances that inhibit the growth of other bacteria. In nature, these substances help protect specific types of bacteria from the harmful chemical substances released by other bacteria. These chemical substances obtained from microorganisms and used in chemotherapy are referred to as **antibiotics.** For example, the mold *Penicillium notatum* produces a substance that inhibits the growth of many gram-positive pathogenic bacteria. This substance, known as penicillin, is the parent compound of some of the most widely used antibiotic drugs. Some antibacterial drugs, such as the sulfonamides, are produced by chemical synthesis. Antibacterial drugs that are obtained by chemical synthesis and not from other microorganisms are referred to generally as **antimicrobial** drugs.

ANTIBACTERIAL SPECTRUM

Very few, if any, antibacterial drugs inhibit the growth of all pathogenic bacteria. Each antibacterial drug is generally effective for only a limited number of pathogenic bacteria. These susceptible bacteria make up the **antibacterial spectrum** for that particular drug. Some drugs are effective against a limited number of bacteria, for example, only some gram-positive or only some gram-negative bacteria. These drugs are characterized as having a narrow antibacterial spectrum. Other drugs are effective against a wide spectrum of both gram-positive and gram-negative bacteria. These drugs are referred to as **broad-spectrum** or extended-spectrum antibiotics.

DRUG RESISTANCE

During chemotherapy, an antibiotic may occasionally lose its effectiveness. This usually occurs when the bacteria undergo some structural or metabolic alteration or mutation that allows the bacteria to survive the actions of the antibiotic. The ability of bacteria to resist the actions of antibiotics is referred to as **bacterial resistance.** One cause of bacterial resistance involves the ability of bacteria to alter the outer cell wall so that antibiotics can no longer penetrate the bacteria. In addition, some bacteria produce enzymes that inactivate the antibiotic (see below). When resistance occurs, the bacteria are able to survive and reproduce in the presence of the drug. A common finding is that a few resistant bacteria are already present within the infection. As the nonresistant bacteria are eliminated by the antibiotic, the resistant bacteria begin to rapidly multiply and are then responsible for continuation of the infection. When drug resistance occurs, another antibacterial drug that the bacteria are sensitive to must be substituted.

Bacterial β-Lactamase Enzymes   Certain bacteria have the ability to produce enzymes that inactivate penicillin and cephalosporin antibiotics. These enzymes are referred to generally as **β-lactamases.** β-Lactamases that inactivate penicillins are referred to as **penicillinases.** β-Lactamases that inactivate cephalosporins are referred to as **cephalosporinases.** Other types of bacterial enzymes are also produced that can inactivate other antibiotics.

Penicillins

Penicillin is an antibiotic obtained from various species of *Penicillium* mold. Alteration of the basic structure and the addition of various salts have provided numerous penicillin preparations. The main differences among the various preparations involve differences in acid stability (in the stomach), resistance to enzymatic destruction by penicillinase, and antibacterial spectrum. The different penicillin preparations are listed in Table 21-2.

MECHANISM OF ACTION

The penicillins are bactericidal to susceptible bacteria that are in the process of reproducing. Penicillin interferes with synthesis of the bacterial cell wall. With a defective cell wall, the bacteria cannot maintain the necessary osmotic concentration with the surrounding body fluids. Consequently, the bacterial cells gain water, swell, and burst apart (lysis).

ANTIBACTERIAL SPECTRUM

The penicillins are divided into several different groups based on their spectrum of activity. The current classification system divides the penicillins into four generations.

Table 21-2

Penicillin Antibiotics

Drug (Trade Name)	Route	Remarks
First generation		
Penicillin G (Pentids)	PO	Inactivated by gastric acid, absorption is unreliable
Penicillin G (Na, K salts)	IM, IV	Produces high plasma levels, has a short duration of action
Penicillin G benzathine (Bicillin)	IM	Penicillin G is slowly released from injection site over 28 days, provides low plasma levels
Penicillin G procaine (Wycillin)	IM	Penicillin G is slowly released from injection site over 12–24 h
Penicillin V potassium K (Pen-Vee K, V-Cillin K)	PO	Resists acid destruction in stomach; used to treat minor throat and ear infections
Penicillinase resistant		
Cloxacillin sodium (Tegopen)	PO	Resistant to the destructive actions of penicillinase; used to treat infections only when penicillinase-producing organisms are causing the infection
Dicloxacillin sodium (Dynapen)	PO	
Methicillin sodium (Staphcillin)	IM, IV	
Nafcillin sodium (Unipen)	IM, IV	
Oxacillin sodium (Prostaphlin)	PO, IM, IV	
Second generation		
Amoxicillin (Amoxil)	PO	Broader spectrum than first-generation drugs; amoxicillin and bacampicillin usually provide higher plasma levels
Ampicillin sodium (Omnipen)	PO, IM, IV	
Bacampicillin hydrochloride (Spectrobid)	PO	
Cyclacillin (Cyclapen-W)	PO	
Third generation		
Carbenicillin indanyl (Geocillin)	PO	For the treatment of urinary tract infections
Ticarcillin disodium (Ticar)	IM, IV	Broad spectrum, generally reserved for pseudomonal and other serious gram-negative infections
Fourth generation		
Mezlocillin sodium (Mezlin)	IM, IV	Increased effectiveness compared to third-generation drugs; indicated for serious gram-negative infections
Piperacillin (Pipracil)	IM, IV	

First-Generation Penicillins   This group includes penicillin G and penicillin V, which have a narrow antibacterial spectrum. They are effective against common gram-positive organisms (streptococci and pneumococci) that are often responsible for causing ear and throat infections and organisms that cause the common venereal diseases such as gonorrhea and syphilis. They are not effective against most gram-negative bacilli (rods) or organisms that produce penicillinase. These drugs are listed in Table 21-2 under first-generation penicillins.

Another subgroup of first-generation penicillins are resistant to penicillinase and are indicated primarily for the treatment of resistant staphylococcal (staph) infections. Staph infections, caused mainly by *Staphylococcus aureus,* cause abscesses and other serious infections (endocarditis and pneumonia). Staph infections are often difficult to treat because there is a high incidence of bacterial resistance as a result of penicillinase production among staph bacteria. These drugs are listed in Table 21-2 as penicillinase resistant.

Second-Generation Penicillins   The second generation includes ampicillin, amoxicillin, and similar drugs that are considered to have an extended, or broad, spectrum. The second-generation drugs are effective against the same organisms as penicillin G plus a number of common gram-negative organisms. These include *Escherichia coli, Proteus mirabilis,* and *Haemophilus influenzae,* which are responsible for common urinary, respiratory, and ear infections. All second-generation penicillins can be taken orally, which is an important advantage in the treatment of a variety of common gram-positive and gram-negative infections. Amoxicillin is widely used because it is well absorbed from the GI tract and produces higher plasma drug levels than ampicillin.

Second-generation penicillins are not effective against penicillinase-producing organisms, and in recent years, greater numbers and percentages of organisms produce penicillinase, which inactivates the penicillin molecule.

Third-Generation Penicillins   The third generation includes carbenicillin and ticarcillin, which have a broader spectrum than do the second-generation drugs. The main indication for these penicillins is in the treatment of more serious urinary, respiratory, and bacteremic infections caused by gram-negative *Pseudomonas aeruginosa* and *Proteus vulgaris.* These infections are often difficult to treat and may require combination therapy with the aminoglycoside antibiotics. Carbenicillin indanyl (Geocillin) is administered orally and is indicated only for the treatment of urinary tract infections. Ticarcillin (Ticar) is administered parenterally (IM, IV) for the treatment of systemic infections. These drugs are not resistant to penicillinase-producing organisms.

Fourth-Generation Penicillins   These drugs have been more recently introduced and generally have a wider antibacterial spectrum than do third-generation penicillins, are more effective (potent), and are administered in the form of monosodium salts. This form reduces the amount of sodium ingested compared to some other penicillins that are disodium salts. This may be important for individuals with hypertension or congestive heart failure, who are usually on sodium-restricted diets.

The fourth-generation drugs are mainly indicated for serious infections caused by *Pseudomonas aeruginosa, Proteus vulgaris, Klebsiella pneumoniae,* and *Bacteroides fragilis* (anaerobe). These infections can also be difficult to treat and may require combination therapy. The fourth-generation penicillins are not resistant to penicillinase-producing organisms, and they require parenteral administration.

ß-Lactamase Inhibitors   There still is not a single penicillin that combines all of the following: can be taken orally, has a broad spectrum, and is resistant to penicillinase. However, several drugs, known as β-lactamase inhibitors, can be administered along with the various penicillins. These drugs inhibit the penicillinase enzymes and allow the penicillin drug to remain effective. These inhibitors include clavulanic acid, sulbactam, and tazobactam. Combinations of the various penicillins plus inhibitor are marketed together. Amoxicillin plus clavulanic acid is marketed as *Augmentin*, ampicillin is combined with sulbactam in *Unasyn*, and piperacillin is combined with tazobactam in *Zosyn*. These antibiotic combinations are indicated when bacterial resistance is suspected.

ADVERSE EFFECTS

As a group, the penicillins are relatively nontoxic. Minor adverse effects, such as nausea or rashes, may occur in some patients. Diarrhea is more common with oral administration. When used in very high doses, the penicillins can cause CNS disturbances, including convulsions.

The most serious adverse effect involves individuals who develop an allergy to penicillin. As a drug class, the penicillins cause the highest incidence of drug allergy. Common allergic symptoms include rashes, fever, and inflammatory conditions. The most serious allergic reaction involves anaphylaxis or anaphylactic shock. All patients must be questioned about the possibility of penicillin allergy. In cases of suspected allergy, skin sensitivity testing can be performed to determine whether patients are allergic to penicillin. Patients allergic to one penicillin are considered allergic to all of the penicillin drugs.

ANTIBIOTICS RELATED TO THE PENICILLINS

Imipenem (Primaxin), meropenem (Merrem), and aztreonam (Azactam) are bactericidal drugs that are structurally related to penicillins and have the same mechanism of action. Imipenem and meropenem are effective against both gram-positive and gram-negative bacteria, including bacteria that are resistant to penicillins. Imipenem and meropenem are administered parenterally. Nausea, vomiting, seizures, and allergic reactions are adverse effects.

Aztreonam is also highly resistant to penicillinase and is mainly used intravenously for resistant gram-negative infections. It can usually be used in individuals who are allergic to penicillin. Gastrointestinal disturbances and rash are common adverse reactions.

Cephalosporins

The cephalosporins are bactericidal antibiotics that have chemical structures similar to those of the penicillins. The mechanism of action of the cephalosporins is the same as that of the penicillins. The cephalosporins are considered to be broad-spectrum drugs. Their two main uses are as substitutes for penicillins in cases of allergy or bacterial resistance and in the treatment of certain gram-negative infections. Some organisms, usually gram negative, can produce cephalosporinase. The cephalosporins are ineffective against organisms that produce these enzymes. The cephalosporins are also classified into four generations and are listed in Table 21-3.

First-Generation Cephalosporins These antibiotics are considered to be the older cephalosporins. They all have a similar antibacterial spectrum, which includes both some gram-positive and some gram-negative organisms. The cephalosporins are the drugs of choice for treating infections caused by gram-negative *Klebsiella pneumoniae*. Of this group, cefazolin (Kefzol) is among the most widely used because of the higher plasma levels that it produces. These drugs are useful for most of the common gram-positive and gram-negative infections that cause ear, throat, and urinary tract infections.

Second-Generation Cephalosporins These cephalosporins have a broader spectrum than the first-generation drugs and are generally more potent. They are indicated when first-generation drugs are ineffective. Cefoxitin (Mefoxin) is especially

Table 21-3
Cephalosporin Antibiotics

Drug (Trade Name)	Route	Remarks
First generation		
Cefadroxil (Duricef)	PO	Used to treat common gram-positive and
Cefazolin (Kefzol)	IM, IV	gram-negative infections, including
Cephalexin (Keflex)	PO	*Klebsiella pneumoniae*
Cephradine (Velosef)	PO, IV	
Second generation		
Cefaclor (Ceclor)	PO	Indicated for gram-negative infections, are
Cefamandole (Mandol)	IM, IV	more resistant to the actions of penicillinase
Cefoxitin (Mefoxin)	IM, IV	and cephalosporinase
Cefonicid (Monocid)	IM, IV	
Cefotetan (Cefotan)	IM, IV	
Third generation		
Cefixime (Suprax)	PO	Indicated for serious gram-negative infections
Cefoperazone (Cefobid)	IM, IV	that are resistant to other cephalosporins;
Cefotaxime (Claforan)	IM, IV	they have longer durations of action and are
Ceftazidime (Fortaz)	IM, IV	more potent without producing any
Ceftriaxone (Rocephin)	IM, IV	additional toxicities compared to the
		first- and second-generation cephalosporins
Fourth generation		
Cefepime (Maxipime)	IM, IV	Similar to third generation, but greater resistance to β-lactamase inactivating enzymes

useful in treating infections caused by *Bacteroides fragilis* and *Serratia marcescens.* Also, these drugs are often effective in treating respiratory and other infections caused by *Haemophilus influenzae* and *Neisseria gonorrhoeae,* including organisms that produce penicillinase and that are often resistant to penicillins.

Third-Generation Cephalosporins   These drugs have a broader spectrum than do the second-generation drugs. They are more potent antibiotics, and they have longer durations of action than do the other cephalosporins. The third-generation cephalosporins are mainly indicated for the treatment of serious gram-negative infections that are not susceptible to second-generation drugs. These drugs are also more lipid soluble and cross the blood–brain barrier more readily than most other penicillins and cephalosporins. Consequently, they are often used for both gram-positive and gram-negative infections involving the brain (meningitis).

Fourth-Generation Cephalosporins   Recently, a new cephalosporin drug, cefepine *(Maxipime),* was approved. This drug has been classified as the first drug of the fourth generation of cephalosporins. It is similar in spectrum to the third-generation drugs; the main feature is greater resistance to β-lactamase-inactivating enzymes. It should be used when the lower generations of cephalosporins are ineffective.

ADVERSE EFFECTS

Oral cephalosporins may cause GI disturbances, especially diarrhea and rashes. Intramuscular injections with the cephalosporins are usually painful and may cause local inflammation. Intravenous administration may cause phlebitis at the infusion site. The first-generation cephalosporins may cause nephrotoxicity, especially in patients with renal impairment or in patients who are dehydrated. In comparison, the newer cephalosporins are associated with a lower incidence of nephrotoxicity.

Cephalosporins that possess the *N*-methylthiotetrazone side chain (cefamandole, cefoperazone, cefotetan, others) may interfere with blood coagulation and cause bleeding problems. In addition, these same drugs can cause a disulfiram reaction when combined with alcohol. This reaction is marked by intense flushing, rapid pulse, pounding heart, and hyperventilation.

Cephalosporins do cause allergic reactions, but the incidence of allergy with cephalosporins is lower than that with the penicillins. Some individuals are allergic to both penicillins and cephalosporins. Usually, cephalosporins can be used in patients allergic to penicillins. The guiding principle is that cephalosporins are not administered to penicillin-allergic individuals who have previously experienced the immediate type of penicillin allergic reaction (hives, anaphylaxis).

Aminoglycosides

The aminoglycosides are a group of bactericidal antibiotics whose antibacterial spectrum mainly includes gram-negative bacilli. The mechanism of action of the aminoglycosides is that the drug passes into the bacterium, where it attaches irreversibly to the ribosomes to cause an irreversible inhibition of bacterial protein synthesis. The bacteria can no longer produce the enzymes and proteins necessary for survival and reproduction.

PHARMACOKINETICS

The aminoglycosides are poorly absorbed from the GI tract, and this effect is used to advantage before intestinal surgery. Large doses are given orally before abdominal surgery to reduce the number of intestinal bacteria and sterilize the bowel. The usual route of administration for systemic effects is either IM or IV. These drugs are effective against most gram-negative organisms and generally reserved for the treatment of serious gram-negative infections in hospitalized patients. The aminoglycosides are not significantly metabolized and are excreted mostly unchanged in the urine. Consequently, high urinary concentrations are attained, contributing to the effectiveness of the aminoglycosides in the treatment of resistant urinary tract infections. The most frequently used aminoglycosides are listed in Table 21-4.

RESPIRATORY USE

Tobramycin is one of the only antibiotics that are given via inhalation by respiratory care practitioners. It is primarily used for patients with cystic fibrosis (CF) to treat resistant *Pseudomonas aeruginosa* pulmonary infections. Sometimes CF patients develop a variant of *Pseudomonas* known as mucoid, and tobramycin treatment can be beneficial. Like other medications that are inhaled, this places the drug directly where it is needed. This avoids parenteral administration, which can be associated with numerous adverse drug effects. There are some adverse effects associated with the inhaled route. These include bronchospasm, hoarseness, fun-

Table 21-4
Aminoglycoside Antibiotics

Drug (Trade Name)	Remarks
Amikacin (Amikin)	Reserved for treatment of serious gram-negative infections, especially with bacteria resistant to tobramycin or gentamicin
Gentamicin (Garamycin)	Reserved for the treatment of serious gram-negative infections; produces a significant incidence of ototoxicity
Kanamycin (Kantrex)	Used in the treatment of gram-negative infections and before intestinal surgery; also used in the treatment of tuberculosis
Neomycin (Neobiotic)	Produces a significant degree of ototoxicity and is usually used only as a topical antibiotic (Myciguent) in the treatment of skin and ocular infections
Streptomycin	Used in the treatment of tuberculosis, plague, and tularemia
Tobramycin (Nebcin)	Reserved for the treatment of serious gram-negative infections, particularly *Pseudomonas aeruginosa*

gal infections, and bacterial resistance. Because giving tobramycin via inhalation concentrates the drug in the lungs, no blood level monitoring is required.

Tobramycin has been used as suppressive therapy as a chronic treatment for CF. It has been shown to decrease the need for hospitalization and parenteral antibiotic therapy.

Until recently, tobramycin for parenteral use has been used for inhalation treatment. There are now several brands of tobramycin that have been developed specifically for inhalation. These preparations are preservative-free. The usual dose is 300 mg twice daily regardless of age or weight.

ADVERSE EFFECTS

When taken orally, the aminoglycosides may cause nausea, vomiting, and diarrhea. When administered parenterally, the two most serious adverse effects are nephrotoxicity (renal toxicity) and ototoxicity. Because of the high urinary levels, the aminoglycosides may interfere with normal renal function. Increased casts, albuminuria (protein in the urine), and oliguria (reduced urine output) may occur. The aminoglycosides interfere with the function of the auditory nerve (cranial VIII). The earliest symptoms are tinnitus (ringing in the ears) and temporary impairment of hearing; this is generally referred to as ototoxicity. In some cases, in which the aminoglycosides were taken for extended periods, irreversible damage and permanent hearing loss has occurred.

CAUTIONS AND CONTRAINDICATIONS

Pregnancy   Aminoglycosides are designated FDA Pregnancy Category D and should not be used during pregnancy. The aminioglycosides have been shown to cause fetal harm, in particular hearing loss and deafness.

DRUG INTERACTIONS

The aminoglycosides possess some peripheral neuromuscular blocking activity. Administration during surgery or other procedures in which general anesthetics or other neuromuscular blockers are also being used may produce excessive degrees of muscular blockade. The most serious effect would be respiratory arrest from paralysis of the diaphragm and the other muscles of respiration.

The ototoxic effect of the aminoglycosides is increased when other ototoxic drugs, such as some diuretics (ethacrynic acid and furosemide), are administered at the same time. Combination therapy using other nephrotoxic drugs may increase nephrotoxicity.

Tetracyclines

The tetracyclines—a group of broad-spectrum antibiotics—are clinically useful in both gram-positive and gram-negative infections. The first tetracycline developed was chlortetracycline (Aureomycin). Other members of this group produce effects similar to chlortetracycline. Tetracyclines interfere with bacterial protein synthesis to produce a bacteriostatic effect.

ADMINISTRATION

The tetracyclines are usually administered orally, but IM and IV injection may be used if necessary. Foods, especially those containing calcium (milk), and substances such as antacids and mineral supplements interfere with the GI absorption of the tetracyclines. Because tetracyclines bind calcium molecules (chelate) and form insoluble compounds, tetracycline should be taken 1 hour before meals or several hours after meals. Doxycycline and minocycline are more completely absorbed from the GI tract than are the other tetracyclines and are least affected by calcium and other mineral-containing substances. The tetracyclines are listed in Table 21-5.

CLINICAL INDICATIONS

The tetracyclines are occasional alternatives to the penicillins for some of the gram-positive and gram-negative infections. However, the most important indications for the tetracyclines are for infections caused by rickettsiae (Rocky Mountain spotted fever, typhus), *Mycoplasma pneumoniae, Vibrio cholerae* (cholera), *Chlamydia trachomatis* (urethritis), and *Borrelia burgdorferi* (Lyme disease). In addition, the tetracyclines are sometimes used to treat lower respiratory infections that often contribute to chronic bronchitis.

ADVERSE EFFECTS

The most common side effects associated with the tetracyclines are nausea, vomiting, and diarrhea. Suppression of normal intestinal bacteria may result in overgrowth of nonsusceptible organisms (superinfection), especially fungi *(Candida albicans)*. These conditions usually produce diarrhea and various skin rashes. The tetracyclines also produce photosensitivity in some individuals. After ingestion of the tetracyclines and exposure to sunlight, an exaggerated sunburn may occur. The

Table 21-5
Tetracycline Antibiotics

Drug (Trade Name)	Usual Adult Oral Dose
Demeclocycline (Declomycin)	150 mg every 6 h
Doxycycline (Vibramycin)	100 mg once per day
Methacycline (Rondomycin)	150 mg every 6 h
Minocycline (Minocin)	100 mg every 12 h
Oxytetracycline (Terramycin)	250–500 mg every 6 h
Tetracycline (Achromycin)	250–500 mg every 6 h

use of outdated tetracycline products may produce a particular type of reaction known as the Fanconi syndrome. The main effects of this syndrome involve the kidneys, where polyuria, proteinuria, and acidosis are most frequently observed.

CAUTIONS AND CONTRAINDICATIONS

Pregnancy   The tetracyclines bind to calcium and therefore should not be administered to children below the age of 8 or to women who are pregnant or nursing. These drugs are deposited in growing bones and teeth, producing a yellow discoloration and possible depression of bone growth. Tetracyclines are designated FDA Pregnancy Category D and have been shown to cause growth retardation in relation to infant skeletal development.

Sulfonamides

The sulfonamides are a group of synthetic drugs that were discovered in 1935 as a by-product of the dye industry. The first sulfonamide was sulfanilamide. Alteration of its basic structure produced many other compounds having similar activities. The sulfonamides were initially effective against many gram-positive and gram-negative organisms. Unfortunately, early widespread use of the sulfonamides led to the development of bacterial resistance. After introduction of the penicillins (early 1940s), use of the sulfonamides rapidly declined. Today, the sulfonamides have limited uses in selected infections. Some of the sulfonamides are used topically, especially in burn cases to prevent and treat infection. Other sulfonamides are used primarily for the treatment of urinary and gastrointestinal tract infections.

MECHANISM OF ACTION

Bacteria have an essential requirement for *para*-aminobenzoic acid, which is used in the synthesis of folic acid. The sulfonamides are competitive antagonists of *para*-aminobenzoic acid. The sulfonamides block the synthesis of folic acid, which subsequently inhibits bacterial growth, producing a bacteriostatic effect.

ADMINISTRATION

The most common route of administration is oral, although a parenteral route may be used. The main pathway of elimination is renal, and the sulfonamides tend to be concentrated in the urine. The various sulfonamides have different durations of action and generally are classified as short-, intermediate-, and long-acting. In addition, because of their poor oral absorption, some sulfonamides are used to reduce intestinal bacteria before intestinal surgery. The sulfonamides are listed in Table 21-6.

ADVERSE EFFECTS

Oral administration frequently causes nausea, vomiting, and diarrhea. One of the more serious adverse effects is crystalluria. In the presence of dehydration and acidic urine, the sulfonamides have a tendency to crystallize in the renal tubules, causing

Table 21-6

Sulfonamide Antimicrobial Drugs

Drug (Trade Name)	Main Uses	Comment
Mafenide (Sulfamylon)	In burn cases to prevent infection	Topical
Silver sulfadiazine	In burn cases to prevent infection	Topical
Sulfacetamide (Sulamyd)	Ocular infections	Topical
Sulfamethoxazole (Gantanol)	Urinary tract infections	Intermediate acting
Sulfasalazine (Azulfidine)	Ulcerative colitis	Long acting
Sulfisoxazole (Gantrisin)	Urinary tract infections	Short acting

cell damage, blood in the urine, and reduced urine output. Therefore, patients must receive adequate fluid intake, and urine should be made alkaline if it is highly acidic.

The sulfonamides also may produce allergic reactions, which usually are limited to the skin and mucous membranes. The most common reactions include rashes, pruritis, and photosensitivity. A very serious type of skin condition, the Stevens-Johnson syndrome, produces a skin reaction that can be fatal. The development of any rash after ingestion of the sulfonamides must receive medical evaluation.

Blood disorders, including anemia, leukopenia, and thrombocytopenia, may develop with sulfonamide therapy. Patients with existing deficiency of glucose-6-phosphate dehydrogenase (G6PD) are particularly susceptible to the development of hemolytic anemia.

DRUG INTERACTIONS

The sulfonamides may produce a number of drug interactions because of their ability to displace other drugs from inactive plasma protein-binding sites. The most frequent drug interactions involve the coumarin anticoagulants (increased anticoagulant effect) and the oral hypoglycemic drugs (hypoglycemia). Patients receiving sulfonamides and any of these drugs should be closely monitored for bleeding tendencies or hypoglycemic effects.

TRIMETHOPRIM-SULFAMETHOXAZOLE

This combination, marketed under the trade names of Septra and Bactrim, has broad-spectrum antimicrobial actions. It is a combination of one of the sulfonamides, sulfamethoxazole, and the drug trimethoprim. Trimethoprim inhibits the enzyme dihydrofolate reductase, which interferes with the further synthesis of folic acid to its activated form. Together, these two drugs exert a synergistic effect to inhibit folic acid production in bacteria that is very effective. Administration is either oral or parenteral in varying concentrations.

Clinical Indications   The sulfamethoxazole-trimethoprim combination is effective against a broad spectrum of gram-positive and gram-negative bacteria. It is often used as an alternative to the penicillins and cephalosporins for respiratory, urinary, gastrointestinal, and other systemic infections. It is frequently the drug of choice for treatment of *Pneumocystis carinii* pneumonial infections and ear, sinus, and pneumonial infections caused by *Haemophilus influenzae.*

The adverse effects of trimethoprim are generally similar to the sulfonamides; however, trimethoprim does not usually cause crystalluria.

Macrolide Antibiotics

The term macrolide refers to the large chemical ring structure that is characteristic of these antibiotics. These antibiotics inhibit bacterial protein synthesis and are considered bacteriostatic. The macrolides include erythromycin and several newer derivatives that cause less gastric irritation and have a wider antibacterial spectrum than erythromycin. The newer derivatives include azithromycin, clarithromycin, and dirithromycin. The most common adverse effect of these drugs is gastrointestinal irritation.

ERYTHROMYCIN (ERYTHROCIN, E-MYCIN)

Erythromycin is a macrolide antibiotic with an antibacterial spectrum similar to that of penicillin G, but with the addition of a few other organisms. The main uses of erythromycin are as a penicillin substitute in the treatment of *Legionella pneumophilia* (Legionaire's disease), *Mycoplasma pneumoniae,* and genital infections caused by *Chlamydia trachomatis.* The usual oral dose is 250 mg every 6 hours. GI disturbances such as nausea, vomiting, and diarrhea and minor skin rashes are usually the common adverse effects associated with erythromycin and the other macrolide drugs.

AZITHROMYCIN (ZITHROMAX)

Azithromycin is administered orally or parenterally; its longer half-life of 65 to 70 hours allows once-a-day dosing. The drug is eliminated mostly in an unmetabolized state via the biliary-intestinal route. Azithromycin has greater activity against gram-negative and anaerobic organisms than erythromycin. It is particularly useful in ear and respiratory infections caused by *Haemophilus influenzae.*

CLARITHROMYCIN (BIAXIN)

Clarithromycin is well absorbed after oral administration. The drug forms an active metabolite during first-pass liver metabolism. Clarithromycin has the same antibacterial spectrum as erythromycin, but it is a more potent drug. The main uses are infections caused by *Haemophilus influenzae, Legionella pneumophilia, Chlamydia trachomatis,* and *Borrelia burgdorferi* (Lyme disease).

DIRITHROMYCIN (DYNABAC)

Dirithromycin is a prodrug (an inert drug that becomes active after biotransformation) that is rapidly converted into an active metabolite that is responsible for the antibacterial effect. Oral absorption is increased by food, and administration with meals is recommended. The main indications for dirithromycin are common staphylococcal and streptococcal infections and gram-negative infections caused by *Mycoplasma pneumoniae, Legionella pneumophilia,* and *Moraxella catarrhalis.*

Fluoroquinolone Antimicrobials

The fluoroquinolones are synthetic antimicrobial agents that have a broad spectrum of antibacterial activity, especially against gram-negative organisms. One of their advantages, over some of the other broad-spectrum antibiotics, is that they are well absorbed after oral administration. The prototype of this drug class is ciprofloxacin. Other fluoroquinolones are listed in Table 21-7.

CIPROFLOXACIN (CIPRO)

The mechanism of action of ciprofloxacin and the other fluoroquinolones is to inhibit an enzyme, DNA gyrase, that is essential to the function of DNA and bacterial replication. These drugs are bactericidal against a wide variety of gram-positive and gram-negative organisms.

Ciprofloxacin is used in the treatment of a wide variety of urinary, gastrointestinal, respiratory, bone and joint, and soft tissue infections, especially those resistant to other antibacterial drugs.

The most common adverse reactions include headache, dizziness, GI disturbances, and rash. Some rashes are related to photosensitivity reactions. The fluoroquinolones are not recommended for children or pregnant women. There is evidence of cartilage defects in animal studies and arthralgias and joint swelling in humans.

Table 21-7
Fluoroquinolone Antimicrobial Drugs

Drug (Trade Name)	Main Uses
Ciprofloxacin (Cipro)	Most potent, used for wide variety of infections
Enoxacin (Penetrex)	Urinary tract infections and gonorrhea
Levofloxacin (Levaquin)	Community–acquired pneumonia
Lomefloxacin (Maxaquin)	Respiratory and urinary tract infections
Norfloxacin (Noroxin)	Urinary tract infections
Ofloxacin (Floxin)	Respiratory, urinary tract, and gonorrheal infections

Miscellaneous Antimicrobial Drugs

CHLORAMPHENICOL (CHLOROMYCETIN)

Chloramphenicol is a broad-spectrum antibiotic that is reserved for serious and life-threatening infections. Two of the main indications for chloramphenicol are typhoid fever and certain types of meningitis. The mechanism of action of chloramphenicol is to inhibit bacterial protein synthesis, which produces a bacteriostatic effect. Absorption of chloramphenicol from the GI tract is excellent. The oral dose is 250 to 500 mg every 6 hours. Chloramphenicol is also used topically in the treatment of ocular infections.

Adverse and Toxic Effects   Common side effects usually involve nausea, vomiting, and diarrhea. Chloramphenicol is potentially a very toxic drug. One of the most serious effects is bone marrow depression, which usually produces anemia or other blood disorders. In most cases, the effects are reversible. However, in some patients the adverse effects are irreversible and may include aplastic anemia. Frequent blood cell counts should be taken while patients are receiving chloramphenicol. As with all broad-spectrum antibiotics, suppression of normal intestinal bacteria may result in superinfections.

Cautions and Contraindications   Chloramphenicol should not be administered to infants less than 2 weeks old. Infant livers are unable to metabolize chloramphenicol, and accumulation leads to toxic blood levels, resulting in a condition known as the gray baby syndrome, which is characterized by abdominal distention, circulatory collapse, and respiratory failure.

CLINDAMYCIN (CLEOCIN)

Clindamycin is a bacteriostatic antibiotic that inhibits bacterial protein synthesis. The drug is effective against most of the common gram-positive organisms and especially against anaerobic organisms, which is its major indication. The most common adverse effects involve the GI tract, usually diarrhea. Occasionally, clindamycin allows the overgrowth of another intestinal organism, *Clostridium difficile.* This can cause a condition known as pseudomembranous colitis, which causes severe diarrhea and abdominal cramps, and can be fatal if untreated. This overgrowth can be seen with all antibodies, but was first noticed in patients receiving clindamycin.

VANCOMYCIN (VANCOCIN)

Vancomycin is a bactericidal antibiotic that interferes with cell wall synthesis. The drug is mainly used to treat resistant staphylococcal infections and pseudomembranous colitis caused by *Clostridium difficile.* Vancomycin may produce some serious adverse effects that include ototoxicity (deafness), nephrotoxicity (kidney), and a flushing redness of the neck and trunk caused by histamine release. This condition is known as "red man syndrome" and occurs when parenteral administration is too rapid or the solution is too concentrated.

Drugs Used to Treat Tuberculosis

Tuberculosis is an infection caused by *Mycobacterium tuberculosis.* The infection usually involves the lung, but can spread to other body organs, including the brain. The infecting organism can lie dormant within the body, only to reemerge and cause infection years later. Reemergence of the organism often occurs when body resistance to infection is lowered. Infection with human immunodeficiency virus (AIDS) has been one of the factors that accounts for the increased incidence of tuberculosis in recent years. One of the biggest problems in treating tuberculosis has been the dramatic increase in bacterial resistance to drug therapy. Drug therapy usually involves administration of three or four different drugs for prolonged periods of time, often a year or more. The most important drugs for treating tuberculosis are isoniazid, rifampin, ethambutol, pyrazinamide, and streptomycin. Streptomycin is one of the aminoglycosides; it is sometimes used in initial therapy for the first few weeks. The major disadvantage is that it requires parenteral administration.

ISONIAZID (INH)

Isoniazid is a synthetic drug that is bactericidal for reproducing organisms. The drug inhibits the production of mycolic acid, which is essential for bacterial cell wall synthesis. Isoniazid is well absorbed orally and metabolized by acetylation. This reaction is highly variable among individuals: some are "fast acetylators," and others are "slow acetylators." Slow acetylators usually experience better antibacterial results but also experience more adverse effects of the drug.

The two most important adverse effects of isoniazid are peripheral neuritis and hepatitis. Peripheral neuritis can usually be prevented by taking pyridoxine (vitamin B_6) supplementation. Hepatitis is more common in individuals over the age of 35 and those who drink alcohol on a regular basis. Other adverse effects include fever, rash, and CNS disturbances.

RIFAMPIN (RIFADIN)

Rifampin is an antibiotic that has a wider antibacterial spectrum than isoniazid. The drug inhibits a bacterial enzyme required for RNA synthesis. Rifampin is taken orally, undergoes enterohepatic cycling, and induces drug-metabolizing enzymes. This leads to a decrease in the duration of action of both itself and other drugs and may require an increase in drug dosage.

Adverse effects include GI disturbances, hepatotoxicity, rash, and headache. A flu-like syndrome, usually fatigue and muscle ache, may occur when the drug is not taken on a regular basis. Rifampin also stains urine, tears (contact lenses), and other body fluids orange-red.

ETHAMBUTOL (MYAMBUTOL)

Ethambutol is a synthetic compound that produces a bacteriostatic effect. The drug is believed to inhibit the incorporation of mycolic acid into the bacterial cell wall. Ethambutol is generally used only in combination with other drugs. The drug is usually well tolerated; fever, rash, and GI disturbances are common side effects. The most serious concern is the loss of visual acuity from optic neuritis. It is recommended that visual eye tests be performed before and during therapy to prevent any permanent loss of vision.

PYRAZINAMIDE

Pyrazinamide is a derivative of nicotinamide. Its antibacterial effects are increased by acidic conditions. The drug is mainly used in initial therapy for the first few months. Its mechanism of action is not well understood. The most serious adverse effect is development of hepatotoxicity. In addition, some patients develop hyperuricemia and symptoms of gout.

Chemoprophylaxis

Chemoprophylaxis refers to the use of antibiotics before bacterial infection has occurred in order to prevent infection. Chemoprophylaxis is indicated before certain surgeries that carry a high risk for infection, for example abdominal surgery, especially after gunshot wounds, where the intestines may be ruptured. In addition, individuals who are susceptible to certain infections that may be life-threatening often take antibiotics on a regular basis to prevent infection. Individuals who have had rheumatic fever, heart valve replacement, knee or hip replacement, and other conditions are particularly susceptible to infections that can cause endocarditis and heart valve damage. These individuals should receive chemoprophylaxis before dental, respiratory, urinary, and other invasive medical procedures. In addition, individuals exposed to patients with tuberculosis, meningitis, and other contagious infections are often given chemoprophylaxis to prevent infection. The selection and timing of antibiotic administration depend on the type of infection that is anticipated, patient characteristics, and other considerations related to the specific clinical situation.

Chapter 21 Review

UNDERSTANDING TERMINOLOGY

Test your understanding of the material in this chapter by answering the following questions.

1. Differentiate between the terms *bactericidal* and *bacteriostatic*.
2. Define *antibacterial spectrum* and *broad-spectrum* drugs.
3. Define the terms *Gram stain*, *gram positive*, and *gram negative*.
4. What is the difference between nonpathogenic bacteria and pathogenic bacteria?

ACQUIRING KNOWLEDGE

Answer the following questions.

5. What are the major sources of antibacterial drugs?

6. Why are Gram stains important?

7. Explain the mechanism of action of the penicillin and cephalosporin antibiotics.

8. What are the main advantages of the third- and fourth-generation penicillins? Third-generation cephalosporins?

9. What are the main uses, adverse effects, and drug interactions associated with the aminoglycosides?

10. Explain how the sulfonamides produce their antibacterial effect. What advantages does trimethoprim-sulfamethoxazole offer?

11. Explain the mechanism of action of the tetracyclines, choramphenicol, and fluoroquinolones.

12. What are the contraindications to the use of the tetracyclines? Chloramphenicol?

13. List some of the drugs used in the treatment of tuberculosis.

14. Explain the mechanism of action of isoniazid and rifampin. What are the major toxicities of these drugs?

APPLYING KNOWLEDGE ON THE JOB

Answer the following questions.

15. Mrs. Randazzo is an elderly woman admitted to the hospital from a nursing home with a diagnosis of sepsis secondary to a urinary tract infection (UTI). She has been receiving piperacillin (Pipracil) for 24 hours, and her temperature chart is showing a downward trend. The lab calls you with the initial results of the blood culture and states that gram-negative rods grew in two of three culture tubes. Do you need to call the attending physician for a change in antibiotic? Why or why not?

16. Mr. Porter is admitted to the hospital with an empirical diagnosis of pneumonia. The emergency room physician prescribed azithromycin 500 mg IV piggyback daily. In the patient's admission history, the patient states he has a penicillin allergy. Is it necessary to call the attending physician for a change in antibiotic because of the penicillin allergy? Why or why not?

17. Mr. Smith has just been diagnosed with a respiratory infection caused by *Pseudomonas aeruginosa*. Which penicillin antibiotic would be appropriate therapy? How is this drug administered?

18. John is a 22-year-old college student who is taking one of the cephalosporins for a throat infection. Last night at a fraternity party he became violently ill after a few beers. What happened?

19. Mrs. Evans is a 45-year-old woman who is on a four-drug regimen for treatment of her tuberculosis. At her recent checkup her liver enzymes were increased, and there were signs of jaundice. Which antitubercular drugs could be causing this condition? What other factors may make her more susceptible to this toxicity?

20. Mrs. Urban was prescribed clindamycin for a minor gram-positive throat infection. After 3 days she was experiencing severe diarrhea and dehydration. The next day she collapsed and was rushed to the hospital. The diagnosis was pseudomembranous colitis. Can you explain how this happened? What drug is indicated for treatment of this condition?

Additional Reading

Aminoglycosides: Is once a day good enough? *Emerg Med* 1997;29(2):83.

Azithromycin versus doxycycline for *Chlamydia*. *Emerg Med* 1996;28(9):100.

Cunha BA. Oral cephalosporins for common infections. *Emerg Med* 1990;15:89.

Double trouble from the deer tick. *Emerg Med* 1997;29(3):44.

Nursing update. Tetracyclines. *Nursing* 1984;14(1):46.

Remington J. Use of third-generation cephalosporins. *Hosp Pract* 1991;26(4):5.

The choice of antibacterial drugs. 1999. *Med Lett* 1999;21:issue 1064.

Internet Activities

Visit the **MecidineNet** Web site (**http://www.medicinenet.com**) and click on the "Diseases and Treatments" heading. Highlight the first letter of the following topics to aquire additional background and clinical information on these antibiotic-related articles: Diarrhea, Antibiotic Induced; Gonorrhea; Infection, Urinary; Neutropenia; Pneumonia; Pseudomembranous Colitis. Incorporate this information with the use of the antibiotics presented in this chapter. Perhaps you and some of your classmates could each take a topic and give a brief presentation to the class.

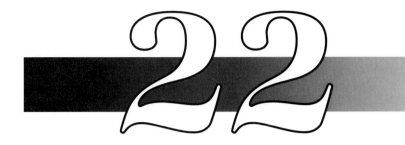

Antiseptics and Disinfectants

HENRY HITNER, PhD
BARBARA NAGLE, PhD

Chapter Focus

This chapter describes chemicals that reduce the potential for acquiring infection. It explains how antiseptics and disinfectants, which are used to control and prevent infection, are different from antibiotics, which are used to treat infection.

Chapter Terminology

antiseptic: Substance that inhibits the growth of microorganisms without totally destroying them; refers to substance used on living tissue.

argyria: Permanent black discoloration of skin and mucous membranes caused by prolonged use of silver protein solutions.

-cidal: Suffix denoting killing, as of microorganisms.

decubitus ulcer: Bedsore.

denaturing: Causing destruction of bacterial protein function; also adulteration of alcohol, rendering it unfit for drinking.

disinfectant: Substance that inhibits the growth of disease-causing microorganisms; refers to substances used on nonliving surfaces.

eschar: Thick crust or scab that develops after skin is burned.

fungicidal: Any agent that kills fungus.

fungistatic: Any agent that inhibits the growth of fungus.

hypersensitivity: Exaggerated response, such as rash, edema, or anaphylaxis, that develops following exposure to certain drugs or chemicals.

iodophor: Compound containing iodine.

irrigation: Washing (lavage) of a wound or cavity with large volumes of fluid.

lyse: To disintegrate or dissolve.

nosocomial: Infection acquired as a result of being in a hospital.

-static: Suffix denoting the inhibition of, as of microorganisms.

sterilization: Process that results in destruction of all microorganisms.

virucidal: Any agent that kills viruses.

Chapter Objectives

After studying this chapter, you should be able to:

- Explain the difference between reducing bacterial growth and inhibiting all bacterial growth (eradication).
- Describe the mechanisms by which antiseptics reduce bacterial function.
- List four common chemicals that inhibit infectious microorganisms.
- Explain why many of these chemicals are not administered by mouth to treat infection.
- Explain to respiratory care patients how to prevent infection by cleansing their breathing apparatus properly.

Antiseptics and disinfectants are used to control and prevent infection. These drugs can be distinguished from other antimicrobials in that they are usually chemical solutions (such as alcohols, aldehydes, or iodophors) that are topically applied to surfaces such as skin, mucous membranes, or inanimate objects (floors, walls, or instruments) where microorganisms may be present. The primary mode of application is via swab, sponge, scrub solution, or occasionally as a mouthwash.

Antiseptics and disinfectants destroy microorganisms on contact. The term **antiseptic,** however, is more frequently associated with the eradication or inhibition of microbial growth on living tissue surfaces. **Disinfectants,** on the other hand, reduce the risk of infection by destroying pathogenic microbes on nonliving surfaces. Neither antiseptics nor disinfectants are intended to be swallowed or injected in order to destroy microorganisms.

Mechanism of Action

Antiseptics and disinfectants destroy bacteria either by interfering with cell metabolism or by **denaturing** bacterial protein. In addition, these agents can decrease the surface tension of bacterial cell walls, causing the cells to swell and **lyse** (disintegrate or dissolve). Chemicals that denature protein or decrease surface tension have a more immediate onset of action than do those that affect cell metabolism. Alcohol, formaldehyde, glutaraldehyde, and chlorhexidine disrupt cell membrane integrity on contact. Solutions of heavy metals (mercury or silver) and hexachlorophene inhibit cell enzyme systems (cell metabolism) and, therefore, require more time to produce a complete effect.

Chemicals that kill microorganisms (**-cidal**) are termed **bactericidal, fungicidal,** or **virucidal,** depending on the type of microorganism they affect. Chemicals that reduce or inhibit growth without eradicating the microorganisms are considered -**static** agents, such as **bacteriostatic** or **fungistatic.** Antiseptics and disinfectant solutions differ in their antimicrobial potency (bactericidal versus bacteriostatic), spectrum of activity, and duration of action. Some of these chemicals are nonselective in their antimicrobial action and have broad-spectrum activity. Formaldehyde, glutaraldehyde, and iodine-containing solutions, which are effective against bacteria, bacterial spores, fungi, viruses, and protozoa, are broad-spectrum agents. More selective chemicals, such as hexachlorophene and benzalkonium chloride, are primarily effective against gram-positive bacteria. Alcohol (40% to 70% ethyl alcohol solution) is bactericidal for vegetative forms of gram-positive and gram-negative bacteria, whereas benzalkonium chloride, cetylpyridinium chloride, and thimerosal may be more bacteriostatic. Examples of commonly used antiseptics and disinfectants are presented in Table 22-1.

Sterilization, the complete eradication of all microorganisms, may be achieved with disinfectants. It is not practical to steam-sterilize large areas, such as an entire operating room. It is often easier to disinfect the area by washing surfaces with a combination of disinfectant solutions (cold sterilization). Because microorganisms vary in their sensitivity to disinfectants, a combination or a sequence of disinfectant solutions usually is applied.

Surfaces, whether walls, fingernails, or open wounds, must be thoroughly cleaned before disinfectants or antiseptics are used. Organic matter (pus, mucus, or protein exudate), dirt, and other foreign material reduce the activity of the disinfectant or antiseptic by complexing (binding) the active ingredient (iodine, hexachlorophene, or formaldehyde) or by simply blocking penetration to an area of microbial activity. Dirt and organic matter can be removed first by washing with medicated soap or detergent. Depending on the nature of the surface to be treated, a combination of alcohol, phenols, or iodophors are then generously washed over the area. Some disinfectant combinations are incompatible; for example, quaternary ammonium compounds are inactivated by contact with soaps or cotton.

Under optimal conditions (that is, application of an appropriate concentration of chemical solutions to a particular surface for a specified length of time), even narrow-spectrum disinfectants may be effective in sterilizing a localized area. Bacterial spores are particularly difficult to destroy but may be eliminated by increasing the disinfectant-to-surface contact time. Various disinfectant-to-surface exposure times have been recommended, particularly before surgical procedures.

Table 22-1

Examples of Antiseptics and Disinfectants

Name (Trade Name)	Primary Antimicrobial Activity
*Alcohols**	
Ethanol, ethyl alcohol; isopropanol, isopropyl alcohol	Vegetative bacteria
*Aldehydes**	
Formaldehyde	Bacteria, spores, fungi, viruses
Glutaraldehyde (Cidex)	
*Biguanides**	
Chlorhexidine (Exidine skin cleanser, Hibiclens liquid)	Bacteria, spores, fungi, viruses
*Halogenated compounds**	
Iodine, tincture of iodine	
Sodium hypochlorite (Dakin's solution)	Bacteria, spores, fungi, viruses
Sodium hypochlorite mixture (Chlorpactin-XCB, Chlorpactin-WCS-90)	
Iodophors†	
Povidone-iodine (Betadine, Isodine)	Vegetative microorganisms and spores
Poloxamer-iodine (Prepodyne, Septodyne)	
Heavy metals†	
Nitromersol (mercurial) (Metaphen)	
Thimerosal (mercurial) (Merthiolate)	
Silver nitrate	Vegetative forms of bacteria and fungi
Silver protein (Argyrol)	
Silver sulfadiazine (Silvadene)	
Oxidizing agents	
Peroxide, hydrogen peroxide	Vegetative microorganisms
Phenols†	
Hexachlorophene (pHisoHex, Septisol)	Vegetative gram-positive bacteria
Triclosan/Irgasan (Septisoft, Septisol)	Vegetative gram-positive and gram-negative bacteriostatic
Quaternary ammonium compounds†	
Benzalkonium chloride (Benz-all, Zephiran)	Vegetative gram-positive bacteria
Cetylpyridinium chloride (Ceepryn, Cepacol)	

* Bactericidal.
† Bacteriostatic.
Note: Antiseptics in general and disinfectants in particular should never be swallowed or injected in order to destroy microorganisms.

These periods include a 2-minute wash with soap followed by a 2-minute alcohol wash followed by a 5- to 10-minute iodophor scrub. The particular ritual for surgical disinfection varies among individual institutions.

Even with an inherently low- or moderate-potency chemical, antimicrobial efficiency can be increased by combining the agent with alcohol. It is not unusual to find ethyl or isopropyl alcohol as an active vehicle for clorhexidine, benzalkonium chloride, hexachlorophene, or iodine. The term "active vehicle" means that the solution used to dissolve or dilute the antiseptic is capable of killing microorganisms by itself. Therefore, the activity of the active vehicle contributes to the overall germ-killing activity.

Main Uses

Microorganisms are ubiquitous and migrate freely on skin, hair, and furniture and in air currents. Given an optimal environment that supports colonization (growth), any microbe can produce an infection. An infectious process that is localized to the skin surface can frequently be treated without the use of systemic antibiotics, thus minimizing the risk of further infection.

A serious consequence of any infection, including one originally localized on the skin surface, is migration of the pathogenic microorganisms to the general circulation. At home, simple wounds and skin abrasions provide potential pathogens an access route to the circulation. In hospitals and other health care institutions, the risk of infection is complicated by the type of wound—**decubitus ulcer** (bedsore), trauma, or surgical—as well as the potential for contracting a nosocomial infection.

Nosocomial infections (hospital-acquired infections) develop while patients are in the hospital and are characteristically virulent and difficult to eradicate. Hospital-acquired infections may result from catheterizations (either urinary tract or intravenous therapy), which provide a pathway for microorganisms to enter the body. These infections develop during prolonged hospitalization or as a result of decreased patient resistance (such as high-risk, elderly, malnourished, burned, or immunosuppressed patients).

In this era of highly effective systemic antibiotics, antiseptics have limited application in the treatment of infections. Antiseptics and disinfectants are useful for reducing microbial growth and contamination, and thus reducing the risk of infection (especially wound infection) from exogenous sources. This is particularly important during surgical procedures, in which local infection could significantly delay wound (incision) healing as well as jeopardize the general patient health should a systemic infection develop.

Antiseptics are used to cleanse and **irrigate** wounds, cuts, and abrasions, to prepare (degerm) patients' skin before surgery or injection, and to prepare the surgical team before surgery. An ideal antiseptic would kill bacteria with a persistent duration of action and would not irritate or sensitize the skin, but it is impossible to sterilize the skin without damaging tissue. Therefore, the objectives of antiseptic treatment are to decrease the opportunity for bacteria to enter the body and to permit normal defense mechanisms to continue uninterrupted in the healing process. Table 22-2 lists examples of antiseptic use.

Iodine is probably superior to all other antiseptics for degerming the skin. Iodine is a rapid-acting, potent germicide effective against bacteria, protozoa, and viruses. Although much more effective than the aqueous solution, iodine tincture

Table 22-2
Indications for the Use of Antiseptics and Disinfectants

Chemical Name	Concentration	Disinfectant Use	Antiseptic Use
Alcohol, ethyl isopropyl	40–70% solution 70–90% solution	Disinfect instruments, ampules	Prepare skin before injection
Benzalkonium chloride	0.02–0.5% solutions	Preservation of instruments, ampules, rubber articles; disinfect operating room equipment	Preoperative treatment of denuded skin, mucous membranes; irrigation of deep wounds, vagina; topical treatment of acne; preservative in ophthalmic products
Chlorhexidine gluconate	1% solution 4% emulsion	—	Cleanse skin wounds, surgical scrub, hand washing, mouthwash for aphthous ulcers; keep out of ears and eyes
Formaldehyde	10–37% solution	Cold sterilization of equipment; tissue always fixative, preserve cadavers	Avoid contact with skin or mucous membranes; dilute 37% solution
Glutaraldehyde	2% solution	Cold sterilization of surgical instruments; fumigation (aerosol) of operating rooms	Use only on inanimate objects
Hexachlorophene	0.25–3% foam, soaps, lotions	—	Surgical scrub, skin cleanser; use with caution in infants and burned patients, where absorption can occur
Hydrogen peroxide	1.5–3% solution	—	Wound cleansing, mouthwash for Vincent's infection; excessive oral use causes hairy tongue

is associated with residual staining and local pain. The stinging sensation is principally related to the alcohol vehicle of the tincture (2% iodine in 50% ethanol). Iodine complexes (**iodophors**) cause less irritation and staining, and although they are only bacteriostatic, they are used frequently as surgical preps. In general, preparations containing iodine are for topical use and are not to be taken orally.

Ethyl alcohol is an effective antiseptic in concentrations of less than 70%, whereas isopropyl alcohol (rubbing alcohol) is bactericidal at all concentrations

Table 22-2 (continued)

Indications for the Use of Antiseptics and Disinfectants

Chemical Name	Concentration	Disinfectant Use	Antiseptic Use
Iodine	2% solution	—	Topical treatment of skin; germicide; stains skin and linens
Nitromersol	0.2% solution 0.5% tincture	Disinfect instruments	Topical treatment of skin abrasions, irrigate mucous membranes
Oxychlorosene calcium	0.5% solution	—	Preoperative skin cleanser, local irrigation during surgery, ophthalmic irrigant
Poloxamer-iodine	1–5% scrub, swab, solution	—	Preoperative skin preparation, cleanse wounds; less irritating than iodine
Povidone-iodine	0.5–10% foam, swab, douche, gel	Disinfect instruments	Preoperative scrub, postoperative antiseptic, often used for bedsores, burns, lacerations; skin preparation prior to injections and hyperalimentation line; whirlpool solution
Silver nitrate	0.1–0.5% solution	—	Treatment of conjunctiva, burned skin
Silver protein	5–25% solution	—	Topical treatment of inflammation of the eye, nose, or throat; prolonged use results in permanent discoloration of skin (argyria)
Silver sulfadiazine	1% cream	—	Topical treatment of wound sepsis in second- and third-degree burns
Sodium hypochlorite	4–6% solution 0.15–0.5% antiseptic	Disinfect walls, floors	Wound irrigation; avoid contact with hair (bleach)
Thimerosal	0.1% cream, ointment 0.02% ophthalmic	—	Preoperative skin preparation, antiseptic for eyes, nose, throat, urethral membranes, wounds; contraindicated in patients sensitive to mercury compounds

(50% to 90%). Alcohol can be used alone or in combination with other topical agents to degerm the skin before surgery or hypodermic injection. Alcohol preparations such as tinctures frequently increase the penetrability of additional antiseptic ingredients, which improves antiseptic efficiency but may lead to increased skin irritation. Most "prep" wipes or swabs contain isopropyl alcohol, which quickly evaporates following topical application. Because isopropyl alcohol causes local vasodilation, increased bleeding at the venipuncture site occasionally occurs. Either ethyl alcohol or isopropyl alcohol is appropriate to chemically disinfect vial tops or membranes on sterile containers before liquid or reconstituted medications are drawn into a syringe. In cases of pulmonary edema, ethyl alcohol diluted with normal saline can be administered through a nebulizer to reduce frothing in the airways.

Hexachlorophene is a bacteriostatic preparation that is primarily effective against gram-positive bacteria. Despite its selectivity, hexachlorophene is useful as a skin cleanser and surgical scrub because potential pathogens that reside on the skin surface are frequently gram-positive bacteria. With repeated use, hexachlorophene accumulates in the skin and maintains its bacterial response.

Hydrogen peroxide, an oxidizing agent, has limited usefulness because it does not penetrate well and rapidly breaks down to molecular oxygen and water. The standard medicinal solution is a weak antiseptic that contains 3% hydrogen peroxide in water. The effervescence may facilitate mechanical cleansing of debris surrounding a superficial wound. Hydrogen peroxide is recommended as a mouthwash for the treatment of Vincent's infection (trench mouth); however, continued use may produce hypertrophied papillae of the tongue, known as "hairy tongue." This effect subsides when treatment is discontinued. Chlorhexidine, a bactericidal surgical preparation, is also useful as a mouthwash for the treatment of aphthous ulcers and to decrease the amount of plaque deposited on teeth.

Among the heavy metal solutions currently available as antiseptics are organic mercurials and inorganic mercurials and inorganic silver complexes. Silver nitrate is commonly used as an ophthalmic antiseptic in newborns to reduce the risk of gonococcal infection. Gonococcal resistance to silver nitrate is unlikely to occur as it might if systemic antibiotics were used. Silver nitrate has also been used in the treatment of burn patients. However, it has been displaced by silver sulfadiazine, which penetrates the crust of burns better and does not produce residual skin staining. Other silver solutions will produce **argyria,** a permanent black discoloration of the skin and mucous membranes.

The bacteriostatic organic mercurials (nitromersol and thimerosal) are not as effective as are other available antiseptics, despite their popularity as over-the-counter first-aid preparations. Some antiseptics, notably benzalkonium chloride, thimerosal, and cetylpyridinium chloride, are also found in eye care and contact lens preparations as preservatives to reduce microflora growth.

Disinfectants are used to clean and store surgical instruments, to disinfect operating room walls and floors, and to sterilize (cold sterilization) objects that cannot tolerate the high temperatures associated with routine sterilization procedures. Common disinfectants include formaldehyde, glutaraldehyde, sodium hypochlorite, alcohol, and nitromersol (see Table 22-2). Certain solutions, such as formaldehyde and glutaraldehyde, are irritating to the skin, eyes, and respiratory tract at any concentration and should be used on inanimate surfaces only. Glutaraldehyde is a commonly used agent to cold sterilize respiratory care equipment and circuits.

Other Methods of Sterilization

Three methods of sterilization available for use with respiratory care equipment are steam sterilization, ethylene oxide sterilization, and plasma sterilization.

Steam sterilization has always been the gold standard (the best) and can be used for equipment that is heat stable. Steam sterilization utilizes moist heat that is also under pressure. Temperatures of 270°F, along with 30 pounds of pressure, are maintained for 4 minutes.

Many parts of respiratory care equipment are plastic or have plastic components. For these items, steam sterilization would destroy the integrity of the equipment. For most of these items, a special sterilizer is available that utilizes a gas called ethylene oxide. Ethylene oxide is a gas that is highly reactive and combines with cellular components to destroy the living cell. It is very toxic and is used in a diluted form for sterilization. In a concentrated form it can cause severe burns to the skin. When ethylene oxide is used for respiratory equipment, there must be an aeration period of 8 to 12 hours before the items can be handled.

A newer form of sterilization is plasma sterilization. The plasma state is the fourth stage of matter, with gas, solid, and liquid being the other three. It is generated by a strong electrical field through hydrogen peroxide and water. This process forms free radicals that, like ethylene oxide, are extremely reactive and combine with cellular components to destroy the living cell. Unlike ethylene oxide, the by-products of the reaction are nontoxic water and oxygen, and so no aeration is required. It is also a low-temperature procedure so it is safe for heat-sensitive equipment.

Adverse and Toxic Effects

The most common side effects associated with the topical use of disinfectants and antiseptics in general are dryness, irritation, rash, and **hypersensitivity** at the contacted surface. Formaldehyde cannot be used as an antiseptic because concentrations large enough to be antimicrobial will damage living tissue. Formaldehyde toxicity is usually limited to local irritation or allergic reaction. However, repeated topical exposure may result in eczematoid dermatitis. Similarly, with topical iodine preparations, individuals occasionally may develop a hypersensitivity reaction. Disinfectants that contain heavy metals such as mercury or zinc have been associated with local swelling and edema when applied to skin and mucous membranes. Iodophors have been reported to penetrate the **eschar** of burn patients, leading to increased absorption of iodine. Iodine toxicity can manifest as erosion of the GI tract or hypothyroidism. In cases of accidental iodine ingestion, sodium thiosulfate is the antidote of choice. It can also be used to remove iodine stains.

Antiseptics and certain disinfectants should not be taken orally. Some agents are toxic when taken internally or absorbed in significant amounts through the skin. Absorption of hexachlorophene via the skin has been reported to cause neurotoxicities, which may manifest as convulsions and can be fatal. Hexachlorophene use should not be prolonged with patients predisposed to absorb the compound through the skin, such as premature infants or burn patients. When taken orally, hexachlorophene can produce anorexia, vomiting, abdominal cramps, convulsions, and death. Although ethanol is a constituent of alcoholic beverages, ingestion of pure ethyl alcohol (99%) can be fatal. Ethyl alcohol and isopropyl alcohol antiseptics are not for consumption because these products contain denaturing agents, methylisobutylketone, and color additives that are poisonous.

Sodium hypochlorite used as a wound irrigant may dissolve blood clots and delay further clotting. In concentrations greater than 0.5% (modified Dakin's solution), sodium hypochlorite may be irritating to the skin.

The protocol for disinfecting large respiratory equipment (not hand-held devices) encountered in the hospital varies with the institution. Machines such as compressors or ventilators are equipped with disposable connectors, tubing, or masks that reduce (or eliminate) the need for sterilization between uses. With the increased dependence on outpatient and home care treatment, however, respiratory care patients must be educated about the care and cleaning of their drug delivery systems (reservoirs and spacers) in order to reduce the potential for infection. Such patient education and instruction is the responsibility of the respiratory care practitioner.

When the patient exhales into a nebulizer or aerosolizer, microorganisms are deposited on the plastic surfaces. The droplets of moisture and microscopic organic matter in the breath provide a perfect medium for bacterial growth. If equipment is not cleaned thoroughly after each use, patients are liable to reinfect themselves with a pathogenic microorganism as they inhale through the contaminated spacer or reservoir. Depending on the age and condition of the patient, reinfection in the respiratory patient may require more than outpatient antibiotic therapy to eradicate the infection. Often, the compromised elderly patient may need to be hospitalized for a complete pulmonary evaluation.

Patients should be reminded to wash their hands before handling their nebulizer and medication. Nebulizers, spacers, and other small parts should be cleaned at least once a day to maintain good bronchial hygiene. The mouthpiece or mask should be separated from the nebulizer before the nebulizer is disassembled. All parts should be washed in a solution of mild dishwashing detergent and thoroughly rinsed under warm running water. Excess water should be removed to avoid microbial growth in the residual fluid. All parts should be soaked in a white vinegar (acetic acid) solution (1 cup of white vinegar to 3 cups of warm water) for 30 to 40 minutes. All parts must be completely submerged in the soaking solution to achieve adequate disinfection. All parts should be completely air dried before being stored or used for another treatment. The patient should be instructed to keep the compressor clean and dust-free, and to check the inlet filter and replace it periodically according to manufacturer recommended instructions.

Chapter 22 Review

UNDERSTANDING TERMINOLOGY

Match the definition or description in the left column with the appropriate term in the right column.

1. Includes responses such as a rash, edema, or anaphylaxis that develop following administration of certain drugs.
2. Compound that contains iodine.
3. A permanent darkening of skin and mucous membranes caused by prolonged use of silver protein solutions.
4. A process that kills all microorganisms.
5. The destruction of bacterial protein function.
6. A scab that develops after skin is burned.

a. argyria
b. denaturing
c. eschar
d. hypersensitivity
e. iodophor
f. sterilization

Test your understanding of the material in this chapter by answering the following questions.

7. Explain the difference between an antiseptic and a disinfectant.
8. Differentiate between a **-static** and a **-cidal** solution.

ACQUIRING KNOWLEDGE

Answer the following questions.

9. How are disinfectants and antiseptics similar in their clinical uses?
10. How do antiseptics differ from antibiotics?
11. What is cold sterilization?
12. What are nosocomial infections?
13. What are two objectives of antiseptic treatment?
14. Why aren't antiseptics given parenterally or by mouth?
15. Why is silver nitrate frequently used for newborns?
16. Why is alcohol frequently a vehicle for other antiseptics such as benzalkonium chloride?

Additional Reading

Gardiner A. Knowledge of disinfection. *Nurs Times* 1995;91(20):59.

Gould D. The significance of hand drying in the prevention of infection. *Nurs Times* 1994;90(47):33.

Kahatib M. Hand washing and the use of gloves while managing patients receiving mechanical ventilation in the ICU. *Chest* 1999;116(1):172.

McLaughlin A. *Infection Control in Respiratory Care,* 2d ed. Gaithersburg, MD: Aspen, 1996.

Wicks J. Handle with care, aldehyde disinfectants. *Nurs Times* 1994;90(12):67.

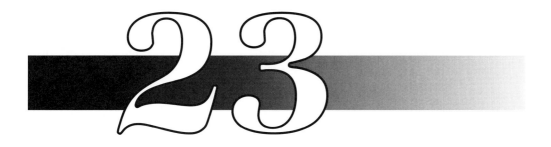

Herbal Remedies for Respiratory Diseases

Ellen Feingold, MD, MPH

Chapter Objectives

After studying this chapter, you should be able to:

- Learn how to use several different, commonly used herbs for the prevention of respiratory diseases.
- Learn the author's method for prevention of viral upper respiratory infections.
- Learn general, good-sense rules when using or recommending herbal remedies.
- Learn advantages of herbal remedies over prescription drugs.

Introduction

Early in the 21st century, we are finding that therapeutic options formally considered "alternative," "complementary," or "unconventional" are becoming mainstream, if not thoroughly conventional. This is a reflection of the popularity of these forms of therapy among patients and their families, if not yet among medical and surgical physicians.

Herbal medicine, as a therapeutic modality, is leading the slow but steady integration between alternative and orthodox medicine. This is because herbal medicine is the most commonly used form of alternative medicine. Sales of herbal remedies in the United States for 1998 reached more than $450 million.

Their popularity is probably a result of four factors: (1) their overall effectiveness, coupled with (2) a perceived gentleness of action, (3) availability without prescription by a health care provider so that self-care is a prominent feature, and (4) moderate pricing in most instances.

Herbal medicines can have side effects as well as drug interactions. They have the potential to harm as well as to help, just as conventional, prescription medicines do; and if we are to use them safely, we must learn their profiles, just as we do other drugs we prescribe for sick people.

Herbal medicines are composed of phytochemicals, pharmacologically active chemicals that are derived from plants, that are used to treat or prevent disease. They often produce a strong effect on bodily tissues and organs. Nonetheless, herbal remedies are labeled as supplements and therefore are not controlled by the Food and Drug Administration (FDA) as long as the manufacturer does not claim that the herb cures any condition. This noncontrol by the FDA also means that the quality and potency of the herbal product actually inside the capsule can and do vary greatly among manufacturers. Not only that, but herbal remedies may be sold without proof of safety and/or efficacy!

Consequently, the consumer, along with the health care practitioner, must learn to rely on his or her own knowledge of safety and efficacy for herbal remedies. The best advice is to purchase herbal remedies from manufacturers that follow the food-processing standards, called Food Good Manufacturing Practices (Food GMPs), or the even higher drug-manufacturing standards, called Drug GMPs.

Some General, Good-Sense Rules to Use When Using or Recommending Herbal Remedies

1. Do not use or recommend any herbal remedies for any purpose if the patient is pregnant or lactating unless prescribed by a herbalist or other health care practitioner.

2. Do not mix herbal remedies with each other or with prescription drugs unless so advised by a herbalist or other health care practitioner.

3. Do disclose which herbal remedies you are taking to your health care practitioner and, more especially, to the surgeon and anesthesiologist. Some herbal remedies should be discontinued 2 weeks before surgery. Some herbal remedies have chemical interactions with commonly prescribed drugs.

4. Develop the same cautionary approach to herbal remedies that you are accustomed to using with prescription medications. Use caution recommending herbal remedies for infants and the elderly.

Some of the Advantages of Using Herbal Remedies Instead of Prescription Drugs

1. When the patient chooses his or her own remedy to treat a disease or symptom(s), the patient chooses the herb, its formulation, dosage, and price. This is called self-care and is often a satisfying experience for the patient.

2. Herbal remedies are often gentler in action than the prescription drug that would be indicated for that same condition. For example, consider St. John's Wort used for mild to moderate depression, in contrast to one of the selective serotonin reuptake inhibitors (SSRIs), such as Prozac.

3. Herbal remedies are sometimes available to treat chronic, relapsing conditions for which no prescription drug exists. For example, consider the use of ginseng for physical or emotional exhaustion.

4. Herbal remedies are often used to prevent the onset of a condition, especially if used at the very first symptoms. For example, echinacea can prevent viral upper respiratory infections (URIs) and influenza if taken at the first sign of a cold or sore throat. Echinacea works even better in combination with goldenseal to prevent URIs.

5. In **my** experience, using a **combination** of homeopathy and herbal remedies is the best therapy for such chronic conditions as asthma, chronic fatigue syndrome, obesity, eating disorders, depression, anxiety, social phobia, panic attacks, and chronic, debilitating headaches.

However, most serious **respiratory diseases** are best treated by prescription medications under the supervision of a medical doctor. These conditions include pneumonia, tuberculosis, *Pneumocystis carinii*, cystic fibrosis, bronchiectasis, respiratory failure from any cause, cancer, and other life-threatening infections and conditions.

The herbal remedies included in Tables 23-1 through 23-4 are only those herbs that are easily obtained in health food stores. The tables do not include Ayurvedic herbal remedies, traditional Chinese medicine herbs, South American herbs, or Native American herbs. For descriptions of these herbal remedies, see Earl Mindell's *New Herb Bible*.

Table 23-1
Herbal Remedies for Prevention of Respiratory Diseases

Common Name	Botanic Name	Actions	Indications
Astragalus	Astragalus membranaceous (huang-qi)	Inhibits replication of viral particles; stimulates the immune system	Viral infections in respiratory and other systems; immune depression
Bee propolis		Stimulates immune system; antimicrobial	Gum and mouth infections
Cat's claw	Uncaria tomentosa (una de gato)	Stimulates immune system; antiinflammatory	HIV
Echinacea	Echinacea purpurea (purple coneflower)	Stimulates immune system; antiviral; antibacterial	Viral URIs, bronchitis, influenza
Garlic	Allium sativum	Antimicrobial; antimycotic	Viral URIs, bronchitis
Goldenseal	Hydrastis canadensis	Antiinflammatory	Viral URIs, bronchitis, influenza
Grapeseed extract	Vitis vinifera	Antiinflammatory; enhances action of vitamin C; proanthocyanidins have antioxidant properties	Infections of respiratory tract
Green tea	Camellia sinensis	Flavonoids may have anticancer properties	May have preventive effect on cancers of the respiratory tract
Olive leaf extract	Olea europaea	Enhances immune system	Viral infections; influenza
Yarrow	Achillea millefolium	Antiinflammatory	Viral URIs, influenza

Note: Table 23-1 includes herbal remedies that have some medically demonstrable **preventive** effect on respiratory diseases and conditions. Certain of the herbs have preventive effects on other conditions, for example, cancer, but these effects are not included. Therefore, the table is not all-inclusive but, instead, limited specifically to respiratory diseases and conditions.

The most efficacious preparation to prevent viral upper respiratory illnesses in the author's experience is to use a combination of echinacea and goldenseal, totaling approximately 450 to 500 mg per capsule. Take three of these capsules at the very first symptom of becoming ill. Taking the first dose at the very first symptom of illness

Table 23-1 (continued)

Herbal Remedies for Prevention of Respiratory Diseases

Side Effects	Cautions/Interactions	Dosage/Forms
None	Do not use in cancer, transplant, or autoimmune patients unless prescribed by a herbalist	400-mg capsules TID
None	None	250-mg capsules once a day; skin creams; salve for gums; lozenges for first sign of cold
May reduce estrogen and progesterone levels	Contraindicated in pregnancy, lactation	500-mg capsules TID
Hypersensitivity	Do not use with cyclosporine or other antirejection drugs or during cancer chemotherapy or with multiple sclerosis, collagen diseases, AIDS, or TB	250-mg capsules TID or QID; do not use more than 6–8 weeks consecutively
Allergic reactions, headache, fatigue, gastrointestinal complaints; risk of postoperative bleeding	Do not use during lactation nor in conjunction with anticoagulants	Odorless capsules, 1 capsule TID
Raises blood pressure	Do not use in pregnancy; do not use in G6PD deficiency, hypertension	250–500-mg capsule TID; do not use more than 2 weeks consecutively
None	None	Daily dosage 150–600 mg
If decaffeinated, none	Pregnant and nursing mothers should use decaffeinated green tea	About 3 cups of tea per day
None	Not for use in persons with gallstones	500-mg tablet once daily
None	Contact dermatitis; do not use in pregnancy	Prepare tea with 1 cup dried herb in 6 cups water and drink half cup every hour

is absolutely essential. Repeat the three capsules in 2 to 3 hours if that very first symptom is still present; otherwise, do not repeat. You may repeat taking the three capsules every 2 to 3 hours for a total of four times the first day. You may continue with two capsules three times a day for the second day if the symptoms of illness persist; otherwise, simply discontinue. Do not take the echinacea and goldenseal combination for more than 2 weeks consecutively.

Table 23-2

Herbal Remedies for Relief of Cough, Cold, and Flu Symptoms

Common Name	Botanic Name	Actions	Indications
Elderberry	Sambucus nigra (European elder)	Antiviral	Cold, cough, bronchitis, flu
Ephedra	Ephedra sinica (Ma-Huang)	Decongestant	This herb is **not recommended** because it has many toxic side effects and contraindications. There have been reports of lethal poisonings with arrhythmia, hyperpyrexia, and shock.
Eucalyptus	Eucalyptus globulus	Expectorant, secretolytic	Cough, bronchitis, asthma, flu, whooping cough
Horseradish	Armoracia rusticana	Antimicrobial	Cough, bronchitis, influenza
Hyssop	Hyssopus officinalis	Antimicrobial, antiviral	Colds, coughs
Iceland moss	Cetraria islandica	Decongestant, demulcent	Cough, bronchitis, stomatitis, pharyngitis, whooping cough
Onion	Allium cepa	Antimicrobial	Cough, bronchitis, cold, asthma
Oregano	Origanum vulgare	Antimicrobial	Cough, bronchitis, colds, flu
Siberian ginseng	Eleutherococcus senticosus	Stimulates immune system, antiviral	Colds, bronchitis, chronic lung problems (tonic)
Yerba santa	Eriodictyon californicum	Decongestant	Asthma, cough

Note: Table 23-2 includes herbal remedies that have antiviral effects on coughs, colds, asthma, and influenza, although they may have other effects as well.

Table 23-2 (continued)
Herbal Remedies for Relief of Cough, Cold, and Flu Symptoms

Side Effects	Cautions/Interactions	Dosage/Forms
None	None	300-mg capsules BID

This herb is **not recommended** for any use.

Side Effects	Cautions/Interactions	Dosage/Forms
Nausea, vomiting, diarrhea; do not take internally with biliary, gastrointestinal, or liver disease	Do not apply the oil to face	Preparations for steam inhalation; cough drops
None	Not for use with ulcers or kidney disease because of irritation of mucous membranes	Take grated root with warm water (strong but effective!)
None	Not for use in pregnancy	Tea from dried herb TID
None	None	Daily dosage 4–6 g dry herb
None	Not recommended for lactating mothers	Prepare fresh onion juice in blender, 1 tsp juice TID or QID
None	None	Cup tea TID or QID
None	Not recommended for persons with hypertension	400–650 mg capsules once daily
None	None	Tea from 1 tbl dry herb in 1 cup water daily

Table 23-3

Herbal Remedies Acting as Expectorants

Common Name	Botanic Name	Indications
Anise	Pimpinella anisum	Common cold, cough, bronchitis, stomatitis, pharyngitis, whooping cough
Bayberry bark	Myrica certifera (southern bayberry)	Coughs, colds
Fennel	Foeniculum vulgare	Cough, bronchitis, colds
Gotu kola	Centella asiatica	Colds, asthma
Horehound	Marrubium vulgare	Cough, colds
Horseradish	Armoracia lapathifolia	Cough, colds
Licorice	Glycyrrhiza glabra	Cough, bronchitis, sore throat, hoarseness
Lungwort	Pulmonaria officinalis	Cough, bronchitis
Marshmallow	Althea officinalis	Cough, bronchitis
Mullein	Verbascum densiflorum	Cough, bronchitis
Parsley	Petroselinum crispum	Cough, cold
Peppermint oil	Mentha piperita	Cough, cold, bronchitis
Pleurisy root	Asclepias tuberosa	Cough, pleurisy, pneumonia
Red clover	Trifolium pratense	Cough, whooping cough

Note: Table 23-3 includes herbal remedies that act as expectorants, although they may have other effects as well.

Table 23-3 (continued)

Herbal Remedies Acting as Expectorants

Side Effects	Cautions/Interactions	Dosage Forms
None	Contraindicated in patients with allergy to anise and anethole	Drink 1 cup tea BID or inhale essential oil
None; at high doses induces vomiting	None	450-mg capsule TID
None	Rare allergic reactions	Tea taken TID or QID
None	Allergic contact dermatitis	400-mg capsule TID
None	Do not use in pregnancy	10–40 drops of extract in water TID
None	Not for use with ulcers or kidney disease because of irritation of mucous membranes	Take grated root with warm water (strong but effective!)
Hypokalemia, hypernatremia, edema, hypertension	Do not use for more than 6 weeks; do not use with liver or kidney disease; do not use in pregnancy	200-mg capsule TID; for hoarseness, use tea
None	None	Tea made from 1 tbl dried herb daily
None	None	450 mg capsule TID
None	None	3–4 g dry herb as tea daily
Rare contact allergies	Not for use in pregnancy, kidney ailments	Tea from fresh herb, BID or TID
None	Do not apply to infant's face	3–4 drops for inhalation BID; chest rub 5–15 drops BID to QID
None	Not to be used during pregnancy	Tea made from 1 tbl dried herb in cup, daily
None	Not to be used during pregnancy	Tea made from 1 tbl dried herb up to TID

Table 23-4

Herbal Remedies for Relief of Sore Throats and Mouth Ulcers

Common Name	Botanic Name	Actions	Preparation
Bayberry bark	Myrica certifera (southern bayberry)	Soothing to mucous membranes	Mouthwash
Elderberry	Sambucus nigra (European elder)	Soothing to mucous membranes	Mouthwash
Horehound	Marrubium vulgare	Soothing to mucous membranes	Lozenge
Hyssop	Hyssopus officinalis	Antimicrobial, antiviral	Gargle, mouthwash
Lemon balm	Melissa officinalis	Treatment for herpes simplex	Cream
Licorice	Glycyrrhiza glabra	Treatment for hoarseness	Tea
Myrrh	Commiphora myrrha	Soothing to mucous membranes	Mouthwash
Raspberry leaves	Rubus idaeus	Soothing to mucous membranes	Tea
Sage	Salvia officinalis	Soothing to sore or bleeding gums	Gargle
Slippery elm bark	Ulmus rubra	Soothing coating	Lozenge
Thyme	Thymus vulgaris	Disinfectant	Gargle

Note: Table 23-4 includes herbal remedies that act to soothe inflamed mucous membranes of the mouth and pharynx, although they may have other effects as well.

Table 23-4 (continued)
Herbal Remedies for Relief of Sore Throats and Mouth Ulcers

Side Effects	Cautions/Interactions	Dosage Forms
None	None	
None	None	
None	Do not use in pregnancy	
None	Not for use in pregnancy	
None	None	
Hypokalemia, hypernatremia, edema, hypertension	Do not use for more than 6 weeks; do not use with liver or kidney disease; do not use in pregnancy	For hoarseness, use tea TID or QID
None	Do not use in pregnancy	2–5 drops extract in water BID or TID
None	None	Tea from 1 tbl dried herb daily
None	Not for use in pregnancy	Tea from 1 tbl dried herb daily
None	None	1 lozenge TID
None	None	Tea from 1 tbl dried herb; use as gargle or drink tea

Additional Reading

Barrett B, Kiefer D, Rabago D. Assessing the risks and benefits of herbal medicine: An overview of scientific evidence. *Alt Ther* 1999;5:40–50.

Blumenthal M, ed. *The Complete German Commission E Monographs Therapeutic Guide to Herbal Medicines.* Boston: Integrative Medicine Communication, 1998;685.

Grieve M. *A Modern Herbal.* New York: Dorset Press, 1994;912.

Gruenwald G, Brendler T, Jaenicke C, eds. *PDR for Herbal Medicines,* 2d ed. Montvale, NJ: Medical Economics Company, 2000;858.

Kemper KJ. Seven herbs every pediatrician should know. *Contemp Pediatr* 1996;13:79–90.

Mindell E. *New Herb Bible.* New York: Fireside, 2000;317.

Ody P. *The Complete Medicinal Herbal.* London: Dorling Kindersley, 1996;192.

O'Hara MA, Kiefer D, Farrell K, Kemper K. A review of 12 commonly used medicinal herbs. *Arch Fam Med* 1998;7:523–536.

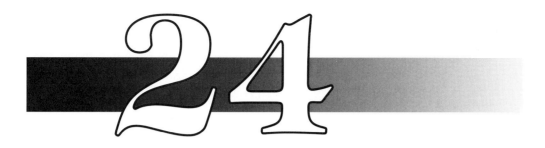

Antiviral Drugs

Henry Hitner, PhD
Barbara Nagle, PhD

Chapter Focus

This chapter describes drugs that inhibit the growth of a variety of viruses that cause infection.

Chapter Terminology

acquired immunity: Protection from viral reinfection in the form of antibodies.

acquired immunodeficiency syndrome (AIDS): Viral-induced disease characterized by multiple opportunistic infections as a result of depleted lymphocytes involved in the cell-mediated immune process.

antigen drift and antigen shift: The ability of viruses to change the composition or structure of their surface proteins (viral coat) responsible for producing disease (pathogenicity).

HIV: Human immunodeficiency virus, responsible for producing AIDS.

immunity: Condition that causes individuals to resist acquiring or developing a disease or infection.

immunosuppressed: Having inhibition of the body's immune response (ability to fight infection), usually induced by drugs or viruses.

opportunistic organism: Microorganism capable of causing disease only when the resistance (immunocompetence) of the host is impaired.

Reye syndrome: A potentially fatal illness characterized by vomiting, an enlarged liver, convulsions, and coma in children and adolescents, linked to the use of salicylates in the management of influenza, usually type B, or chickenpox.
thrush: Candidal infection of the oral mucosa.

Chapter Objectives

After studying this chapter, you should be able to:

- Describe two different treatment options that are effective against influenza.
- Describe the mechanism of action of drugs effective against viral infections, especially drugs used in the treatment of influenza.
- Explain how the treatment of viral infection is different from treatment that kills microorganisms such as bacteria.
- List three side effects associated with antiviral drugs.

Viral Diseases and Antiviral Drugs

INFLUENZA

Flu viruses (such as Asian influenza) primarily affect the upper (nasal passages and pharynx) and lower (lungs) respiratory tract. The virus is spread in the aerosolized droplets from a sneeze or cough of an infected person. The inoculated droplets are inhaled directly or transmitted by contact with the uninfected person who inadvertently delivers the virus into the mouth or respiratory tract (as by sucking on contaminated pencils, pens, and fingers). Influenza is a family of viruses categorized as types A, B, and C. Influenza A and B infect humans, although the alternate host for type A is often birds, such as chickens, or pigs before human inoculation. Influenza outbreaks occur every year in the Northern Hemisphere between November and April (and May to October in the Southern Hemisphere) coincident with the winter season. A localized wave of infection confirmed as a high incidence (20%) in the general population is considered an epidemic. Influenza A epidemics typically begin suddenly, last for several months as the wave of infection spreads throughout the population, and end as abruptly as they began. In contrast, influenza B is less severe and more localized, often occurring in schools and nursing homes. When an outbreak of influenza occurs worldwide, it is considered to be "pandemic." Pandemics, like the influenza outbreak of 1918 that killed 675,000 Americans alone (more than in all the wars of the 20th century), are facilitated by global travel but, fortunately, occur over a greater cycle of 15 to 20 years. (Go to the Internet, **www.pbs.org/wgbh/amex/influenza/maps,** for a fantastic presentation on the epidemiology of the influenza pandemic.)

Clinical Profile In the general population (relatively healthy individuals), flu viruses usually produce headache, fever, intense fatigue, dry cough, muscle ache, and sensitivity of the eyes to light. The reaction to viral infection is usually mild or moderate, with symptom onset within 24 to 72 hours of incubation and resolution after a short period of infection of 7 to 14 days. Flu and its accompanying symptoms are not the same as the constellation of symptoms that occur from "cold" viruses (rhinoviruses). As shown in Table 24-1, the clinical profile of the common cold differs from flu in that a cold develops gradually, over days, characterized by nasal secretion (rhinorrhea), congestion, and sneezing. Fever and muscle and joint aches are usually not associated with a cold.

The problem with flu, especially in children and elderly patients, is that secondary complications may occur, such as bacterial infections, otitis media, or bronchitis, that prolong the duration of illness in spite of treatment. Moreover, in the elderly and chronically ill, the same flu viruses may produce a more difficult or more intense infection such as pneumonia. Because the immune systems of these patients are often less competent to fight the infection, severe reactions such as dehydration, convulsions, and death may occur.

Virus Exposure and Immunity Many viral diseases such as chickenpox, measles, and mumps occur during childhood. Usually, these diseases occur only once because antibodies are produced against viral antigens that protect individuals from reinfection. This protection is referred to as **acquired immunity. Immunity** also may be acquired without experiencing the disease through vaccination. For example, with viruses such as smallpox and polio, vaccination exposes individuals to a weakened (attenuated) virus, which stimulates antibody production without producing the full spectrum of disease symptoms.

Influenza Vaccine A vaccine is available for influenza. The influenza vaccine is formulated each year to produce flu within the population for the following win-

Table 24-1

Characteristics of Infection: Influenza versus the Common Cold

Characteristic Symptom	Influenza	Common Cold
Sudden onset of symptoms	Yes	No
Headache	Prominent	Mild or absent
Myalgia or arthralgia	Prominent	Mild or absent
Fatigue	Prominent	Uncommon
Fever (>100.5°F)	Yes	Uncommon
Chills	Yes	Uncommon
Cough (nonproductive)	Common	Uncommon
Rhinorrhea, nasal congestion, sneezing	Uncommon	Prominent
Sore throat	Yes	Yes

ter. The viruses are grown in highly purified chicken eggs. Usually, three strains of virus are included in the vaccine, two type A and one type B. To be optimally effective, vaccinations are given in the United States between October and mid-November. Following a single-dose intramuscular injection, antibody production is initiated and continues over a 2-week period, just in time for the onset of the flu season. The immunity conferred by the antibody response is only effective for the strains contained in the vaccine. Occasionally, despite vaccination, the population succumbs to the wave of influenza or suffers a more severe course than expected. This may occur because a strain of virus (in the wild) has changed its antigentic nature during the year when the vaccine was in production. As a result the antibodies produced from the vaccination no longer recognize the wild virus on infection.

Despite the variability in effectiveness, vaccination is recommended by the Centers for Disease Control for persons over 6 months of age who are at high risk for complications from the flu or who are in a position to transmit the virus to high-risk patients (such as health care providers or household members). High-risk persons include those over 65 years of age, frail elderly, residents of nursing homes or long-term care facilities, and adults and children who have chronic pulmonary (asthma, COPD) or cardiovascular disorders or who are immunosuppressed, have HIV, and/or require hospitalization. Other high-risk groups include women who would be in the second or third trimester of pregnancy during the flu season and children who require long-term aspirin (salicylates) therapy and are at risk for **Reye's syndrome.**

Vaccination in healthy young adults is up to 90% effective in preventing or minimizing the clinical symptoms of flu. Vaccination is recommended for healthy individuals to minimize the incidence of febrile upper respiratory tract illness and to reduce the economic burden from days of lost work and wages, lost productivity, and visits to health care providers.

The most common adverse reaction to vaccination is soreness at the injection site; however, mild fever and myalgia may also occur. Although hypersensitivity reactions such as hives or systemic anaphylaxis are rare, the influenza vaccine should never be given to persons with a history of allergy to eggs.

Resistance to Antiviral Therapy   Resistance (vaccine ineffectiveness) occurs with influenza, primarily with influenza type A. During the replication process the virus is able to make subtle changes in its surface proteins so that antibodies specific to its former biochemistry cannot completely recognize the virus in order to inactivate it. Small changes in viral surface proteins are known as **antigenic drift** and result in decreased vaccine effectiveness. When the virus undergoes a major change in its surface proteins such as hemagglutinin and neuraminidase, it is considered an **antigenic shift.** This could obliterate antibody recognition and has been shown to reduce antiviral drug effectiveness of the neuraminidase inhibitors in laboratory experiments.

RESPIRATORY SYNCYTIAL VIRUS

Respiratory syncytial virus (RSV) infects more than 95% of children by the age of 2 years. It also reinfects more than 50% of children each year. RSV accounts for the majority of cases of severe bronchitis and pneumonia in infants and children. Severe cases of RSV result in hospitalization of fewer than 2% of children. Although that number may seem small, this is a tremendous national medical expense. Risk factors for severe RSV infections include:

1. Prematurity (gestational age <35 weeks at birth)
2. Chronic lung disease such as bronchopulmonary dysplasia
3. Congenital heart disease
4. Body weight <5 kg

Prevention has been the primary approach to controlling RSV infections. In the mid-1990s, a RSV immune globulin, Respigam, was marketed to prevent RSV infections and thereby prevent hospitalizations. This preparation was a product of pooled blood and was sometimes difficult to obtain because of a shortage in blood supply. The antibodies in the immune globulin provided passive immunity transferred from others to the child. Antibodies in the immune globulin would fight against the respiratory syncytial virus. It was administered as an IV infusion, over several hours, usually in a hospital setting. The hospital setting provided establishment of an IV line for infusion and a means of monitoring adverse effects. These adverse effects included fever, chills, and on rare occasions anaphylaxis. Although this was an expensive treatment, it was believed to be cost effective in preventing hospitalization. As a means of controlling the cost to healthcare, the immune globulin was limited to the risk groups listed above. It was administered monthly during the first and perhaps the second RSV season of the child's life. The RSV season runs from winter to early spring.

In the late 1990s the same company that brought Respigam to market marketed a monoclonal antibody, known as palivizumab (Synagis). This is a combination of both human and mouse antibodies that bind with proteins on the virus and prevent it from fusing with the host cells, preventing entry. This preparation, which has a higher cost, provided a medication that could be given IM and could be administered in a doctor's office. Palivizumab reduces the rate of severe RSV infection in high-risk infants. It has resulted in a 55% decrease in hospitalization rate. In addition to reducing the rate of hospitalization, it reduces the duration of hospital stay of those admitted versus those who have not received any treatment. The adverse effects of palivizumab are mostly minor. They include fever, irritability, and redness at the injection site. A 6-month treatment, during RSV season, costs approximately $7,000.

Neither of the two medications used for prophylaxis of RSV is effective as a treatment of existing RSV infection. Ribavirin is the only antiviral that has been used in the treatment of pediatric RSV infections. It is converted to a compound that inhibits certain viral enzymes involved in producing viral DNA and RNA. It works on messenger RNA produced by the virus. Ribavirin is administered by inhalation through a special type of aerosol generator, known as a SPAG-2 unit. The use of ribavirin for the treatment of RSV is controversial, based on its efficacy and expense. A 7-day course can cost the patient $10,000.

Ribavirin has a number of adverse effects. Respiratory function worsening has occurred, sometimes suddenly during ribavirin inhalation therapy in infants with RSV. It has also been associated with apnea and physical dependence on assisted respiration. Other respiratory problems include bronchospasm, pulmonary edema, hypoventilation, cyanosis, difficulty breathing, bacterial pneumonia, and pneumothorax. There are also adverse cardiovascular effects including cardiac arrest, hypotension, decreased heart rate, and arrhythmias.

Adverse effects to health care workers are also a concern. Although there is little definitive information on long-term effects, based on animal evidence of ribavirin, many recommend that pregnant women and possibly those women who may become pregnant should avoid exposure to ribavirin.

Frequent adverse effects have been reported in respiratory care practitioners who administered ribavirin to patients, including eye irritation and headache. These were usually mild and reversible after discontinuing exposure. Other effects include nasal or throat irritation, pharyngitis, tearing, nausea, dizziness, fatigue, rash, bronchospasm, chest pain, and nasal congestion. Contact lenses should not be worn while administering ribavirin aerosol because they may increase the likelihood of eye irritation and conjunctivitis should the drug leak around the protective goggles and precipitate on the lenses. Patient's visitors should also be advised on the risks of ribavirin therapy.

Respiratory care practitioners must consider a number of important points regarding the correct method of administering ribavirin therapy. Ribavirin must be administered extremely cautiously to patients requiring ventilatory assistance because the drug may precipitate in the ventilatory apparatus. Adverse reactions in patients include worsening respiratory status, bacterial pneumonia, apnea, pneumothorax, and ventilator dependency. Administration of the drug should be, whenever possible, in a room with negative-pressure ventilation. Caregivers must wear gowns, masks, gloves, and eye protection during administration of the drug.

Also, the flowmeter should be turned off when mist tent, oxyhood, or aerosol appliances are opened. Any equipment modification for administration of ribavirin to patients on ventilators must be in accordance with the manufacturer's recommendations.

The dose of ribavirin is 600 mg placed in a total volume of 300 mL of sterile water. If there is any drug left in the reservoir after 24 hours, it should be discarded.

HERPES

The family of herpes viruses includes herpes simplex (types 1 and 2) and herpes (varicella) zoster. Herpes simplex type 1 is responsible for producing innocuous though unpleasant skin lesions known as fever blisters, yet the same virus can produce encephalitis and severe changes in the eye that can lead to blindness (keratitis and corneal scarring). Herpes simplex type 2 is associated with adult genital infections and neonatal (generalized) infections, and herpes zoster causes inflammation of nerve roots resulting in severe pain. Herpes zoster (the same virus that causes chickenpox) produces lesions on the skin surface in adults known as "shingles." All of these viral diseases are characterized by their high incidence of recurrence either through seasonal exposure (flu) or because the virus remains within human tissue for years (herpes zoster). Although the elderly and immunocompromised patients may die from complications associated with the flu, most people who have been exposed to flu or herpes viruses survive seasonal attacks because the clinical symptoms are usually self-limiting. However, *this is not the case with HIV.*

AIDS

Incidence of Infection   Today, one of the most notorious virus-induced diseases is **acquired immunodeficiency syndrome (AIDS).** AIDS is caused by the **human immunodeficiency virus (HIV).** The spread of this disease is still escalating worldwide, and more than 50,000 new infections occur in the United States each year. HIV/AIDS is the leading cause of death among young adults in the United States, and the virus is reaching younger people each year. More than 80% of all people who developed AIDS have died within 10 years of diagnosis. As of 1995, one in four new infections occur in someone under 21 years of age. The incidence among men has declined slightly since HIV was first identified in 1981; however, the incidence in women continues to escalate. The virus is transmitted through sexual contact, perinatally from an infected mother to the neonate, through infected blood during transfusion, or through injection into the blood due to IV drug use. Among all AIDS cases in women in the United States, almost half are from nonmedicinal IV drug use. Fortunately, measures to protect against blood bank contamination have succeeded in virtually eliminating this route of infection. Although the route of transmission varies among communities, more than 95% of HIV infection today occurs through sexual contact and/or needle-borne infection.

Clinical Profile   After exposure to the virus a person may test HIV-positive. This only indicates that the person was infected by the virus at some time. It does not give any indication what the virus is currently doing. The typical course of infection has an acute clinical illness that varies in severity, followed by a prolonged period of clinical latency. Hence, the infected individual may go for years (3 to 10 years) without signs or symptoms associated with active infection. During the clinical latency period, the virus is active within the host preparing conditions for the onset of AIDS. Finally, patients develop opportunistic infections or cancers that manifest a constellation of clinical symptoms announcing the progression to AIDS. Only 5% to 10% of HIV-infected people remain asymptomatic 10 years after the initial infection.

HIV and Immune System Competence   Human immunodeficiency virus has made a significant negative impact on the health of young adults because there is no acquired immunity or vaccine that can prevent or interrupt the devastating effects of the chronic infection. HIV is significantly different from other viruses already mentioned. Protection from reinfection is conferred by the final outcome of the disease process—death. HIV attacks the heart of the cell-mediated immune system (lymphocytes) so that the human host is progressively **immunosuppressed** and cannot fight disease. As a result, patients become susceptible to multiple infections such as candidiasis, **thrush,** pneumonia, tuberculosis, and toxoplasmosis. Because these patients are incapable of efficiently fighting infection, they are always susceptible to **opportunistic organisms** such as *Pneumocystis carinii*, which leads to pneumonia.

The incompetent immune system, specifically a deterioration of cell-mediated immunity, permits patients to develop secondary cancers such as Kaposi sarcoma, non-Hodgkin lymphoma, or primary lymphoma of the brain.

A common pathogen of concern for respiratory care practitioners is *Pneumocystis carinii*. Therapy is aimed at both treatment and prophylaxis of this pathogen. The drug administered by the respiratory care provider is pentamidine, an antiprotozoal agent that is reviewed in Chapter 26.

PROPAGATION OF VIRUSES

Unlike other microorganisms, viruses are totally dependent on the metabolic system of the host's cells. In order to multiply, viruses must enter the host-cell nucleus. Viruses have surface proteins (such as hemagglutinins) that enable them to attach to the host-cell membrane by binding to specialized structures called receptors. After attaching to the cells, the viruses inject their nucleoprotein (DNA or RNA) into the cells. The viral nucleoproteins direct the production of more virus particles by using the host's substances (host DNA, amino acids, enzymes, bases, and ions) present in the cells; therefore, the cells become efficient factories for production of new viruses. Periodically the cells are triggered to rupture, expelling new viruses into the circulation so that more host cells become infected.

The goal of antiviral therapy is destruction of the microorganisms, thereby reducing the severity and length of infection. Attempts have been made to synthesize drugs that arrest the infection after the symptoms have developed. Because viruses are so closely involved with host cells, it is difficult to find a drug that will kill the virus without destroying the cells. Despite the lethal nature of HIV, you might be surprised that outside of a living cell, HIV is considered a "fragile" virus. When left outside living tissue, a dilute solution of household bleach is sufficient to kill the HIV virus. This is the recommended disinfectant when cleaning or wiping a surface that has been exposed to fluids containing HIV (such as infected blood spilled on a countertop).

Antiviral Drugs

MECHANISMS OF ACTION

Theoretically, inhibiting the initial attachment of the virus to the human host cells, blocking the injection of viral contents into the host cell, inhibiting enzymes that transcribe or synthesize viral proteins, or interrupting virus shedding and reinfection of other cells could inhibit viral activity. Two of these routes (virus attachment and interference with viral protein transcription or synthesis) have proved profitable in the development of antiviral drugs. The discussion of mechanism and site of antiviral drug action that follows may seem confusing because there are no simple terms for the nucleoproteins. To make it more confusing, the current cadre of antiviral drugs all sound alike. Don't be discouraged! Remember, for the viruses under discussion (influenza, HSV, HIV, CMV), antiviral drugs are effective because they block virus attachment to human cells or they mess up the viral proteins at transcription or synthesis.

Inhibition of Cell Penetration   Amantadine *(Symmetrel)* prevents the Asian (A2) virus that causes influenza from penetrating human cells and releasing viral DNA into the cell. When given prophylactically (within 20 hours after exposure to the flu), amantadine reduces the severity of the infection. It has no effect on other viral infections or influenza viruses other than type A. Therefore, this drug has limited utility and is usually recommended only for high-risk patients (chronically ill, infants, and elderly) who would suffer most from an influenza attack.

In contrast, the neuraminidase inhibitors, the newest group of antiinfluenza drugs, are expected to have a wide range of therapeutic antiviral effectiveness. Drugs in this class include oseltamivir *(Tamiflu)* and zanamivir *(Relenza)*. Neuraminidase and hemagglutinin are present on the surface of *all* influenza viruses. Hemagglutinin is responsible for docking the virus onto host cell membranes by bonding to sialic acid molecules (components of glycoproteins and mucoproteins) and inducing cell penetration. After replication, the viral clones are coated with sialic acid as they emerge from the ruptured cells. During the exodus, neuraminidase on the surface of the viral clones releases the sialic acid connections. This critical step directly affects (increases) viral pathogenicity because it frees the hemagglutinin for docking with new sialic acid molecules on the next host cells to be invaded (and not with the sialic acid–coated viruses).

Neuraminidase inhibitors are designed as sialic acid analogs so that the drug preferentially attaches to the virus surface protein but cannot be released by the enzymatic action of neuraminidase. As a result, the bound sialic acid drug causes the viruses to aggregate and clump together, attaching to each other: sialic acid drug to new virus hemagglutinin. In the end, host-cell penetration is inhibited, and infection (pathogenicity) is reduced, because the "virus-clot" cannot be released from the cell and is unable to connect with host-cell receptors. Because the sialic acid–binding site is the same for all influenza virus strains, neuraminidase inhibitors are expected to offer a greater therapeutic advantage in the treatment of influenza. Table 24-2 reviews drugs used for the treatment or prophylaxis of influenza.

Transcription of Viral Proteins   Other antiviral drugs interfere with one or more sites of viral enzyme activity. For example, HIV infection is initiated when the virus binds to a select group of white blood cells known as T lymphocytes, helper T

Table 24-2
Drugs Effective in the Treatment or Prophylaxis of Influenza

Drug (Product Name)	Outcome	Use	Adult Dose
Amantadine (Symmetrel)	Inhibits release of viral DNA into host cells	Influenza A	200 mg PO daily as single dose or 100 mg BID for at least 10 days
Rimantadine (Fluvadine)	Inhibits early viral replication through uncoating the virus	Influenza A	100 mg BID PO for 7 days
Oseltamivir (Tamiflu)	Inhibits neuraminidase by blocking sialic acid binding sites	Influenza A and B	75 mg PO BID, within 2 days of symptom onset, for 5 days
Zanamivir (Trelenza)	Inhibits neuraminidase by blocking sialic acid binding sites	Influenza A and B	Two 5-mg blisters by oral inhalation with a Diskhaler BID, within 2 days of symptom onset, for 5 days

cells, or CD4-positive lymphocytes. HIV preferentially attaches to a glycoprotein, known as CD4, present on the membranes of lymphocytes and some macrophages. It is believed that after this fusion on the outside viral coat (lipid envelope), the internal contents of the virus enter the human lymphocyte cytoplasm. HIV is a retrovirus, which means it uses its single strand of RNA to manipulate the host cell's DNA into making more retroviruses. To accomplish this, a specific enzyme, known as reverse transcriptase, is required. Eventually, the newly produced viral-coded DNA enters the human nuclei so that production of new viruses can begin. As the new HIV are shed into the cytoplasm and meet other helper T cells, reinfection occurs.

Although cells other than T lymphocytes may be the target of the virus—for example, herpes (nervous tissue), cytomegalovirus (retina, liver, lung), or influenza viruses (respiratory tract)—the route of access to host-cell nuclei and propagation of viruses is similar. This is simplistically illustrated in Figure 24-1.

CLINICAL INDICATIONS

Herpes Simplex Virus (HSV) Drugs available in the United States have selective antiviral activity, which means the drug is effective against one specific virus. Occasionally, these drugs may have activity against two viruses. Idoxuridine *(Herplex),* vidarabine *(Ara-A, Vira-A),* and trifluridine *(Viroptic)* are used in the treatment of herpes simplex infections of the eye, keratoconjunctivitis, and epithelial keratitis. These compounds may be administered topically (ocular instillation) for treatment of acute viral infections of the cornea and conjunctiva. Acyclovir *(Zovirax)* is approved for the treatment of cutaneous and genital herpes infections. Acyclovir is

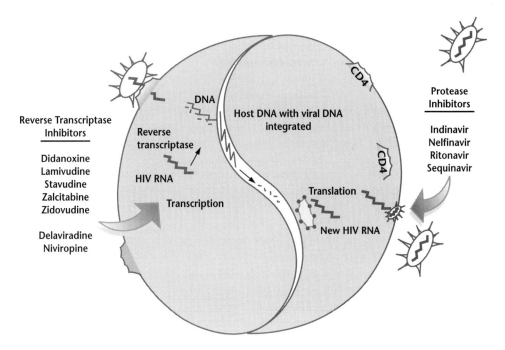

Figure 24-1
Propagation of HIV and sites of drug action.

also used to treat infections of herpes and cytomegalovirus which occur after bone marrow or renal transplant. Valacyclovir *(Valtrex)* is an analog of acylovir that is rapidly converted to acyclovir in the tissues.

Cytomegalovirus (CMV)   Cidofovir *(Vistide),* foscarnet *(Foscavir),* and ganciclovir *(Cytovene)* are approved for use in the treatment of CMV retinitis in patients with AIDS, CMV disease in transplant recipients, and acyclovir-resistant HSV infections in immunocompromised patients. CMV is a member of the herpes group of viruses. In susceptible patients of any age, CMV may cause hepatitis and encephalitis. Exposure during pregnancy may result in abortion or severe brain damage in newborns.

Influenza   Amantadine *(Symadine, Symmetrel)* and rimantadine (Fluvadine) are used prophylactically to reduce the severity of influenza attacks, specifically the influenza A virus, in susceptible groups. These include the elderly, immunocompromised patients, and patients with chronic diseases predisposing to infection. Because of the limited spectrum of antiviral activity, these drugs are often given in addition to vaccination during the flu season. Zanamivir (Relenza) and oseltamivir (Tamiflu) are FDA approved for the treatment of uncomplicated influenza (any influenza strain type A or B) in adults who have been symptomatic for less than 3 days. These drugs are not substitutes for annual vaccination and are compatible adjunct therapy in addition to vaccination.

Respiratory Syncytial Virus (RSV)   This virus causes severe bronchitis and pneumonia in infants and children, often leading to death. Prophylactic medication, such as palivizumab (Synagis) in the high-risk population, is the best approach to prevent severe illness associated with RSV.

HIV   A significant number of drugs have recently been approved for use alone or in combination for the management of HIV infection. These drugs are indicated for treatment of advanced infection and are not approved for prophylaxis. The frequency of virus mutation results in drug resistance and poor clinical response.

ADMINISTRATION AND PHARMACOKINETICS

All of the antiviral drugs presented in this chapter are available as oral formulations except for those used against CMV, ophthalmic herpes, and zanamivir *(Relenza)*. Oral administration facilitates patient adherence to therapy, particularly because the treatment of recurrent genital herpes and HIV may be several months to life-long. In general, these drugs are well absorbed after oral administration, attaining peak blood drug levels within 1 to 2 hours, are metabolized to some extent, and are excreted in the urine.

Zanamivir *(Relenza)* is a dry powder administered through a breath-actuated Diskhaler. Drug is distributed to the pharynx and lower tracheobronchial tree for an immediate onset of action.

Absorption   Most of the drugs presented in this chapter are absorbed as the active antiviral agent. A few, however, must be converted to the active moiety. Oseltamivir *(Tamiflu)*, which has no antiviral activity, is readily absorbed following oral administration and converted in the liver to the active neuraminidase inhibitor.

Among the other oral antiviral drugs for herpes, acyclovir *(Zovirax)*, famciclovir *(Famvir)*, valacyclovir *(Valtrex)*, or for influenza, oseltamivir *(Tamiflu)*, oral absorption is good and unaffected by food or meal content.

Renal Excretion   Inhibition of glomerular filtration and tubular secretion by any means (drugs, renal impairment) will cause certain antiviral drugs to accumulate. Almost all of the active moieties of their metabolites are excreted via urine. All of the drugs used in the treatment of herpes and CMV, as well as amantadine, stavudine, and zalcitabine, must be dose adjusted in the presence of renal impairment. Anything that decreases renal clearance as evidenced by a creatinine clearance less than 50 mL/min will obligate a reduction in the antiviral dose. Both oral and intravenous doses are reduced. Amantadine and rimantadine are also dose-adjusted for patients over 65 years of age in whom renal clearance is decreased with age. This is to avoid precipitation of CNS adverse effects including seizures.

ADVERSE EFFECTS

Influenza   The incidence of adverse effects associated with amantadine is relatively low. The most common adverse effects include slurred speech, ataxia, lethargy, dizziness, nausea, and irritability. Hypotension and congestive heart failure have also been reported. Because amantadine produces anticholinergic effects within the CNS, this drug should be used with caution in the presence of other anticholinergic medication (potentiation). Amantadine *(Symmeterel)* is not indicated for patients who have impaired liver or renal function, epilepsy, or psychosis, and it is not recommended for administration during pregnancy. Rimantadine *(Fluvadine)* has a similar profile, and with both drugs, elderly patients appear to experience adverse effects more frequently. This does not preclude the use of these drugs in the elderly. The neuraminidase inhibitors are generally well tolerated. The incidence of adverse effects (nausea, vomiting, diarrhea, abdominal pain, and headache) reported during oseltamivir *(Tamiflu)* treatment is very low and indistinguishable from the clinical course of flu. In addition to the type of adverse effects seen with oseltamivir, zanamivir *(Relenza)* has some unique warnings. Zanamivir is not generally recommended for the treatment of patients with underlying airway disease such as asthma or chronic obstructive pulmonary disease (COPD). Bronchospasm and decline in lung function has occurred. This was not limited to patients with underlying airway disease. There have also been reports of allergic-like reactions and a potential for serious bacterial infections that appear with influenza-like symptoms or as a complication of influenza.

SPECIAL CONSIDERATIONS AND CONTRAINDICATIONS

Except for the drugs used in the prophylaxis of influenza and treatment of herpes zoster, there is little experience in the use of the other antiviral drugs in elderly patients. Specifically for HIV, CMV, and genital herpes, the patient population has been primarily young adults. With the success of the newer treatment strategies and remarkable protease inhibitors, patients may be surviving longer before the onset of AIDS, and this will contribute critical information on long-term safety.

The respiratory care practitioner often encounters the complications of providing respiratory care to patients who have acute or chronic viral infections. The treatment of HIV, especially advanced stages or with opportunistic infections, warrants close monitoring of the patient's vital signs, body temperature, and frequent evaluation of serum chemistry and hematology profiles.

ADVERSE EFFECTS THAT AFFECT RESPIRATORY CARE

Amantadine *(Symmetrel)* may decrease alertness and cause blurred vision, which may interfere with tasks requiring concentration. Idoxuridine (Herplex) may cause sensitivity to bright light. Both of these effects can interfere, especially in older patients, with the patient's ability to read instructions or properly perform inhalation techniques for respiratory care.

Notifying the Physician   With any of these drugs, including those for the prophy-laxis of cold and flu, patients should receive clear instructions that swelling, edema, shortness of breath, or dizziness should be reported to the prescribing physician.

Use in Pregnancy   In general, antiviral drugs are designated FDA Pregnancy Cate-gory B or C because they have not been adequately studied in pregnant women. Among the systemic drugs, safe use in pregnancy has not been established in hu-mans. Nevertheless, there are situations where their use is clearly indicated, and they may be used with caution and close patient monitoring. There are registry centers that encourage physicians to provide information on antiviral (HIV, her-pes) use during pregnancy in order to accumulate information on maternal-fetal outcome. These centers are supported by the specific drug manufacturers.

Zanamivir (Relenza) has been changed from a category B to a category C based on animal toxicity data.

Chapter 24 Review

UNDERSTANDING TERMINOLOGY

Match the definition or description in the left column with the appropriate term in the right column.

1. A medication used for treatment/prophylaxis for *Pneumocystis carinii* that is commonly administered by the respiratory therapist.

2. Condition that causes individuals to resist acquiring or developing a disease or infection.

3. A microorganism capable of causing disease only when the resistance of the host is impaired.

4. An incurable disease caused by a virus and characterized by multiple opportunistic infections.

a. AIDS
b. pentamidine
c. immunity
d. opportunistic organism

ACQUIRING KNOWLEDGE

Test your understanding of the material in this chapter by answering the following questions.

5. What is the best way to prevent infection with the influenza virus?
6. Are vaccines available to treat any virus infection?

7. Do patients exposed to HIV always test HIV positive?
8. Why are viral infections difficult to treat with drugs?
9. How do amantadine and idoxuridine affect viruses without damaging the human cells?

Additional Reading

1995 drugs for AIDS and associated infections. *Med Lett* 1995;37:Oct 13.

Bartlett J, Finkbeiner A. *The Guide to Living with HIV Infections*. Baltimore: The Johns Hopkins University Press, 1996.

Cox NJ. New options for the prevention of influenza. *N Engl J Med* 1999;341:1387.

Danner SA. A short-term study of the safety, pharmacokinetics and efficacy of ritonavir, an inhibitor of HIV-1 protease. *N Engl J Med* 1995;333(23):1528.

Laver G. Disarming flu viruses. *Sci Am* 1999;280:78.

Petrow S, ed. *The HIV Drug Book*. New York: Project Information, Pocket Books, 1998.

Internet Activities

There are a tremendous number of government, private, and public organizations that maintain Web pages specifically to educate and inform the public about virally transmitted diseases. The topics cover cold viruses, guidelines to minimize seasonal symptoms of flu, AIDS databases with computer response to posted questions, daily summary of AIDS news, and coping with herpes through management of herpes during pregnancy. The format of these presentations includes tutorials, colored pictures of lesions, interactive chat rooms, and sometimes an accompanying audio narrative. Access to information is as easy as entering "AIDS" or "herpes" at the search prompt or using search engines such as Yahoo or AltaVista to reach preset health and medicine categories. Try any of the following paths as instructed and expand your knowledge of the viruses covered in this chapter. All of the information in these exercises can be printed using on-screen prompts.

1. Flu Viruses

    a. Enter **www.yahoo.com.** At the home page type "influenza" into the search box. From the list of flu-related topics, double-click on "Patient Information Sheet." Physicians from the University of Florida have provided instructions for surviving the flu.

    b. While in **yahoo.com.health,** select "influenza virus replication." An illustration appears on screen that describes the process by which a virus invades the host cell and uses it to reproduce its own genetic material.

    c. Test review: Case studies in influenza are provided through the University of Florida at **www.medinfo.ufl.edu/cme/flu/flu.html.**

2. Herpes Viruses

   a. Enter **www.yahoo.com/health,** then enter "herpes" into the search box or scroll down the preset list of health topics to the herpes category. This will bring a list of relevant Web pages, which can be accessed by double-clicking on the topic of interest. Continue to request additional information until you reach the category "Health: Diseases and Condition: Herpes." Select "Herpes Site" to review a current update on HSV and support information for people with herpes.

   b. Return to the list of topics by clicking the right mouse button and selecting "back." Then click on "FAQ" (frequently asked questions) to see what information is of most interest to students, patients, and health care providers. Presentations include transmission, treatment, diagnostic tests, and management of herpes during pregnancy. Note the side panels identify how to obtain a video cassette on herpes management. If you wish to return to this Web site, it can be accessed directly by entering the URL: **www.advicecenter.com.**

   c. Another Web site, "Herpes Zone," is an excellent tutorial with schematic cartoons showing how the virus gets into cells and makes more viral proteins. Enter **www.herpeszone.com,** then select "Introduction" for the viral-cell interaction. In herpeszone, select "medications of choice" or "nutritional therapy." Did you know that the lysine:arginine amino acid ratio in the diet of herpes patients can trigger exacerbations of lesions? To review nutritional therapy and the lysine and arginine levels in specific foods, select the "nutritional therapy" category.

   d. Enter **www.yahoo.com** and select "Health: Diseases and Conditions" and scroll down until you reach "Shingles" (you can also type "Shingles" or "Herpes zoster" into the search box). This brings you into an online journal club that discusses the clinical course of herpes zoster.

3. HIV/AIDS Viruses

   a. Enter **www.AIDS.com** to enter "NetHealth" (also accessible through **www.nethealth.com**). This is a service with more than 500 Web sites specifically dedicated to sorting and identifying information on AIDS, depression, and Alzheimer disease available on the Internet.

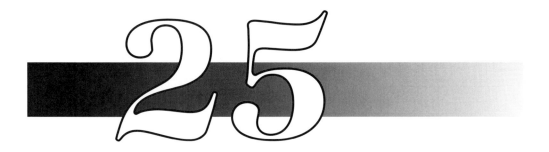

Mechanical Ventilation*

Vinay Nadkarni, MD
Stuart Levine, PharmD

Chapter Focus

Patients requiring respiratory support on a mechanical ventilator frequently develop sudden respiratory distress and are characterized as "out of phase with the ventilator" or "fighting the ventilator." Respiratory distress is common following intubation and ventilatory support and is largely related to anxiety and stress associated with both the reason for the ventilation and the ventilatory support itself.

The four primary groups of drugs used to facilitate mechanical ventilation are sedatives, neuroleptics, analgesics, and neuromuscular blocking agents. Although these have been reviewed in previous chapters, this chapter brings those agents together and presents the rationale for their use.

Chapter Terminology

ileus: An intestinal obstruction.
neuroleptics: Agents or drugs that modify psychotic behavior.

*Adapted from Essentials of Mechanical Ventilation by Dean Hess, PhD, RRT, FAARC, and Robert Kacmarek, PhD, RRT, FAARC.

Chapter Objectives

After studying this chapter, you should be able to:

- Describe four groups of drugs used to support the patient on mechanical ventilation.
- Describe the indication for use of each of the four drug groups.
- Name the drugs of choice for each drug group.
- Describe the method used to monitor the effectiveness of neuromuscular blockers.

Most patients requiring acute ventilatory support also require sedation and analgesia. Mechanical control of ventilation is a frightening experience, highlighting a life-threatening problem that can be expected to produce fear and anxiety. The four primary groups of drug that are used to facilitate mechanical ventilatory support are sedatives, neuroleptics, analgesics, and neuromuscular blocking agents.

Sedatives

The term sedative can be applied to a number of categories of drugs: benzodiazepines (diazepam, lorazepam, midazolam), barbiturates, and propofol. In general, all of these agents are anxiolytic and hypnotic, and they produce muscle relaxation and amnesia but do not relieve pain. Many of these drugs are also anticonvulsants but have little depressant effect on the cardiovascular system. The exceptions to this are midazolam and propofol, which may produce some cardiovascular depression. Of concern is the lengthy half-life of many of these agents. Diazepam (Valium) and the long-acting barbiturates are of particular concern because they have half-lives of 1 to 3 days. In addition, because these drugs are highly lipid soluble and metabolized by the liver and kidney, accumulation and prolonged effects are common in the critically ill, especially the elderly. This is a particular concern during weaning. As a result, lorazepam (Ativan), because of its shorter half-life (6 to 15 hours), is more appropriate during weaning than is diazepam. Midazolam (Versed) is the most rapidly acting and has the shortest half-life (1 hour) of the benzodiazepines. As a result, finer control of the level of sedation is possible as compared to the other agents in this class of drugs.

Benzodiazepines can be reversed by the specific antagonist flumazenil. However, the use of this agent in the intensive care unit (ICU) has not been well evaluated, and its half-life is very short (1 hour), requiring continuous infusion lest periodic respiratory depression occur.

Propofol (Diprivan) has become the sedative of choice for rapid induction of anesthesia in the ICU. It is particularly useful for minor surgery and other invasive procedures (bronchoscopy, line placements). It has a very rapid onset of action

Table 25-1

Sedatives Used in the ICU*

	Lorazepam	*Midazolam*	*Propofol*
Onset of action	>3–5 min	2–2.5 min	1 min
Loading dose	0.05 mg/kg	0.03 mg/kg	0.5–1.0 mg/kg
Infusion rate	0.05–0.3 mg/kg/h	0.05–0.3 mg/kg/h	1–9 mg/kg/h
Cost	Low	Moderate	High

*Use lower end for adults.

and short half-life (<30 minutes). However, it frequently causes hypotension (occasionally profound) and is very expensive (Table 25-1).

Neuroleptics

Delirium is common in critically ill adults and usually manifests as reduced ability to respond appropriately to external stimuli. Disorganized thinking, rambling, incoherent or irrelevant speech, decreased levels of consciousness, altered sensory perception, and disorientation are common clinical findings in the delirious patient. The use of narcotics and sedatives generally worsens the symptoms of delirium because these agents further alter sensory perception. The drug of choice in treating delirium is haloperidol (Haldol), a butyrophenone neuroleptic drug. Usual dosing is 2 to 10 mg administered intravenously every 2 to 4 hours. Generally, clinical effects are observed within 30 to 60 minutes.

Analgesics

All patients acutely requiring mechanical ventilation experience pain. Unfortunately, practitioners are so focused on correcting pathophysiological problems that they frequently overlook the fact that acutely ill patients are experiencing physical pain. Sedatives modify the emotional component of pain but do nothing to affect the physical component. Analgesics are required to control pain.

In the acutely ill, mechanically ventilated patient, intravenous narcotic analgesics are the drugs of choice. Three primary agents used in this setting are morphine, fentanyl (Sublimaze), and hydromorphone (Dilaudid). Morphine is generally considered the preferred agent unless cardiovascular instability exists. Morphine administration is associated with transient hypotension because of histamine release. In the setting of hemodynamic instability, fentanyl is the drug of choice, although hydromorphone is considered an acceptable substitution for morphine.

Of concern with large-dose intermittent or continuous infusion of narcotic

Table 25-2

Narcotics Used in the ICU*

	Morphine	Fentanyl	Hydromorphone
Onset of action	Fast	Fast	Fast
Loading dose	0.05–0.10 mg/kg	1–2 μg/kg	0.015 mg/kg
Infusion rate	0.1–0.2 mg/kg/h	≥1–2 μg/kg/h	1–2 mg/h
Cost	Low	Low	Moderate

*Use lower end for adults.

analgesics is ileus, causing intolerance to enteral feeding and aggravation of pancreatic inflammation. In spite of these concerns, narcotic analgesics are the drugs of choice for pain relief and respiratory depression in the mechanically ventilated, critically ill patient (Table 25-2).

Paralytic Agents

Paralytic agents are reviewed in Chapter 9. There are two basic types, depolarizing and nondepolarizing. They all render patients paralyzed, but none has any analgesic or sedative properties and *must* always be administered with appropriate levels of either sedatives or narcotics. The depolarizing agents, because of their short duration of action (5 minutes), are used only for short-term paralysis to allow intubation, whereas the nondepolarizing type may be used for prolonged paralysis to ensure controlled ventilation. As a result of the longer period that paralysis is maintained in the ICU, the sicker the patient being paralyzed and the higher doses used over time, numerous problems have occurred in the ICU that have not been observed in the operating room. As compared with use in the operating room, marked tolerance develops in the ICU over several days. Frequently, the required dose is increased three- to fourfold because of up-regulation of the nicotinic receptors. As a result, the use of these agents in the ICU should be avoided. They should be used only when sedatives and analgesics have failed to facilitate controlled ventilation. In addition, their use for longer than 24 hours should be avoided in patients with sepsis or renal failure and those who are receiving high-dose steroids (Table 25-3).

Because there is a wide individual variation in the response to neuromuscular blocking agents, careful monitoring of their effects is essential. Observation of the patient is normally the most direct method of evaluating the level of paralysis. Spontaneous breathing efforts, chewing on the endotracheal tube, and coughing may indicate inadequate blockade. Although direct observation is the most common method of assessing blockade, it is crude. A more precise method is to assess motor nerve response to a supramaximal stimulus applied over the ulnar nerve at the wrist. This form of stimulation is referred to as a *train of four,* as four rapid and independent stimuli are applied. The level of initial and subsequent response to the four stimuli indicates the magnitude of blockade.

Table 25-3
Neuromuscular Blocking Agents Used in the ICU*

	Pancuronium	*Vecuronium*	*Rocuroniuim*
Loading dose	0.04–0.1 mg/kg	0.1–0.4 mg/kg	0.6–1.2 mg/kg
Infusion rate	0.1 mg/kg/h	0.3–0.9 mg/kg/h	0.3–0.9 mg/kg/h
Cost	Low	Moderate	Moderate

*Use lower end for adults.

Practical Guide to Pharmacologic Therapy

All patients receiving acute invasive ventilatory support require some level of sedation. Most patients can be adequately sedated with benzodiazepines or propofol. Those experiencing pain should receive narcotics, titrated to the minimal level of comfort to avoid ventilatory dyssynchrony. In patients experiencing delirium, haloperidol should be added. Dosages of sedatives and narcotics should be increased in patients fighting the ventilator once other causes of respiratory distress have been ruled out. It is only in the exceptionally difficult to sedate patient, where patient activity is interfering with gas exchange and hemodynamics, that neuromuscular blocking agents should be considered. If they are used, the duration of use should be limited.

Chapter 25 Review

UNDERSTANDING TERMINOLOGY

Test your understanding of the material in this chapter by answering the following questions.

1. Review the progression of drugs used to control a patient who is "fighting the ventilator."

2. What are the indications of the four types of medications used to control a patient on the ventilator?

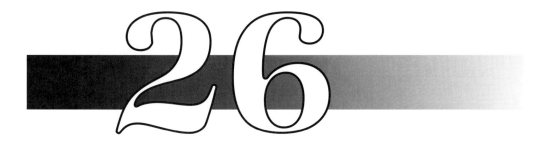

New Treatments in Respiratory Care Pharmacology

Barbara Nagle, PhD
Stuart Levine, PharmD

Chapter Focus

This chapter focuses on three drug categories that have unique implications to the respiratory care practitioner(RCP). These medications do not really fall into a specific heading, so we thought we would group them together.

Surfactants are medications that treat respiratory distress syndrome related to a deficiency in lung surfactant. Nitric oxide is a recently approved therapy for children with pulmonary hypertension. It is becoming a drug the RCP must have knowledge of for the care of the patient. Finally, pentamidine is a medication used in the treatment of opportunistic infections commonly seen in the AIDS population. Although it is an important drug in the care of those patients, it can put the health of the RCP at risk.

Chapter Terminology

alveoli: Small sacs in the lung parenchyma where gas exchange occurs.

apnea: Cessation of breathing.

asphyxia: Condition resulting from an insufficient intake of oxygen, resulting in death.

atelectasis: Incomplete expansion of the lung or a portion of the lung.

conjunctivitis: Inflammation of the membrane that lines the eyelid and covers the white part of the eye (sclera).

hypoglycemia: Low blood sugar.

opportunistic infections: Infections from microorganisms that do not ordinarily cause disease but under some circumstances (eg, impaired immune response) can cause disease.

protozoa: The simplest single-celled member of the animal kingdom.

Chapter Objectives

After studying this chapter, you should be able to:

- List the types of surfactants and their components.
- Describe the administration technique of surfactants.
- Describe the function of surfactants.
- List the indications for using nitric oxide.
- List the toxicities that may limit the use of nitric oxide.
- Describe the indication for use of pentamidine.
- Describe the adverse effects commonly seen in the patient when receiving aerosolized pentamidine therapy.
- Describe the common adverse effects seen in RCP who administer pentamidine.
- Describe methods to reduce the risk of exposure of the RCP.

Surfactants

WHAT IS RESPIRATORY DISTRESS SYNDROME (RDS)?

Respiratory distress syndrome, once called hyaline membrane disease, is a problem associated with a deficiency in lung surfactant. It is the most frequent problem encountered in preterm infants and is one of the most important causes of death and illness in this group. This occurs in 60,000 to 70,000 preterm infants each year and is responsible for 5000 deaths.

RDS arises as a result of a delay in production or deficiency in lung surfactant. Infants born before 35 weeks' gestation are at a high risk of RDS. This is because production of surfactant does not start until after this time. Factors that increase or decrease the risk of RDS are listed in Table 26-1.

Surfactant is a mixture of fats (phospholipids in this case), proteins, and complex sugars. Surfactant forms the lining of the small air sacs in the lungs known as alveoli, where it reduces the surface tension. Think of having some plastic wrap

Table 26-1

Factors Affecting Risk of Respiratory Distress Syndrome

Increase Risk	*Decrease Risk*
Male sex	Female sex
Caucasian race	African-American race
Acute perinatal asphyxia	Prenatal exposure to steroids
Infants born to diabetic mothers	Prolonged rupture of membranes

and bunching it up together. Try opening the wrap. You can see it takes a lot of work to pull it apart. That is surface tension holding the wrap together. Surfactant reduces that surface tension, and it therefore takes less energy to open, and keep open, the alveoli sacs.

When the alveoli cannot open, less oxygen can be absorbed through the lungs. The infant's breathing rate increases (tachypnea), and it starts to use some additional chest muscles to help in breathing and to grunt on expiration, and the skin turn blue (cyanosis). Over time all of this leads to damage to the lungs and can lead to the infant's death.

PREVENTION OF RDS

Our goal is to minimize the effects of RDS. If possible, birth should be delayed to allow time for the lungs to mature with support of the mother including supporting blood pressure and reducing bleeding. Support of the infant includes providing warmth and additional oxygen.

For mothers with less than 32 weeks of gestation, corticosteroids have been given to accelerate the maturity of the lungs and prevent RDS. Beclomethasone increases the production of surfactant and increases the presence of antioxidants, which help to protect the lungs from damage.

TREATMENT OF RDS

All children at less than 28 weeks of gestation should receive surfactant prophylactically. For those beyond 28 weeks, the physician will determine if it is needed. Surfactant is a very costly therapy, and decisions need to be made regarding the cost-effectiveness of the therapy.

TYPES OF SURFACTANTS

There are four surfactants on the market today. They represent two types of surfactants: modified natural biological surfactant and synthetic surfactant.

Modified natural surfactant is derived from the washings (lavage) of alveoli of calves (bovine) and adding and/or removing some components. This substance is marketed under the name beractant (Survanta). Calfactant (Infasurf) is also a lavage of calf lung tissue and was recently marketed. Another recently marketed surfactant, poractant alfa (Curosurf), is from a lavage of lung tissue from pigs (porcine).

Finally, there are artificial or synthetic compounds that may or may not be components of natural surfactant. Exosurf is the only synthetic surfactant approved for marketing.

ADMINISTRATION OF SURFACTANTS

The administration technique for surfactants is unique and critical to the outcome of the treatment. If you think about the theraputic goal that you are attempting to accomplish, the technique makes sense. Your goal is to coat the lining of the lungs with surfactant. Think about trying to coat the inside of a bottle. You can't just pour liquid in to coat all of the surfaces. You can't shake a baby to coat the inside of the lungs. You need to slowly roll the infant into four different positions to coat the lungs with surfactant: head and body down to the right, down to the left, body up to the right, and then up to the left.

ADVERSE EFFECTS OF SURFACTANTS

There are several undesirable adverse effects associated with surfactants. There may be a substantial drop in the oxygenation of up to 20%. This may be the result of the presence of mucus plugs, apnea, or bleeding in the lungs. In addition, decreased heart rate (bradycardia) sometimes occurs. If bradycardia and decreased oxygen saturation occur, then the procedure should be stopped. Once the surfactant is given, the oxygenation should improve.

CONCLUSION

RDS is a serious, life-threatening disease of premature infants. Four different surfactants are now available that will improve oxygenation in these patients. Questions still remain about which is the best agent to use and the best time for administration.

Nitric Oxide

OVERVIEW

Nitric oxide (NO) is a unique medication that reduces pulmonary hypertension. It began as an investigational drug in the 1980s, expanded its use well into the 1990s, and finally became available commercially in December 1999. Its availability provides another option for treatment that can be administered by the respiratory care practitioner.

MECHANISM OF ACTION

Inhaled nitric oxide is the only drug that is a specific pulmonary vasodilator. It works as a vasodilator by relaxing smooth muscle in the lungs. It has the ability to affect smooth muscle throughout the body, but, because of its short half-life, it does not reach the main circulation of the body.

The body actually produces a small amount of its own nitric oxide. Levels of 10 parts per billion (ppb) are found in cells that line the blood vessels. During times of shock, the body increases the level of nitric oxide throughout the vascular system, and this contributes to the hypotension seen as part of shock.

Other actions of nitric oxide include acting as bronchodilator and platelet aggregation inhibitor.

TOXICITY

Nitric oxide is not excreted by the kidneys and, acting as a free radical, binds with hemoglobin to produce methemoglobin. This is a toxic product because it has little ability to transport oxygen compared to free hemoglobin.

Nitric oxide also changes to nitrogen dioxide during its metabolism. Nitrogen dioxide converts to nitric acid and nitrous acid, which are directly toxic to tissue. It has also been identified as a carcinogen.

All of the abovementioned problems may limit its use in the future.

INDICATIONS AND POTENTIAL USES

Nitric oxide is approved for use in the treatment of persistent pulmonary hypertension in neonates with respiratory failure. It has also been used to reduce the pressure in the lungs during neonatal cardiac surgery and to reduce pulmonary hypertension after lung transplantation. About 60% of patients given nitric oxide benefit from its use.

ADMINISTRATION AND DOSAGE

The initial dose of nitric oxide is 20 parts per million (ppm). Ordinarily doses are not greater than 20 ppm because of increased risk of methemoglobinemia and increased nitrogen dioxide levels. A patient successfully treated at 20 ppm should be reduced to 5 ppm if tolerated. Nitric oxide is administered via inhalation with complex equipment that can constantly monitor levels of nitric oxide in the inhaled gas and ensure that the concentration, during the breathing cycle, is consistent.

WARNINGS

Nitric oxide should never be abruptly discontinued. This may result in worsening of oxygen diffusion into the arterial blood and an increase in pulmonary hypertension. Patients receiving nitric oxide therapy should be weaned slowly.

CAUTIONS FOR THE RESPIRATORY CARE PRACTITIONER

Low levels of NO do not appear to be toxic. The gas is present in many environments. The Occupational Safety and Health Administration (OSHA) states that breathing up to 25 ppm of NO in the workplace is acceptable, with brief exposures up to 100 ppm being allowed. These data were supported by reports of animal exposure of 40 to 100 ppm for 6 days that showed no evidence of toxicity. The exposure limit set by OSHA is 25 ppm for nitric oxide and 5 ppm for nitrogen dioxide.

PREGNANCY

It is not known whether nitric oxide can cause fetal harm when administered to a pregnant woman or can affect reproduction. Nitric oxide is currently listed as a category C medication.

Pentamidine Isethionate

Pentamidine isethionate, or pentamidine as we will refer to it, is a medication used for the treatment of opportunistic infections as we talked about in Chapter 24 on antivirals and HIV infections. The use of pentamidine requires more than a brief discussion, so we include a section for it in this chapter.

ACTIVITY

Pentamidine is an antimicrobial that is used to kill organisms called protozoa. It is used by the respiratory care practitioner for the treatment and prophylaxis of the protozoa *Pneumocystis carinii*. There are other reasons that it is ordered, and they include leishmania and trypanosoma infections. For these indications, and sometimes for *Pneumocystis carinii*, pentamidine is used as an IV or IM preparation.

MECHANISM OF ACTION

As for many drugs, the exact way pentamidine works is not fully known. It may work by affecting the synthesis of RNA and DNA, and/or it may work by reducing the production of energy the organism needs to survive.

SOME BASIC PHARMACOKINETICS

When pentamidine is given by inhalation, it reaches levels five to ten times those seen when similar doses are administered IV. As with the inhaled steroids, where we saw that it made more sense to administer the drug directly into the area where it is needed rather than giving it IV, IM, or orally, we place the drug directly into the lung, where the pneumonia occurs.

When given by inhalation, the drug is distributed throughout the body. However, the extent to which it goes into other tissues varies greatly among people and is related to many factors. Those factors include:

1. Delivery device
2. Particle size of the aerosolized drug
3. Dose
4. Patient position (distribution is more uniform from a supine than from a sitting position)
5. Efficiency of the nebulizer

ADVERSE REACTIONS

Pentamidine is very toxic when given IV or IM and can lead to death from severe hypotension, cardiac arrhythmias, and hypoglycemia. Infusing pentamidine over 1 to 2 hours can reduce the risk of hypotension. The most common adverse effects include nephrotoxicity, cough, and bronchospasm. Nephrotoxicity occurs in about 25% of the patients. This is an important consideration in regard to possible drug interactions. Other medications that are nephrotoxic may contribute to toxicity and should be avoided if possible.

Reactions to inhalation are far less severe than those seen with IV or IM routes of administration. The most common adverse effects are the same as those seen with IV or IM use, which include nephrotoxicity, cough, and bronchospasm. A list of adverse reactions appears in Table 26-2.

Hypoglycemia can occur with any route of administration. It usually appears within 5 to 7 days of beginning therapy but may occur up to several days after pentamidine has been discontinued. Reactions can be severe, and deaths have been reported.

Conjunctivitis can occur but is usually associated with removal of the nebulization mouthpiece and misdirecting the aerosol mist toward the face. The RCP should monitor the patient carefully during this procedure in order to avoid this potential problem.

Table 26-2
Adverse Effects of Pentamidine Inhalation

Most common
Nephrotoxicity, cough, bronchospasm

Rare

Nausea	Gastric ulcers
Vomiting	Dry mouth
Diarrhea	Chapped lips
Abdominal discomfort	Increased saliva production
Pain	Hepatitis
Loss of or decreased appetite	Liver dysfunction
Metallic taste	Tremors
Hypotension	Confusion
Hypertension	Anxiety
Tachycardia	Memory loss
Palpitations	Seizures
Fainting	Hallucinations
Dizziness	Conjunctivitis
Lightheadedness	Blurred vision
Sweating	Contact lens discomfort
Stroke	Chills
Anemias	Gout
Rashes	Body odor
Itching	Headaches
Hypoglycemia	Edema
Gingivitis	Incontinence
Gagging	

PLACE IN THERAPY

We have said a few times that pentamidine is used for the treatment and prophylaxis of *Pneumocystis carinii.* However, it is not the first choice. For the primary prevention of *Pneumocystis carinii,* co-trimoxazole (a combination of the sulfa sulfamethoxazole and trimethoprim) is used. This is an oral agent and therefore much easier to administer. Pentamidine is used commonly even though it is not the drug of choice because HIV patients tend to have a high rate of adverse reactions to co-trimoxazole. These reactions include fever, skin reactions, and blood reactions, which become so severe that therapy must be stopped. It is at that point that pentamidine is used.

DOSAGE, RECONSTITUTION, AND ADMINISTRATION

Pentamidine can be used for both the treatment and prophylaxis of *Pneumocystis carinii* (see Table 26-3). Solutions for oral inhalation are prepared by adding 6 mL of sterile water to reconstitute 300 mg of pentamidine. Once you have prepared the solution, it is stable for 48 hours. To administer pentamidine you should use a nebulizer called a Respiguard II jet nebulizer. No other medications should be placed in the reservoir, and this is not the type of device used for bronchodilator therapy.

ENVIRONMENTAL CONCERNS

A RCP who administers pentamidine inhalation to an HIV-infected patient should be aware of the possibility of exposure to tuberculosis. Administering pentamidine by inhalation can result in coughing as a side effect. A patient with an undiagnosed tuberculosis infection can inadvertently infect the therapist. Antituberculosis therapy should be started before initiating pentamidine inhalation therapy in patients with a confirmed or suspected diagnosis of tuberculosis.

There are numerous other adverse reactions seen in RCP's who are exposed to aerosolized pentamidine. Their reactions are listed in Table 26-4.

Pentamidine must be administered in a room equipped with a negative-pressure ventilation system, and RCPs must wear gloves, gown, mask, and goggles during administration of the drug.

The dose is diluted in 6 mL of preservative-free sterile water. ***Do not*** dilute with 0.9% sodium chloride solution. Delivery systems other than the Respirigard II are not currently recommended.

Table 26-3

Pentamidine Dosing via Inhalation

Indication	Adult Dose	Pediatric Dose (>5 Years Old)	Frequency
Prophylaxis	300 mg	300 mg	Every 4 weeks
Treatment	600 mg	4–8 mg/kg	Daily for 21 days

Table 26-4

Adverse Reactions Seen in Respiratory Care Practitioners Exposed to Aerosolized Pentamidine

Eye irritation	Cough
Conjunctivitis	Tightness in the chest
Numbness of the nose and mouth	Bronchospasm
Bitter metallic taste	Wheezing
Burning eyes, nose, and throat	Hoarseness
Sinus irritation	Fatigue
Nasal stuffiness and increased mucus	Headache
Sneezing	Lightheadedness
Shortness of breath	

Patients should be instructed to wear nose clips during treatment, and efforts should be made to prevent leakage of aerosol. The flowmeter must be turned off when the mouthpiece is removed from the patient's mouth, even during coughing.

Bacterial filters should be used to filter both the source gas and the patients' exhaled gas. A separate nebulizer must be used in order to administer any other medications.

PREGNANCY

Because of unknown risk, environmental exposure to aerosolized pentamidine by pregnant women and those planning to become pregnant should be avoided. This applies to the RCPs as well as patient visitors. This medication is a category C pregnancy risk.

INSULIN—A LOOK TO THE FUTURE

Up to the present time, all medications and pharmacology learned by respiratory care practitioners have revolved around the treatment of respiratory diseases or diseases that have a respiratory component. With the new millennium comes a change in the types of patients you will treat. Within the next two years, you will begin to see diabetic patients.

Diabetic patients have been treated for many years by the injection of insulin, oral hypoglycemics, and recently implantable insulin pumps. Within the next few years, we will see the marketing of inhaled insulin. This will be a great challenge for the respiratory care practitioner to learn about the treatment of a completely unique disease state. Handheld nebulizers will be utilized to aerosolize insulin and allow for administration of this drug without the need of needles or syringes.

In the future, respiratory care practitioners will learn about different types of insulin and their onset and duration of action. Knowledge of a new disease state will be required so that respiratory care practitioners can aid in patient education as well as monitor care. The future holds expanded roles and new ways to assist in the care of our patients.

Chapter 26 Review

ACQUIRING KNOWLEDGE

Test your understanding of the material in this chapter by answering the following questions.

1. You are working on the obstetrics unit, and there is a women 31 weeks pregnant. Her obstetrician is concerned about the baby's health. The obstetrician thinks the baby might be born prematurely. What do you think will be recommended to prevent RDS?

2. On the same unit you are able to observe the administration of surfactant. Can you describe the administration technique?

3. You are working on a neonatal unit, and one of the neonatologists is describing some of the toxicities associated with NO therapy. What does the neonatologist describe?

4. On a med/surg patient care unit you receive an order for pentamidine. Why do you think the physician has prescribed this aerosol?

Additional Reading

AHFS Drug Information 2000. Published by American Society of Health Systems Pharmacists. ISBN 1-58528004-6.

Micromedix System—Online drug information data bases. Copyright 2000.

Dorland's Medical Dictionary. Published by WB Saunders. Copyright 1988. ISBN 072163154-1.

Appendix I

Regulatory Issues in the Practice of Respiratory Care

ROBERTO PALERMO, MBA, RRT
ARTHUR J. MCLAUGHLIN, JR, MS, CRT

After completing their respiratory care education programs, respiratory care practitioners (RCPs), when interviewing for jobs, frequently learn that individual health care institutions and companies may not permit them to perform procedures that they have been trained to perform. Likewise, they may be expected to perform procedures that they may have been taught only in theory. In the second situation, continued employment may well be based on successful completion of prescribed training courses. Increasingly, the questions of what drugs RCPs are permitted to administer, as well as the methods of administration of the drugs that RCPs are permitted to employ, have come to be very important for the profession.

Currently, some of the procedures in question for RCPs include: emergency endotracheal intubation, arterial punctures, and injection of medications subcutaneously or directly into airways. The amount of discretion allowed regarding RCPs in adjusting medication dosage, choice of oxygen appliances, or settings on ventilators can vary greatly from hospital to hospital and among other health care organizations.

In virtually every case, the final determination regarding approval of RCP duties is made by the Medical Director of the Respiratory Care Services. The Medical Director makes this decision based on many practical factors including: the type of patients that the department or company serves and the expressed needs of Physician Directors of other departments, as well as the Medical Director's opinion of the capabilities of the RCP staff.

In addition, many regulatory groups make decisions regarding how medical care will be given and under what circumstances. Regulations created by these

367

groups, both governmental and nongovernmental, often affect the way in which RCPs can practice their profession. Some of these groups include the Occupational Safety and Health Administration, the Federal Drug Administration, Medicare, and the Joint Commission for the Accreditation of Health Care Organizations.

So, in addition to Medical Directors having to interpret those regulations, most Medical Directors who supervise RCPs today are familiar with, and take into account, the American Association for Respiratory Care's (AARC) Model Practice Act when deciding just what procedures RCPs will be permitted to perform in a given situation. Following the AARC Model Practice Act assures that Medical as well as Technical Directors of Respiratory Care Services throughout the United States will eventually reach the standards of practice intended by the RCPs and Medical Directors who wrote the act in 1993, twice amending it in 1994.

Licensure

The AARC Model Practice Act has made it possible for state AARC Affiliates to develop licensure acts that follow standard levels of practice in a general manner.

Today, most states have either successfully established, or are in the process of establishing, legislation regarding the professional role of the RCP by passing licensing bills. Although the professional roles of RCPs described in state laws vary from state to state, because all laws must be developed and passed through political forces in each state, the general trend toward licensure is a very good one for the profession. Every RCP should carefully read and keep a copy of the law in applicable states.

Some of the differences in practice among states are well illustrated in the responses to an AARC questionnaire on the status of RCPs regarding the administration of IV medication, done in 1997 (Table AP-1). Standards of practice should always be regarded as "works in progress."

Table AP-1

Administration of IV Medications

Below are the results of a survey conducted in 1997 by the AARC of State Boards and Advisory Committees for Respiratory Care on whether state law allows respiratory therapists to administer IV medications.

State	Response	Comments
Alabama		(No law)
Alaska		(No law)
Arizona	**YES**	(RCPs may administer IV medicines or any other medicines that relate to the cardiopulmonary system or to keep the IV open.)
Arkansas	NO	(Chartered affiliate said yes.)
California	**YES**	
Colorado		(No law)
Connecticut	NO	
Delaware		(Delaware's rules are not approved yet. If approved as proposed, they would allow IV medications under direct physician supervision.)
District of Columbia		(No response)
Florida	NO	(It is not specifically prohibited. IV medications are not mentioned in the law or rules.)
Georgia		(Law is currently being rewritten.)
Hawaii		(No law)
Idaho	NO	
Illinois	NO	
Indiana	NO	(Current rules and statutes covering the practice of respiratory care do not specifically address this issue.)
Iowa	NO	
Kansas	NO	
Kentucky	NO	
Louisiana	**YES**	(Only under direct orders of a physician. The law is unclear.)
Maine	**YES**	(Title 32, Chapter 97-9706-A, #1)
Maryland	NO	
Massachusetts		(Only those licensed to administer)
Michigan		(No law)
Minnesota	**YES**	(If related to cardiorespiratory care)
Mississippi	**YES**	(If related to respiratory care procedures)
Missouri	**YES**	(Administration of IV medications by RCPs is allowed for those who have had special training.)
Montana	**YES**	
Nebraska	NO	
Nevada	**YES**	
New Hampshire		(The practice act does not directly address this issue.)
New Jersey	**YES**	(Scope of practice: 13:44F-3.1)

Continued

Table AP-1 *(continued)*

Administration of IV Medications

New Mexico	NO	
New York	**YES**	(If related to cardiorespiratory care)
North Carolina		(No law)
North Dakota	NO	(Chartered affiliate said yes.)
Ohio	**YES**	(If intravenous line insertion and intravenous line medication administration meet the conditions of a service that can be legally performed by RCPs, as defined under section 4761.01 of the Revised Code, then it would appear to be a legally acceptable function for RCPs. All areas of respiratory care practice are based on the proviso that the provider is clearly trained and competent to deliver a service.)
Oklahoma		(The state licensure law neither includes nor prohibits administration of IV medications by RCPs.)
Oregon	**YES**	(When done under the direct orders of a physician)
Pennsylvania	**YES**	
Rhode Island	NO	
South Carolina	**YES**	(With medical director's approval)
South Dakota	NO	
Tennessee	NO	
Texas	NO	(Could be administered under the delegated authority of a physician licensed by the board of medical examiners.)
Utah	**YES**	(With physician orders)
Vermont		(No law)
Virginia	**YES**	(Chartered affiliate said no.)
Washington	**YES**	(If related to respiratory care)
West Virginia	**YES**	(If related to respiratory care)
Wisconsin		(Only as delegated medical acts by a physician)
Wyoming		(No law)

SOURCE: Reprinted by permission, American Association for Respiratory Care, Dallas, Texas.

Appendix II

Compatibility Chart for Nebulized Respiratory Medications

Table AP-2

Drug	L-Albuterol[1]	Racemic Albuterol	Budesonide[2]	Cromolyn Sodium	Dexamethasone	Dornase Alfa	Furosemide	Glycopyrrolate	Ipratropium	Tobramycin
L-Albuterol[1]			N/A	P & C_{8H}	P	P	P	P	P & C_{8H}	P
Racemic Albuterol	N/A		P & $C_{0.5H}$	P	P	PI_{4H}	$PI_{0.5H}$	P	P	P
Budesonide[2]	N/A	P & $C_{0.5H}$		P & $C_{0.5H}$	N/A	N/A	N/A	N/A	P & $C_{0.5H}$	N/A
Cromolyn Sodium	P & C_{8H}	P	P & $C_{0.5H}$		P	P	P	P	P	PI_{0H}
Dexamethasone	P	P	N/A	P		P	P	P	P	P
Dornase Alfa	P	PI_{4H}	N/A	P	P		P	$PI_{0.5H}$	P	P
Furosemide	P	$PI_{0.5H}$	N/A	P	P	P		$PI_{0.5H}$	P	PI_{0H}
Glycopyrrolate	P	P	N/A	P	P	$PI_{0.5H}$	$PI_{0.5H}$		P	P
Ipratropium	P & C_{8H}	P	P & $C_{0.5H}$	P	P	P	P	P		P
Tobramycin	P	P	N/A	PI_{0H}	P	P	PI_{0H}	P	P	

Chemical Compatibility Notes:
[1]Murphy, M, et al. *Resp Care* 1999;44:1288.
[2]Data on file, AstraZeneca, LP.

(Courtesy of Kevin Hillegass, Pharm.D. Candidate)

Abbreviations: **C:** Chemically compatible; **N/A:** Not available; **P:** Physically compatible; **PI₀H:** Incompatible immediately upon mixture; **PI₀.₅H:** Incompatible after a half-hour; **PI₄H:** Incompatible after 4 hours; **P & C₈H:** Compatible for 8 hours; **P & C₀.₅H:** Compatible for 1/2 hour.

Index

A

Abbreviations
  drug, 66, 67t
  medication errors and, 66, 67t
Absorption, drug, 17, 19, 19f, 25–26.
  See also specific drugs
  pediatric, 35
Abstinence syndrome, 192
Acetylcholine (ACh), 69, 75, 116
  in nerve endings, 96–97, 97f
Acetylcholinesterase, 95, 97, 97f
Acid drugs, 25–26
Acquired immunity, 335, 337
Acquired immunodeficiency syndrome (AIDS).
  See AIDS
Activated partial thromboplastin time (APTT),
  228
Acyclovir, 344–345
Addiction
  drug, 17, 38, 192
  narcotic, 192
Addison disease, 272–273, 274–275
Additive effects, 37t
Adenosine triphosphatase (ATPase), 209, 211
Adipose tissue, 167, 173
Administration, drug, 22–23, 24t.
  See also specific drugs
  five rights of, 67–68
  of IV medicines, 369t–370t
  pediatric, 358
  routes of, 22–23, 24t (*See also* specific routes,
    e.g., Intravenous (IV))
Adrenal cortex, hormones of, 271–286, 272t
Adrenal steroids, 271–286, 272t
  contraindications and precautions with, 284
  drug interactions with, 284–285, 285t
  glucocorticoids, 273–282 (*See also* Glucocorti-
    coids)
  mineralocorticoids, 282–283
  in pregnancy, 285–286
  in respiratory care practice, 286
  special considerations with, 283–284
Adrenergic blocking drugs. *See also* specific
    types, e.g., Alpha-adrenergic blockers
  ganglionic, 111–112, 112t
  sites of action of, 90f

Adrenergic drugs, 78
  ganglionic, 111–112, 112t
  sites of action of, 89, 90f
Adrenergic nerve endings, 78–79, 79f
Adrenergic neuronal blockers, 77, 81, 87–89,
  88f
Adrenergic receptors, 69, 75, 79–81, 80t
  sites of, 90f
Adverse effects, 1, 5, 6, 10–11
Advice for the Patient, 12
Aerosolizers, disinfection of, 320
Aerosols, 21
Afferent nerve, 69
Age, 31
  drugs and, 35–36
Agonists, 1, 7, 7f
Agranulocytosis, 217
AIDS, 335, 341–342
  drugs for, 345
  propagation of, 343, 344t, 345f
  sites of drug action in, 343, 344t, 345f
Alcohol, 160–163, 316, 316t, 318, 319
  adverse effects of, 162
  aerosolized, 198
  cautions and contraindications with, 162–163
  clinical indications for, 163
  in cold medicine, 198
  in expectorants, 198
  metabolism of, 161–162
  nutritional effects of, 161
  pharmacological effects of, 160–161
  in pregnancy, 163
Alcoholic preparations, 20
Alcoholism, disulfiram for, 163
Aldosterone, 272t, 282–283
Allergic rhinitis, corticosteroids for, 248, 249t
Allergy
  drug, 11
  treatment of (*See* Antiallergic agents; Antihist-
    amines; Corticosteroids)
Alopecia, 217
  from heparin, 222
α-adrenergic blockers, 77, 81, 84–85
  sites of action of, 90f
α-adrenergic drugs, 80, 81–82, 82t
  sites of action of, 90f

373

α-adrenergic receptors, 77, 80t
Alteplase, 229–230
Alternate-day therapy (ADT), steroid, 282
Alveoli, 357
Amantadine, 343, 344t, 345
    adverse effects of, 347
Ambien, 158
Amide local anesthetic, 131, 134, 135t
    adverse effects of, 136–137
    routes of administration of, 135–136
Aminocaproic acid, 230
Aminoglycosides, 298–300, 299t
Amobarbital, 155
Amytal, 155
Analgesia, 167, 169
Analgesic, 181
Analgesic drugs, 183
    in ICU, 353–354, 354t
Anaphylaxis, 236
Anesthesia
    caudal, 131, 136
    dissociative, 167, 174
    epidural, 131, 136
    infiltration, 131, 136
    intradermal, 131, 136
    spinal, 132, 136
Anesthesia, general, 167, 168–171
    adjuncts to, 175–176, 175t
    cautions and drug interactions in, 176–177
    induction of, 167, 170
    maintenance of, 168, 170
    physiological effects of, 170–171
    respiratory care practice and, 177–178
    route of administration of, 170
    signs and stages of, 169–170, 169f
Anesthetics, general, 131, 132, 171–177
    inhalation, 171–173, 172t
    injectable, 172t, 173–175
    use of, 168–169
Anesthetics, local, 131–141
    amide, 131, 134, 135t
    cautions and contraindications with, 138
    clinical application of, 137–138
    defined, 131, 132
    drug interactions of, 139–140, 139t
    epinephrine in, 138
    ester, 131, 134, 135t
    mechanism of action of, 132–134, 133f, 134t
    patient instructions with, 140
    pharmacology of, 134, 135t
    physician notification with, 140
    in pregnancy, 141
    special considerations with, 138–139
Angina pectoris, 201, 205
Anise, 330t–331t
Anistreplase, 229–230
Antabuse, 163
Antagonism, 37t
Antagonists, 1, 7, 7f
Antiallergic, 235

Antiallergic agents, 237, 238–240, 239f, 240t
    adverse effects of, 247–248
    dosing for, 247
    patient instructions with, 247
    physician notification with, 248
Antibacterial agents, 289–308
    aminoglycosides, 298–300, 299t
    cephalosporins, 296–298, 297t
    chemoprophylaxis with, 308
    in chemotherapy, 290, 292–293
    chloramphenicol, 306
    clindamycin, 306
    drug resistance of, 293
    fluoroquinolone antimicrobials, 305, 305t
    macrolide, 304–305
    penicillin-related, 296
    penicillins, 293–296, 294t (*See also* Penicillins)
    sources of, 292
    spectrum of, 292
    sulfonamides, 302–304, 303t
    tetracyclines, 300–302, 301t
    for tuberculosis, 307–308
    vancomycin, 306
Antibacterial spectrum, 289, 292
Antibiotic, 289, 292
Antibiotic susceptibility, 289
Anticholinergic, 95
Anticholinergic drugs, 103–106, 104t
    administration of, 106
    adverse and toxic effects of, 106
    for asthma, 260–261
    on cardiovascular system, 103
    on CNS, 105
    ganglionic, 111–112, 112t
    on genitourinary system, 105
    on GI system, 105
    ocular effects of, 106
    patient monitoring with, 106
    on respiratory system, 103–104, 105t
Anticholinesterase drugs, 100–101, 100t. *See also*
        Cholinergic drugs
    clinical indications for, 102–103
Anticoagulants, 219t, 221–228
    aspirin, 225
    chelators, 224
    clinical indications for, 225
    coumarin derivatives, 222–224, 223t
    dipyridamole, 225
    drug interactions with, 225–227,
        226t–227t
    heparin, 221–222, 223t
    monitoring effects of, 228–229
    on respiratory care, 231
    special considerations with, 227–228
    vitamin K derivatives, 224
Anticytokine therapy, for asthma, 265
Antidiuretic hormone (ADH), 181, 190
Antigen, 235, 236
Antigen drift, 335, 338
Antigen shift, 335, 338

Antihistamines, 235, 237, 241–247, 241t–242t
  adverse reactions to, 243–245, 247–248
  cautions and contraindications to, 245, 246t
  clinical indications for, 243, 244t
  in cold and allergy preparations, 243, 244t
  dosing for, 247
  drug interactions with, 246, 246t
  guidelines for use of, 247
  patient instructions with, 247
  physician notification with, 248
  in pregnancy, 248
Antihistaminic antiallergic drugs, 238–240,
    239f, 240t
Antiinfluenza drugs, 342–343
Antileukotriene drugs, 263, 263t
Antimicrobials, 289, 292
  fluoroquinolone, 305, 305t
Antiseptics, 311, 312, 314t
  adverse and toxic effects of, 319–321
  indications for, 315–319, 316t–317t
  mechanism of action of, 312–315, 314t
Antitussives, 181, 183
  narcotic, 188t, 189, 196–198, 196t
Antiviral drugs, 342–348. *See also* Viral diseases
  administration and pharmacokinetics of, 346
  adverse effects of, 347
    in pregnancy, 348
    in respiratory care, 347–348
  clinical indications for, 344–346
  for influenza, 344t
  mechanisms of action of, 342–344, 345f
  pharmacokinetics of, 346
  in pregnancy, 348
  resistance to, 338
  special considerations and contraindications
    to, 347
Anuria, 181, 190
Apnea, 357
Apothecary system, 50
Aqueous preparations, 20
Ara-A, 344
Argyria, 311
Arrhythmia, cardiac, 131
  from local anesthetics, 137
Arteriosclerosis, 201, 205
Asphyxia, 357
Aspirin
  as anticoagulant, 225
  asthma from, 255–256
  chemical structure of, 5f
Asthma, 235, 236–237, 253, 255–256
  anticytokine therapy for, 265
  autonomic nervous system in, 257–258
  bronchodilator drugs for, 258–261, 259t (*See
    also* Bronchodilator drugs)
  corticosteroids for, 261–262, 262t
  expectorants for, 265
  furosemide for, 265
  immunoglobulin E for, 265
  investigational therapies for, 265

isoflurane for, 265
magnesium sulfate for, 265
mucolytics for, 264
NAEPP guidelines for, 265–266
NSAIDs for, 262–263, 263t
Astragalus, 326t–327t
Atelectasis, 358
Atherosclerosis, 201, 205
ATPase (adenosine triphosphatase), 209, 211
Atrioventricular (AV) node, 202
Atrovent, 261
Automatism, 151, 156
Autonomic ganglia, drugs affecting, 109–112
  blockers, 109, 111–112, 111t, 112t
  stimulants, 109, 110–111
Autonomic nervous system (ANS), 69–76, 71
  in asthma, 257–258
  parasympathetic and sympathetic divisions of,
    72–75, 73f, 73t, 74f
  physiology and pharmacology of, 71
AV, 201, 202
Azactam, 296
Azithromycin, 304
Aztreonam, 296

B
Bacteria, 289, 290
  morphology of, 291–292, 291t
Bacterial diseases. *See* Antibacterial agents
Bacterial resistance, 289, 293
Bactericidal, 289, 292, 313
Bacteriostatic, 289, 292, 311, 313
Bactrim, 303–304
Bandage system, 21
Barbiturates, 154–157
  addiction liability of, 156
  adverse effects of, 156
  cautions and contraindications with, 157
  defined, 151, 152
  doses of, 153t
  drug interactions of, 157
  mechanism of action of, 154–155
  pharmacokinetics of, 155
  poisoning with, 156–157
  in pregnancy, 157
  specific drugs, 155
Basal ganglia, 143, 146
Base drugs, 25–26
Bayberry bark
  as expectorant, 330t–331t
  for sore throat, 332t–333t
Bee propolis, 326t–327t
Benzalonium chloride, 316t, 318
Benzodiazepines, 151, 152–153, 158–160
  advantages of, 159–160
  adverse effects of, 160
  drug interactions of, 160
  mechanism of action of, 158–159
  pharmacokinetics of, 159

Benzodiazepines *(contd.)*
  in pregnancy, 160
  on sleep cycle, 159
β-adrenergic blockers, 85–87, 86t, 90f
  nonselective, 78, 81
  sites of action of, 90f
$β_1$-adrenergic blockers, selective, 78, 81, 90f
$β_2$-adrenergic drug, selective, 78, 81, 90f
β-adrenergic drugs, 80–81, 82–84, 83t
  for asthma, 258–259, 259t
  sites of action of, 90f
β-adrenergic receptors, 77, 80, 80t
$β_1$-adrenergic receptors, 80t
$β_2$-adrenergic receptors, 80t
β drug effects, 82–83
β-lactamase, 290, 293
β-lactamase enzymes, bacterial, 293
β-lactamase inhibitors, 296
Bethanechol, 99–100, 100t
Biaxin, 304
Bioavailability, 17, 31
Biological factors, in drug action, 17–38
  bioavailability, 31
  blood drug levels, 29–30, 29f, 30f
  drug absorption, 25–26
  drug abuse and chronic use terminology,
    37–38, 37t
  drug distribution, 26–27
  drug excretion, 28
  drug forms, 20–21
  drug interaction, 36
  drug metabolism, 27
  in geriatrics, 36
  half-life, 28–29
  individual variation, 31–33
  in infant nursing, 33–34, 34t
  in pediatrics, 35
  in pregnancy, 33, 33t, 34t
  routes of administration, 22–23, 24t
Blockers, 78. *See also* specific types, e.g., α-adren-
    ergic blockers
  depolarizing, 115, 118
  nondepolarizing, 115, 118
Blood drug levels, 29–30, 29f, 30f
Blood flow, in drug distribution, 26–27
Blood–brain barrier, 27
Body fat, percent, 31
Body surface area rule, 55–56
Body weight, in dosage calculations, 56–57
Brainstem, 147
Breast milk, drugs in, 33–34, 34t
Broad-spectrum, 290, 292
Bronchitis, chronic, 253, 255
Bronchodilator drugs, 258–261, 259t
  anticholinergics, 260–261
  β-adrenergic, 258–259, 259t
  theophylline, 260
Bronchodilators, 253, 254
BSA rule, 57
Buccal administration, 24t

C
CAD, 201, 204
Calculation errors, 67
Calculations, dosage, 48–49, 54–57
  body weight in, 56–57
  pediatric, 55–57
Capsules, 20
  absorption of, 26
Cardiac. *See also* Heart
Cardiac arrhythmia, 131
  from local anesthetics, 137
Cardiac disease, 204–205
Cardiac function, 202–204, 203f
Cardiac glycosides, 209, 210–213
  adverse and toxic effects of, 213
  clinical indications for, 213
  drug interactions with, 213
  mechanism of action of, 211
  pharmacokinetics of, 211–212
  pharmacologic effects of, 211
  serum electrolyte levels and action of, 212
Cardiac muscle, 202, 203f
Catabolism, 271, 274
Catecholamines, 77, 78
Cat's claw, 326t–327t
Caudal anesthesia, 131, 136
Ceiling effect, 8, 8f
Central nervous system (CNS), 70, 143–148
  basal ganglia, 146
  brainstem, 147
  cerebellum, 146f, 147
  cerebral cortex, 145–146
  cerebral medulla, 146
  cerebrum, 145–146, 146f
  functional components of, 148
  hypothalamus, 146f, 147
  limbic system in, 148
  medulla oblongata, 146f, 147
  pons, 146f, 147
  reticular formation in, 148
  role of, 152
  spinal cord, 147–148
  thalamus, 146f, 147
Centrally acting skeletal muscle relaxants, 115,
    117, 117f, 122–124, 123t
Cephalosporinases, 290, 293
Cephalosporins, 296–298, 297t
  adverse effects of, 298
  first-generation, 297, 297t
  fourth-generation, 297t, 298
  second-generation, 297–298, 297t
  third-generation, 297t, 298
Cerebellum, 143, 146f, 147
Cerebral cortex, 143, 145–146
Cerebral medulla, 143, 146
Cerebrum, 143, 145–146, 146f
Cetylpyridinium chloride, 318
Chelators, as anticoagulants, 224
Chemical mediators, 253, 256–257
Chemical name, 1, 11, 11f

Chemical structure, 4, 5f
Chemoprophylaxis, 290
　antibiotic, 308
Chemoreceptor trigger zone, 188, 189f
Chemotherapy, 290, 292–293
CHF. *See* Congestive heart failure
Chloral hydrate, 158
Chloramphenicol, 306
Chlorhexidine gluconate, 316t, 318
Chloromycetin, 306
Chlorpromazine, structure of, 5f
Cholinergic, 95
Cholinergic crisis, 101–102
Cholinergic drugs, 96, 99–103
　adverse and toxic effects of, 101–102
　direct-acting, 99–100, 100t
　ganglionic, 111–112, 112t
　indirect-acting, 100–101, 100t
Cholinergic nerve endings, 96–97, 97f
Cholinergic receptors, 69, 75, 97–99, 98f
Chronic drug use, terminology for, 37–38, 37t
Chronic obstructive pulmonary disease
　　(COPD), 253, 255
Chronotropic action, 203–204
-cidal, 313
Cidofovir, 345
Ciprofloxacin, 305, 305t
Clarithromycin, 304
Clark's Rule, 55, 56
Cleocin, 306
Clindamycin, 306
Clover, red, 330t–331t
Coagulants, 230
Coagulation, 217, 218–220, 220f
　anticoagulants for, 218, 219t
　monitoring of, 228–229
Cocaine, 136. *See also* Anesthetics, local
Codeine, as antitussive, 196–197, 196t
Cold preparations, narcotic antitussives in, 188t
Compliance, patient, 32–33
Conduction, nerve, 132
Conduction system, 201, 202–203, 203f
Congestive heart failure (CHF), 201, 204–205, 209
　diuretic therapy for, 213–214, 214t
Conjunctivitis, 358
Contraindications, 1, 4
Controlled substances, 1, 13, 13t
Controlled substances act, 13, 13t
Controllers, 239, 253, 258
Conversions, of measures, 49–52
　examples, 51–53
　household, 51
　volumes, 50–51
　weights, 50
COPD (chronic obstructive pulmonary disease),
　　253, 255
Coronary artery disease (CAD), 205
Corticosteroids
　for asthma, 261–262, 262t
　intranasal, 248–249, 249t

Cortisol, 272t
　effects of, 273–274
　regulation of secretion of, 273
　on sleep-wake cycle, 273
　in stress, 273
Cortisone, 272t
Cosyntropin, 275
Coughing reflex
　narcotics on, 189
Coumarin derivatives, 222–224, 223t
Craniosacral division. *See* Parasympathetic
Cromolyn sodium, 238–240, 239f, 240t, 262
　compatibility of, 372t
Cross-tolerance, 37
Cushing disease, 273
Cytomegalovirus (CMV), drugs for, 345
Cytovene, 345

D

Dalmane (flurazepam), 159
Decimals, 43, 46–47
Decongestants, nasal, 249–250
Decubitus ulcer, 311, 315
Delayed-release products, 20–21
Denaturing, 312, 313
Denominator, 43, 44, 45f
Dependence
　drug, 17, 37–38
　physical, 182, 192
Depolarizing blockers, 115, 118
Dermatitis, 235
　eczematoid, 235, 245
Diazepam, structure of, 5f
Dicumarol, 222–224, 223t
Digitalization, 209, 211–212
Digitoxin, 212, 212t. *See also* Cardiac glycosides
Digoxin, 212, 212t. *See also* Cardiac glycosides
Dipyridamole, 225
Direct-acting skeletal muscle relaxants, 122
Dirithromycin, 305
Disease presence, 32
Disinfectants, 311, 312.318–319, 314t
　adverse and toxic effects of, 319–321
　indications for, 315–319, 316t–317t
　mechanism of action of, 312–315, 314t
Disinfection
　of aerosolizers, 320
　of large respiratory equipment, 320
　of nebulizers, 320–321
Dissociative anesthesia, 167, 174
Distribution, drug, 17, 19, 19f, 26–27. *See also*
　　specific drugs
　pediatric, 35
Disulfiram, 163
Diuretic therapy, for congestive heart failure,
　　213–214, 214t
DMMS (drug microsomal metabolizing system),
　　17, 27
　on barbiturates, 155

Dosage calculations, 48–49, 54–57
  body weight in, 56–57
  pediatric, 55–57
Dose, 1, 8, 8f
  loading, 18, 30
  maintenance, 18, 30
  pediatric, 35
Dose-response curve, 8–9, 8f
Downregulation, 37
Drug(s), 1, 3
  sources of, 3–4
Drug abbreviations, 66, 67t
Drug absorption, 17, 19, 19f, 25–26. *See also* specific drugs
  pediatric, 35
Drug abuse, terminology for, 37–38, 37t
Drug addiction, 17, 38
Drug administration, 22–23, 24t. *See also* specific drugs
  five rights of, 67–68
  IV, 18, 22, 24t, 57–58
    regulations on, 369t–370t
  pediatric, 358
  routes of, 22–23, 24t (*See also* specific routes, e.g., Intravenous; specific routes, e.g., Intravenous (IV))
Drug allergy, 11
Drug dependence, 17, 37–38
Drug distribution, 17, 19, 19f, 26–27. *See also* specific drugs
  pediatric, 35
Drug effects, terminology on, 4–6
Drug excretion, 28. *See also* specific drugs
  pediatric, 35
Drug Facts and Comparisons, 12
Drug fever, 235, 245
Drug forms, 20–21. *See also* specific forms, e.g., Delayed-release products
Drug formulation, 26
Drug indications, 1, 4
Drug Information for the Health Care Professional, 12
Drug Information–American Hospital Formulary Service, 12
Drug interactions, 36. *See also* specific agents, e.g., Skeletal muscle relaxants, drug interactions of
Drug ionization, 25–26
Drug levels, blood, 29–30, 29f, 30f
Drug metabolism, 27
  pediatric, 35
Drug microsomal metabolizing system (DMMS), 17, 27
  on barbiturates, 155
Drug names, sound-alike, 64, 64t
Drug nomenclature, 11, 11f
Drug particles, absorption of, 26
Drug references, 12–13
  pediatric, 13

Drug resistance, antibacterial, 293
Drug safety, 10–11
Drug schedules, 2, 13t, 187t
Duration of action, 9, 9f
Dynabac, 305
Dysphoria, 181, 188

E
E-Mycin, 304
Echinacea, 326t–327t
Ectopic beats, 209, 213
Eczematoid dermatitis, 235, 245
ED50, 2, 8–9, 8f
Edetic acid (EDTA), 224
EDTA, 224
Efferent nerve, 69, 73–74, 74f
Elderberry
  as expectorant, 328t–329t
  for sore throat, 332t–333t
Elderly, 31
  drugs in, 36
Electrocardiogram (ECG), 201, 203, 204f
Electroencephalogram (EEG), 143, 146
Elixirs, 20
Emesis, 182, 188–189, 189f
Emotional state, 32
Emphysema, 253, 255
Endogenous, 182
Endogenous opioids, 185
Endorphins, 185
Enteric-coated products, 21
Enzyme induction, 18, 27
  in tolerance, 37
Eosinophilic chemotactic factor of anaphylaxis (ECF-A), 256
Ephedra, 328t–329t
Epidural anesthesia, 131, 136
Epinephrine (EPI), 69
  adverse effects of, 83–84
  for asthmatic attacks, 258–259
  clinical indications for, 83
  contraindications to, 138
  in local anesthetics, 138
  vs. norepinephrine, 79
Erythema, 235
Erythrocin, 304
Erythromycin, 304
Eschar, 311, 319–320
Ester local anesthetic, 131, 134, 135t
Ethambutol, 307–308
Ethanol. *See* Alcohol
Ethyl alcohol, 316, 316t, 318
  toxicity of, 320
Ethylene oxide sterilization, 319
Eucalyptus, 328t–329t
Euphoria, 167, 169, 187–188
Excretion, drug, 28. *See also* specific drugs
  pediatric, 35

Exercise-induced asthma, 255
Expectorants, 182, 197–198
   for asthma, 265
Extremes, 49

F

False transmitter, 78, 88
Fasciculations, 115, 118
FDA pregnancy categories, 33, 33t
Federal Comprehensive Drug Abuse Prevention
    and Control Act of 1970, 13, 13t, 187t
Fennel, 330t–331t
Fentanyl
   in ICU, 353, 353t
   transmucosal, 193
Fibrin, 219, 220t
Fight-or-flight reaction, 70, 73
Five rights of drug administration, 67–68
Flu, 336–338, 337t
Fludrocortisone, 283
Fluid extracts, 20
Fluid retention, glucocorticoids on, 274
Fluoroquinolone antimicrobials, 305, 305t
Flurazepam, 159
Fluvadine, 344t, 345
   adverse effects of, 347
Food and Drug Administration, web site of, 16
Formaldehyde, 316t, 318–319
   toxicity of, 319
Forms, drug, 20–21
Formulation, drug, 26
Foscarnet, 345
Foscavir, 345
Fraction(s), 43, 44–46, 45f
   improper, 43, 45
   proper, 43, 44
Fried's Rule, 55, 56
Fungicidal, 311, 313
Fungistatic, 312, 313
Furosemide
   for asthma, 265
   compatibility of, 372t

G

GABA (γ-aminobutyric acid), 151, 154, 158–159
Ganciclovir, 345
Ganglion, 74, 74f
Ganglionic blockers, 109, 111–112, 111t, 112t
Ganglionic stimulants, 109, 110–111
Garlic, 326t–327t
Gases, 21, 23
Gastrointestinal excretion, 28
Gelatin capsules, 20
General anesthesia. *See* Anesthesia, general
General anesthetic. *See* Anesthetics, general
Generic name, 2, 11

Genetic variation, 32
Geriatrics, drugs in, 36
GI therapeutic system (GITS), 21
Ginseng, Siberian, 328t–329t
GITS, 21
Glucocorticoids, 271, 273–282
   addiction to, 282
   administration and doses of, 278–281, 278t,
      279t–280t
   adverse effects of, 281–282, 281t
   alternate-day therapy with, 282
   on blood cells, 274
   clinical indications for, 277–278, 279t–280t
   on cortisol secretion, 273
   drug interactions with, 284–286, 285t
   extended-release injectable, 278, 278t
   in fluid retention, 274
   in gluconeogenesis, 274
   metabolism and excretion of, 281
   natural *vs.* synthetic, 275, 275t
   pharmacological effects of, 274–277
      in antiinflammatory therapy, 276f, 277
      in inflammation, 275–277, 276f
      in replacement therapy, 274–275
   in pregnancy, 286
   in protein catabolism, 274
   topical, over-the-counter, 278–279, 280t
   withdrawal from, 282
Gluconeogenesis, cortisol in, 274
Glutaraldehyde, 316t, 318–319
Glycosides, 210. *See also* Cardiac glycosides
Goldenseal, 326t–327t
Gotu kola, 330t–331t
Grain (gr), 50
Gram (g), 49
Gram negative, 290, 291
Gram positive, 290, 291
Gram stain, 290, 291
Grapeseed extract, 326t–327t
Green tea, 326t–327t
Guanadrel, 89
Guanethidine, 89

H

Halcion (triazolam), 159
Half-life, 18, 28–29
Halogenated hydrocarbons, 167, 171–173,
    172t
Handwriting, medication errors and, 66
Heart. *See also* Cardiac
   nerve supply to, 203–204
Heart attack, 205
Heart diseases, 204–205
Hematuria, 217, 223
Hemorrhage, 217
   from heparin, 222
Hemorrhagic disease of the newborn (HDN),
    217, 224

Hemostatic sponges, 230
Hemostatics, 230
Heparins, 221–222, 223t
    drug interactions with, 225–227, 226t–227t
Herbal remedies, 323–333
    advantages of, 325
    composition of, 324
    for cough, cold, and flu symptoms, 328t–329t
    as expectorants, 330t–331t
    popularity of, 324
    for prevention of respiratory diseases, 326t–327t
    rules for using or recommending, 324
    for sore throats and mouth ulcers, 332t–333t
Heroin, 183, 184t. *See also* Narcotic (opioid) analgesics
Herpes simplex virus (HSV), 340–341
    drugs for, 344–345
Herplex, 344
    adverse effects of, 347
Hexachlorophene, 316t, 318
    toxicity of, 320
Histamine, 236, 237–238, 238t, 256. *See also* Antihistamines
Histamine cephalgia, 236
HIV, 335, 341–342
    drugs for, 346
    propagation of, 343–344, 344t, 345f
    sites of drug action in, 344, 344t, 345f
Homeostasis, 70, 71
Horehound
    as expectorant, 330t–331t
    for sore throat, 332t–333t
Horseradish, 330t–331t
Household system, 50
    conversions of, 51
Huang-qi (astragalus), 326t–327t
Human immunodeficiency virus. *See* HIV
Hydrocarbons, halogenated, 167, 171–173, 172t
Hydrogen peroxide, 316t, 318
Hydromorphone, in ICU, 353, 353t
Hypercalcemia, 209, 212
Hyperkalemia, 209, 212
Hypersensitivity, 131, 312
    to disinfectants and antiseptics, 319–320
    to local anesthetics, 138
Hyperthermia, 115
    malignant, 115
        from skeletal muscle relaxants, 120
Hypnotics, 151. *See also* Sedative-hypnotic drugs; specific types, e.g., Benzodiazepines
    use of, 152
Hypoaldosteronism, 282–283
Hypoglycemia, 358
Hypokalemia, 210, 212
Hypothalamus, 143, 146f, 147, 167, 169
Hypoxia, 167, 172
Hyssop
    for coughs and colds, 328t–329t
    for sore throat and mouth ulcers, 332t–333t

I
Ibuprofen, structure of, 5f
Iceland moss, 328t–329t
Idoxuridine, 344
    adverse effects of, 347
Ileus, 351
Imipenem, 296
Immunity, 335, 337
    acquired, 335, 337
Immunoglobulin E (IgE), for asthma, 265
Immunosuppressed, 335, 342
Improper fraction, 43, 45
Incompatibility, 37t, 115
Indications, drug, 1, 4. *See also* specific drugs
Individual variation, 18, 19–20, 31–33
Induction, 155
    of general anesthesia, 167, 170
Infant nursing, drugs in, 33–34, 34t
Infarction, 217. *See also* Myocardial infarction (MI)
Infiltration anesthesia, 131, 136
Influenza, 336–338, 337t
    drugs for, 345
Influenza vaccine, 337–338
INH, 307
Inhalation, 22–23
Inhalation administration, 24t
Inhalation anesthetics, 171–173, 172t
Injectable anesthetics, 172t, 173–175
Inotropic action, 204
Insulin, inhaled, 365
Interactions, drug, 36. *See also* specific drugs
International normalized ratio (INR), 228
Intraarterial administration, 24t
Intradermal anesthesia, 131, 136
Intramuscular (IM) injections, 18, 22, 24t
Intranasal administration, 23
Intrathecal administration, 24t
Intravenous (IV) administration, 18, 22, 24t, 369t–370t
    monitoring rates in, 57–58
Iodine, 315–318, 317t
    toxicity of, 319–320
Iodophors, 312, 316
    toxicity of, 319–320
Ionization, drug, 25–26
Ipratropium bromide, 261
    compatibility of, 372t
Irreversible inhibitors, 101
Irrigation, 312, 315
Ischemia, myocardial, 205
Isoflurane, for asthma, 265
Isoniazid, 307
Isopropyl alcohol, 316t, 318
    toxicity of, 320

L
Labeling, look-alike, 65, 66f
Law of Diffusion, 25

LD50, 2, 10
Lemon balm, 332t–333t
Leukotrienes, 254, 256, 257
    drugs against, 263, 263t
Licensure, 368
Licorice
    as expectorant, 330t–331t
    for sore throat, 332t–333t
Lidocaine. *See also* Anesthetics, local
    as cough suppressant, 140
Limbic system, 143, 148
Lipid solubility, 25
Liquid, absorption of, 26
Liter (L), 49
Loading dose, 18, 29
Local anesthetics. *See* Anesthetics, local
Look-alike drugs, 65, 66f
Lorazepam, in ICU, 352–353, 353t
Low-molecular-weight heparins, 221–222
Lozenges, 20
Luminal (phenobarbital), 155
Lungwort, 330t–331t
Lyse, 312, 313
Lysosome, 271

M

Ma-Huang (ephedra), 328t–329t
Macrolide, 304
Macrolide antibiotics, 304–305
Magnesium sulfate, for asthma, 265
Maintenance, of general anesthesia, 168, 170
Maintenance dose, 18, 30
Malignant hyperthermia, 115
    from skeletal muscle relaxants, 120
Marshmallow, 330t–331t
Means, 49
Measurement, systems of, 49–53
    apothecary, 50
    conversion examples in, 51–53
    conversion tables for, 50–51
    household, 50
    metric, 49–50
Mecamylamine, 111, 111t
Mechanical ventilation, 351–355. *See also* Ventilation, mechanical
Mechanism of action, 2, 6. *See also* specific drugs
Mediators, chemical, 256–257
Medication errors, 64
    prevention of, 63–67
        abbreviations, 66, 67t
        calculation errors, 67
        drug names, sound-alike, 64, 64t
        handwriting, 66
        look-alike drugs and labeling, 65, 66t
        multiple concentrations, 65, 65t
        rights of drug administration, 67–68
Medulla oblongata, 143, 146f, 147
Medullary depression, 168, 169
Medullary paralysis, 168, 170

Menadiol, 224
Menadione, 224
Meropenem, 296
Merrem, 296
Metabolic tolerance, 37
Metabolism, drug, 27
    pediatric, 35
Meter (m), 49
Metered-dose inhalers, 21, 23
    for bronchodilators, 258–259
Methacholine, 99–100, 100t
Methadone, 192–193
Methyldopa, 88
Metric system, 49–50
Midazolam, in ICU, 352–353, 353t
Milk, breast, drugs in, 33–34, 34t
Mineralocorticoids, 271, 282–283
Mixed number, 43, 45
Morphine, 183, 184t. *See also* Narcotic (opioid) analgesics
    in ICU, 353, 353t
Mucolytics, 254, 264
    for asthma, 264
    as expectorants, 197
Mucopolysaccharide, 217, 221
Mullein, 330t–331t
Muscarinic receptors, 95, 97
Muscle relaxants, skeletal
    centrally acting, 115, 117, 117f, 122–124 (*See also* Skeletal muscle relaxants, centrally acting)
    peripheral, 116, 117, 117f, 118–121, 119t (*See also* Skeletal muscle relaxants, peripheral)
Myambutol, 307–308
Myocardial infarction (MI), 201, 205
    thrombolytic enzymes for, 229–230
Myocardium, 202, 203f
Myrrh, 332t–333t

N

Nalmefene, 193, 195, 196t
Naloxone, 193, 195, 196t
Names
    chemical, 1, 11, 11f
    generic, 2, 11
    trade, 2, 11
Narcotic, 182
Narcotic antagonists, 182, 192–193, 195, 196t
Narcotic (opioid) analgesics, 183–193
    absorption and metabolism of, 191
    adverse effects of, 192–193
    cautions and contraindications with, 193–194
    clinical indications for, 191
    doses of, 184t–185t
    drug interactions with, 194
    in ICU, 353–354, 353t, 354t
    overdose or poisoning with, 193

Narcotic (opioid) analgesics *(contd.)*
  pharmacologic effects of, 183, 186t, 187–191
    on cardiovascular system, 190
    on CNS, 187–190
    on eyes, 190–191
    on smooth muscle, 190
  in pregnancy, 195
  receptors for, 185–187
  in respiratory care practice, 194–195
  site and mechanism of action of, 185–187
  source of, 183
  special formulations of, 193
Narcotic (opioid) antitussives, 188t, 189, 196t, 197–198
  in combination cold preparations, 188t
Nasal administration, 23
Nasal congestion, medications causing, 249–250, 250t
Nasal decongestants, 249–250
Nasal sprays, 21
National Asthma Education and Prevention Program (NAEPP) guidelines, 265–266
Nausea, 188
Nebulized respiratory medications, compatibility of, 372t
Nebulized saline, 196
Nebulizers, 21, 23
  disinfection of, 320–321
Nembutal, 155
Nerve conduction, 132
  local anesthetics on, 133, 133f
Nerve endings, adrenergic, 78–79, 79f
Nerve supply, to heart, 203–204
Nervous system, organization of, 70–71
Neuraminidase inhibitors, 343
Neuroleptanalgesia, 168, 175
Neuroleptanesthesia, 168, 175
Neuroleptics, 351
  in ICU, 353
Neuromuscular blocking agents, in ICU, 354, 355t
Neuromuscular junction (NMJ), 115, 116
Neurotransmitters, 70, 75
  in brain, 144–145
Nicorette, 110
Nicotine, 109, 110–111
  in chewing gum, 110
Nicotinic-1 (NI) receptor, 95, 97–99, 98f, 109, 110
Nicotinic-2 (NII) receptor, 95, 98f, 99, 116
Nitric oxide (NO), 360–362
Nitromersol, 317t, 318–319
Noctec, 158
Nomenclature, drug, 11
Nonbarbiturate sedative-hypnotics, 153t, 157–158
Nonbarbiturates, 151, 152
Nondepolarizing blockers, 115, 118
Nonprescription drug, 2, 11
Nonselective β-adrenergic blockers, 78, 81

Nonsteroidal antiinflammatory drugs (NSAIDs), for asthma, 262–263, 263t
Norepinephrine (NE), 70, 75
  adrenergic nerve endings for, 78–79, 79f
  adverse effects of, 82
  chemical structure of, 5f
  clinical indications for, 81
  vs. epinephrine, 79
  synthesis of, 88f
Nosocomial, 312, 315
NREM sleep, 151, 153–154
Numerator, 43, 44, 45f
Nursing, drugs in, 33–34, 34t

O

Ointments, 21
Oliguria, 182, 190
Olive leaf extract, 326t–327t
Onion, 328t–329t
Onset of action, 9, 9f
Opiates, 182, 183. *See also* Narcotic (opioid) analgesics
Opioids, 182, 183. *See also* Narcotic (opioid) analgesics
Opportunistic infections, 358
Opportunistic organisms, 335, 342
Oral administration, 18, 22, 24t
Oregano, 328t–329t
Oseltamivir, 343, 344t, 345–346, 346
  adverse effects of, 347
Over-the-counter (OTC) drug, 2, 11
Oxalic acid, 224
Oxychlorosene calcium, 317t

P

Palivizumab, 339, 346
Pancuronium, in ICU, 354, 355t
Paralytic agents, in ICU, 354, 355t
Parasympathetic, 70
Parasympathetic nervous system, 72–75, 73f, 73t, 74f
  anticholinergic drugs on, 103–106, 104t
    administration of, 106
    adverse and toxic effects of, 106
    on cardiovascular system, 103
    on CNS, 105
    on genitourinary system, 105
    on GI system, 105
    ocular effects of, 106
    patient monitoring with, 106
    on respiratory system, 103–104, 105t
  anticholinesterase drugs on, 102–103
  cholinergic drugs on, 99–103
    adverse and toxic effects of, 101–102
    direct-acting, 99–100, 100t
    indirect-acting, 100–101, 100t
  cholinergic nerve endings in, 96–97, 97f
  cholinergic receptors in, 97–99, 98f

Parasympatholytic, 96, 103. *See also* Anticholinergic drugs
Parasympathomimetic, 96, 99
Parenteral administration, 18, 22
Parsley, 330t–331t
Partial thromboplastin time (PTT), 228
Patch system, 21
Pathogenic, 290
Patient compliance, 32–33
Patient-controlled analgesia (PCA), 185, 191
Pediatric drug considerations, 33–36
Pediatric drug references, 13
Penicillinases, 290, 293
Penicillins, 293–296, 294t
    adverse effects of, 296
    antibiotics related to, 296
    β-lactamase inhibitors, 296
    first-generation, 294–295, 294t
    fourth-generation, 294t, 295
    mechanism of action of, 293
    second-generation, 294t, 295
    third-generation, 294t, 295
Pentamidine isethionate, 362–365, 363t, 364t
    activity of, 362
    adverse reactions to, 362–363, 363t
    dosage and administration of, 364, 364t
    environmental concerns with, 364–365, 365t
    mechanism of action of, 362
    pharmacokinetics of, 362
    in pregnancy, 365
    therapy with, 364
Pentobarbital, 155
Peppermint oil, 330t–331t
Percents, 43, 48
Peripheral nerves, 73–74, 182
    in pain, 185
Peripheral skeletal muscle relaxants, 116, 117,
        117f, 118–121, 119t. *See also* Skeletal muscle relaxants, peripheral
Petechiae, from heparin, 222
Phagocytes, 271
Pharmacodynamic tolerance, 37
Pharmacodynamics, 3t. *See also* specific drugs
Pharmacokinetics, 3t. *See also* specific drugs
Pharmacology
    defined, 2, 3
    major areas of, 3t
Pharmacotherapeutics, 3t
Pharmacy, 3t
Phenobarbital, 155
Phenytoin, structure of, 5f
Phlegm, 182
Physical dependence, 182, 192
Physician's Desk Reference (PDR), 12
Phytochemicals, 324
Phytonadione, 224
Placebo effect, 20, 32
Plasma protein binding, 26
Plasma sterilization, 319
Platelet, 217

Pleurisy root, 330t–331t
Pneumocystis carinii, 342
    pentamidine isethionate for, 364
Poloxamer-iodine, 317t, 318
Pons, 144, 146f, 147
Positive-pressure breathing apparatus, 21
Posology, 3t
Potency, 2, 8
Potentiates, 116
Povidone-iodine, 317t, 318
Powders, 20
Pregnancy. *See also under* specific drugs, e.g.,
        Barbiturates, in pregnancy
    drug exposure in, 33–34, 34t
    drugs in, 33, 33t, 34t
    FDA drug categories in, 33, 33t
Premature ventricular contractions (PVCs), 213
Prescription, elements of, 12t
Prescription drug, 2, 11
Primaxin, 296
Proper fraction, 43, 44
Prophylactic, 236
Propofol, in ICU, 352–353, 353t
Proportion, 43, 48–49
Prostaglandins, 254, 257
Protease inhibitors, 343, 344t
Protein catabolism, cortisol in, 274
Protime (PT), 228
Protozoa, 358
Pyrazinamide, 308

Q
QD, 66, 67t
QID, 66, 67t
QOD, 66, 67t
Quantal, 9
Quarternary ammonium ions, 111

R
Raspberry leaves, 332t–333t
Ratio, 44, 48
Receptor site, 6–7, 7f
Receptors, 2. *See also* specific types, e.g., Cholinergic receptors
    adrenergic, 79–81, 80t
Rectal administration, 24t
Red clover, 330t–331t
References, drug, 12–13
    pediatric, 13
Regulatory issues, in respiratory care, 367–370
    IV medicine administration, 369t–370t
    licensure, 368
Relenza, 343, 345–346
    adverse effects of, 347
Relievers, 254, 258
REM sleep, 152, 153–154
Renal excretion, 28

Replacement therapy, 271, 273
  adrenal steroid, 274–275
Repository preparations, 272, 278
Reserpine, 88–89
Resistance
  to antiviral therapy, 338
  bacterial, 289, 293
Respigam, 339
Respiratory diseases, 254–257
  asthma, 255–256
  chemical mediators, 256–257
  chronic obstructive pulmonary disease, 255
  emphysema, 255
Respiratory distress syndrome (RSD), 358–360,
    359t
Respiratory equipment, disinfection of, 320–321
Respiratory excretion, 28
Respiratory syncytial virus (RSV), 339–340
  drugs for, 346
Response, 2, 8, 8f
Restoril, 159
Reteplase, 229–230
Reticular formation, 144, 148
Reverse transcriptase, 343
Reverse transcriptase inhibitors, 343, 344t
Reversible inhibitors, 101
Reye syndrome, 336, 338
Rhinitis, 236
  corticosteroids for, 248, 249t
Rhinitis medicamentosa, 236, 249–250, 250t
Ribavirin, 339–340
Rifadin, 307
Rifampin, 307
Rights of drug administration, 67–68
Rimantadine, 344t, 345
  adverse effects of, 347
Rocuronium, in ICU, 354, 355t
Rotadisks, 23
Rotohaler, 23
Routes of administration, 22–23, 24t. *See also*
    specific routes, e.g., Intravenous (IV)
  pediatric, 358
Rx List, 15–16

S

SA, 201, 202
Sage, 332t–333t
Saline, nebulized, 198
Salves, 21
Schedule I drug, 2, 13t, 187t
Schedule II drug, 2, 13t, 187t
Schedule III drug, 2, 13t, 187t
Schedule IV drug, 2, 13t, 187t
Schedule V drug, 2, 13t, 187t
Secobarbital, 155
Sedative-hypnotic drugs, 154–160. *See also* Sleep
    cycle

barbiturate, 154–157 (*See also* Barbiturates)
benzodiazepines, 158–160
doses of, 153t
nonbarbiturates, 157–158
Sedatives, 152
  in ICU, 352–353, 353t
  use of, 152
Semisolid preparations, 20
Sensitize, 236
Septra, 303–304
Sex, 31
Siberian ginseng, 328t–329t
Side effects, 2, 5, 6
Silver nitrate, 317t, 318
Silver protein, 317t, 318
Silver sulfadiazine, 317t, 318
Sinoatrial (SA) node, 202
Site of action, 2, 6
SK-Chloral (chloral hydrate), 158
Skeletal muscle, innervation of, 116, 117f
Skeletal muscle relaxants, 115–126
  centrally acting, 115, 117, 117f, 122–124
    adverse effects of, 124
    doses of, 123t
    drug interactions of, 124
    mechanism of action of, 123–124
    route of administration of, 124
  clinical indications for, 117
  direct-acting, 122
  drug interactions of, 120, 121t
  peripheral, 116, 117, 117f, 118–121, 119t
    adverse and toxic effects of, 119–120
    on cardiopulmonary systems, 118–119
    cautions on, 120
    clinical indications for, 120–121
    doses of, 119t
    mechanism of action of, 118
    route of administration of, 118, 119t
  in pregnancy, 125
  in respiratory care practice, 124–125
  use of, 117
Sleep
  NREM, 151, 153–154
  REM, 152, 153–154
Sleep cycle, 153–154
  benzodiazepines on, 159
Sleep-wake cycle, cortisol on, 273
Slippery elm bark, 332t–333t
SODAS, 21
Sodium hypochlorite, 317t, 318–319
  toxicity of, 320
Sodium-potassium exchange, 282–283
Solid preparations, 20
Solute, 44
Solutions, 44, 53
Solvent, 44
Somatic division, 71
Sonata, 158

Sound-alike drug names, 64, 64t
Sources, of drugs, 3–4
Spasmogenic, 182
Spasmogenic activity, 190
Spheroidal oral drug-absorption system (SO-DAS), 21
Spinal anesthesia, 132, 136
Spinal cord, 147–148
Spinhaler, 23
Spirits, 20
Sprays, 21
-static, 312, 313
Steady state, 30, 30f
Steam sterilization, 319
Sterilization, 312, 313–315
    ethylene oxide, 319
    plasma, 319
    steam, 319
Steroids, 272. *See also* specific types, e.g., Adrenal steroids, Glucocorticoids
    contraindications and precautions with, 283–284
    drug interactions with, 284–286, 285t
    in pregnancy, 286
    special considerations with, 283–284
Streptokinase, 229–230
Stress, cortisol in, 273
Subcutaneous (SC) administration, 24t
Sublingual administration, 24t
Sulfonamides, 302–304, 303t
Summation, 37t
Suppositories, 21
Surfactants, 358–360
Symadine, 342–343, 344t, 345
    adverse effects of, 347
Symmetrel, 343, 344t, 345
    adverse effects of, 347
Sympathetic, 70
Sympathetic nervous system, 72–75, 73f, 73t, 74f
    drugs affecting, 77–90
        α-adrenergic blocking drugs, 84–85
        α-adrenergic drugs, 81–82, 82t
        adrenergic nerve endings and, 78–79, 79f
        adrenergic neuronal blocking drugs, 81, 87–89, 88f
        adrenergic receptors, 79–81, 80t
        β-adrenergic blocking drugs, 85–87, 86t
        β-adrenergic drugs, 82–84, 83t
        norepinephrine *vs.* epinephrine, 79
        sites of action of, 89, 90f
Sympatholytics, 78, 81
Sympathomimetic amines, in cold medicines, 198
Sympathomimetics, 78, 80
Synagis, 339, 346
Synaptic connections, 145, 145f
Synergism, 37t
Synergistic, 168, 175

Synthetic drug, 182, 183
Syrups, 20
Systems of measurement, 49–53. *See also* Measurement, systems of

T
Tablets, 20
    absorption of, 26
Tamiflu, 343, 344t, 345–346, 346
    adverse effects of, 347
Temazepam, 159
Teratogens, 34t
Terminology
    on drug abuse, 37–38, 37t
    on drug effects, 4–6
Tetracyclines, 300–302, 301t
Thalamus, 144, 146f, 147
Theophylline, 260
Therapeutic drug range, 29, 29f
Therapeutic effect, 2, 4
Therapeutic index (TI), 2, 10
Thiazide diuretics, 214
Thimersol, 317t, 318–319
Thoracolumbar division. *See* Sympathetic
Thrombin, 230
Thrombocytes, 217, 219
Thromboembolism, 217
Thrombolytic enzymes, 229–230
Thrombophlebitis, 218, 221
Thromboplastin, 219, 219t, 220f
Thrombus, 218, 230
Thrush, 336, 342
Thyme, 332t–333t
Time-response curve, 9, 9f
Tinctures, 20
Tissue plasminogen activator (tPA), 229–230
Tolerance, 37, 182, 192
    enzyme induction in, 37
    metabolic, 37
Topical application, 18, 22, 24t, 132
Toxic effects, 2, 5, 6
Toxicology, 3t
tPA (tissue plasminogen activator), 229–230
Trade name, 2, 11
Transdermal administration, 24t
Transdermal products, 21
Transmitter, false, 78, 88
Transport mechanisms, for drugs, 25
Trelenza, 343, 344t, 345–346
    adverse effects of, 347
Triazolam, 159
Trifluridine, 344
Trimethaphan, 111, 111t
Trimethoprim-sulfamethoxazole, 303–304
Troches, 20
Tropic, 272
Tuberculosis, drugs for, 307–308
Turbuhalers, 23

U

United States Pharmacopoeia Dispensing Information (USP DI), 12
United States Pharmacopoeia/National Formulary (USP/NF), 12
Urokinase, 229–230

V

Vaginal administration, 24t
Vagolytics, 116
  skeletal muscle relaxants as, 118
Valacyclovir, 345
Valtrex, 345
Vancocin, 306
Vancomycin, 306
Variation, individual, 18, 19–20, 31–33
Vasoconstriction, 132
  by local anesthetics, 136
Vasodilation, 132
  by local anesthetics, 136
Vasodilators, 116
  diuretic therapy for, 214, 214t
  as ganglionic blockers, 111–112, 112t
  skeletal muscle relaxants as, 118
ecuronium, in ICU, 354, 355t
Ventilation, mechanical, pharmacological, 351–355
  analgesics, 353–354, 354t
  neuroleptics, 353
  paralytic agents, 354, 355t
  practical guide to, 355
  sedatives, 352–353, 353t
Vidarabine, 344
Vira-A, 344
Viral diseases, 336–342. *See also* Antiviral drugs
  AIDS, 341–342
  herpes, 340–341
  influenza, 336–338, 337t
  propagation of, 342
  respiratory syncytial virus, 339–340
Viroptic, 344
Virucidal, 312, 313

Visceral division, 71
Vistide, 345
Vitamin K_1, 224
Vitamin K_3, 224
Vitamin K_4, 224
Vitamin K derivatives, 224
Volume in volume (V/V) solution, 53
Volumes, conversions of, 50–51
Vomiting center, 188–189, 189f
Vomiting reflex, 188–189, 189f

W

Warfarin sodium, 222–224, 223t
Water soluble drugs, 25
Weight, 31
Weight(s)
  body, in dosage calculations, 56–57
  conversions of, 50
Weight in volume (W/V) solution, 53
Weight in weight (W/W) solution, 53
Withdrawal, from narcotics, 192–193

X

Xerostomia, 236, 243

Y

Yarrow, 326t–327t
Yerba santa, 328t–329t
Young's Rule, 55, 56

Z

Zaleplon, 158
Zanamivir, 343, 344t, 345–346
  adverse effects of, 347
Zithromax, 304
Zolpidem, 158
Zovirax, 344–345

ISBN 0-07-134727-5

90000